CHALLENGES IN NEUROLOGY

CHALLENGES IN NEUROLOGY

Edited by

VLADIMIR C. HACHINSKI, M.D.,
FRCP(C), M.Sc(DME),
D.Sc.(Med)

Richard and Beryl Ivey Professor and Chairman
Department of Clinical Neurological Sciences
The University of Western Ontario

Chief, Department of Clinical Neurological
Sciences
University Hospital

Director, Stroke and Aging Research
The John P. Robarts Research Institute
London, Ontario, Canada

 F. A. DAVIS COMPANY • Philadelphia

Printed in the United States of America

Last digit indicates print number: 10 9 8 7 6 5 4 3 2 1

aquisitions editor: Robert H. Craven
developmental editor: Bernice Wissler
production editor: Crystal S. McNichol
cover design: Donald B. Freggens

As new scientific information becomes available through basic and clinical research, recommended treatments and drug therapies undergo changes. The author(s) and publisher have done everything possible to make this book accurate, up to date, and in accord with accepted standards at the time of publication. The authors, editors, and publisher are not responsible for errors or omissions or for consequences from application of the book, and make no warranty, expressed or implied, in regard to the contents of the book. Any practice described in this book should be applied by the reader in accordance with professional standards of care used in regard to the unique circumstances that may apply in each situation. The reader is advised always to check product information (package inserts) for changes and new information regarding dose and contraindications before administering any drug. Caution is especially urged when using new or infrequently ordered drugs.

Library of Congress Cataloging-in-Publication Data

Challenges in neurology / edited by Vladimir C. Hachinski.
    p. cm.
    Includes bibliographical references and index.
    ISBN 0-8036-4504-X (hardbound : alk. paper)
    1. Nervous system — Diseases. 2. Neurology. I. Hachinski,
Vladimir.
    [DNLM: 1. Nervous System Diseases. 2. Nervous System Diseases —
therapy. WL 100 C437]
  RC346.C44 1992
  616.8 — dc20
  DNLM/DLC
  for Library of Congress
                             91-42517
                             CIP

Challenges in Neurology is dedicated to Dr. H.J.M. Barnett, on the occasion of his 70th birthday, and to Dr. Charles G. Drake, co-founders of the Department of Clinical Neurological Sciences at the University of Western Ontario, in London, Canada.

PREFACE

Neurology has an undeserved reputation for diagnostic precision and therapeutic impotence. Although increasingly effective drugs for epilepsy, parkinsonism, and stroke prevention belie such nihilism, many challenges remain. The mounting burden of degenerative disorders, the bane of chronic pain, and the blurry borderlands between functional and organic disorders are but three examples.

This book attempts to address common and troubling problems for which no agreed approach exists. Each contributor has been asked to identify the nature and magnitude of the problem, explain what pathophysiology is understood, outline a practical approach, and indicate what research would cleave each challenge into soluble parts.

Although this book was inspired by the popularity of the "Controversies" section of the *Archives of Neurology*, the adversarial format has only been retained in the most contentious challenges, since most issues suffer not from polarization but from lack of clear formulation. The problems are discussed in greater depth than are possible in a journal, and the contributors have been asked to provide illustrations, tables, and key references. I have tried to achieve cohesion through introductions and comments on the contributions.

Each challenge in neurology represents not only a problem but also an opportunity to clarify our thinking, acquire new knowledge, and help patients.

Vladimir C. Hachinski

ACKNOWLEDGMENTS

I thank Robert J. Joynt, Editor-in-Chief, *Archives of Neurology*, for giving me the opportunity to edit the section "Controversies and Consensus in Neurology," the direct ancestor of this book. I am grateful to Fred Plum for suggesting the title and for an early discussion on topics and format. I thank Sylvia Fields from F. A. Davis for her enthusiasm, common sense, and friendship. My secretary, Peggy Radcliff, deserves my gratitude for her devotion and effectiveness. As Career Investigator of the Heart and Stroke Foundation of Ontario, I have enjoyed direct and indirect support for all my scholarly activities, for which I am grateful. Lastly and warmly, I thank the contributors, for this is their book.

CONTRIBUTORS

Robert W. Baloh, M.D., Professor of Neurology and Surgery (Head and Neck Division), University of California School of Medicine; Director, Neurotology Laboratory, University of California Medical Center, Los Angeles, California

Warren T. Blume, M.D., FRCP(C), Professor of Neurology and Paediatrics, Department of Clinical Neurological Sciences, The University of Western Ontario, London, Ontario, Canada

Thomas H. Burnstine, M.D., Clinical Fellow, Department of Neurology, The Johns Hopkins Hospital, Baltimore, Maryland

Lisa M. DeAngelis, M.D., Associate Professor of Neurology, Cornell University Medical College; Assistant Attending Neurologist, Memorial Sloan-Kettering Cancer Center, New York, New York

Edward J. Dropcho, M.D., Assistant Professor of Neurology, University of Alabama at Birmingham and the Birmingham Veterans Affairs Medical Center; Director, Neuro-Oncology Program, Comprehensive Cancer Center, The University of Alabama, Birmingham, Alabama

René Drucker-Colín, M.D., Ph.D., Professor and Chairman, Department of Neurosciences, Instituto de Fisiologia Celular, Universidad Nacional Autonoma de Mexico, Mexico, D.F. Mexico

Fernando García-Hernández, Ph.D., Assistant Researcher, Department of Neurosciences, Instituto de Fisiologia Celular, Universidad Nacional Autonoma de Mexico, Mexico, D.F. Mexico

John P. Girvin, M.D., Ph.D., FRCS(C), Co-director, Epilepsy Unit, Department of Clinical Neurological Sciences, University Hospital, London, Ontario, Canada

Timothy C. Hain, M.D., Associate Professor, Departments of Neurology and Otolaryngology, Northwestern University Medical School, Chicago, Illinois

Ronald P. Lesser, M.D., Associate Professor of Neurology and Neurosurgery, The Johns Hopkins University School of Medicine; Director, The Johns Hopkins Epilepsy Center and The Johns Hopkins EEG Laboratories, The Johns Hopkins Hospital, Baltimore, Maryland

Michael W. McDermott, M.D., FRCS(C), Assistant Professor, Division of Neurosurgery, University of British Columbia, Vancouver, British Columbia, Canada

Richard S. McLachlan, M.D., FRCP(C), Associate Professor, Departments of Clinical Neurological Sciences and Physiology, The University of Western Ontario, London, Ontario, Canada

Roger J. Porter, M.D., Deputy Director, National Institute of Neurological Disorders and Stroke, National Institutes of Health, Bethesda, Maryland

Andres M. Salazar, M.D., Col, M.C., USA; Director, Army Head Injury Unit, Department of Clinical Investigation, Walter Reed Army Medical Center, Washington, DC; Professor of Neurology, Uniformed Services University of the Health Sciences, Bethesda, Maryland

Martin A. Samuels, M.D., Associate Professor of Neurology, Harvard Medical School; Director, Harvard-Longwood Neurology Training Program; Chief of Neurology, Brigham and Women's Hospital, Boston, Massachusetts

Barbara Scherokman, M.D., Associate Professor of Neurology, Department of Neurology, Uniformed Services University of the Health Sciences, Bethesda, Maryland

A. Jon Stoessl, M.D., FRCP(C), Assistant Professor, Department of Clinical Neurological Sciences, The University of Western Ontario, London, Ontario, Canada

Robert W. Teasell, B.Sc., M.D. FRCP(C), Assistant Professor, Department of Physical Medicine and Rehabilitation, The University of Western Ontario; Chief, Department of Physical Medicine and Rehabilitation, University Hospital, London, Ontario, Canada

Alan R. Tessler, M.D., Research Associate Professor of Anatomy, Department of Anatomy, Medical College of Pennsylvania; Associate Professor of Neurology, Department of Neurology, Philadelphia Veterans Administration Medical Center and Medical College of Pennsylvania, Philadelphia, Pennsylvania

L. James Willmore, M.D., Professor of Neurology and Director, Texas Comprehensive Epilepsy Program, Department of Neurology, University of Texas Medical School, Houston, Texas

David S. Zee, M.D., Professor, Departments of Neurology, Ophthalmology, Otolaryngology – Head and Neck Surgery, and Neuroscience, The Wilmer Ophthalmological Institute, The Johns Hopkins University, School of Medicine, Baltimore, Maryland

CONTENTS

3 THE WHIPLASH PATIENT: A SYMPATHETIC APPROACH _____ 29

Robert W. Teasell, B.Sc., M.D., FRCP(C)

SECTION TWO: INTENSIVE CARE NEUROLOGY ___ 53

4 TRAUMATIC BRAIN INJURY: THE CONTINUING EPIDEMIC _____ 55

Andres M. Salazar, M.D., Col., M.C., USA

12 CURRENT INDICATIONS FOR SURGICAL MANAGEMENT OF EPILEPSY _____ 149

John P. Girvin, M.D., Ph.D., FRCS(C)

SECTION FIVE: MOVEMENT DISORDERS _____ 163

13 CAN WE TREAT PARKINSON'S DISEASE USING ADRENAL TRANSPLANTS? _____ 165

René Drucker-Colín, M.D., Ph.D., and Fernando García-Hernández, Ph.D.

14 DOES NEURAL TRANSPLANTATION AID THE RECOVERY OF CNS FUNCTION? —————— 183

Alan R. Tessler, M.D.

15 MANAGING THE REFRACTIVE PARKINSONIAN PATIENT —————————————————— 195

A. Jon Stoessl, M.D., FRCP(C)

18 MANAGEMENT OF MULTIPLE BRAIN METASTASES

Edward J. Dropcho, M.D.

Index

SECTION ONE

. . . .

CHALLENGING PATIENTS

EDITOR'S COMMENTARY

Physicians need not seek humility. Some of their patients will bring it to them. Patients complaining of dizziness are near the top of the list. This is such a common and puzzling problem that two chapters have been invited on the topic. Hain and Zee emphasize the bedside examination and Baloh stresses management, but both chapters find common ground in approaching the dizzy patient.

While some problems baffle physicians, others inflame them. Few subjects have the power to arouse as much emotion among physicians as a discussion of the whiplash patient. To some extent their views can be predicted from their specialty and from the side of a litigation on which they tend to testify. Teasell (Chapter 3) is a physiatrist working closely with members of a department of clinical neurological sciences. He offers a comprehensive and sympathetic approach to the whiplash-injured patient. Experts hardened by their experience with malingerers and compensation seekers may think him too sympathetic. Surely, however, physician and patient must begin on the same side.

VCH

CHAPTER 1

• •

THE DIZZY PATIENT: DIAGNOSTIC APPROACHES

Timothy C. Hain, M.D. and David S. Zee, M.D.

Some people have trouble walking and chewing gum at the same time, and yet Hain and Zee tell us that our vestibular system constantly tracks and integrates activity in six motion coordinates successfully! The authors make most vestibular disorders intelligible by classifying them as disorders of tone or gain, and they provide an approach to the dizzy patient firmly based on the bedside examination.

A minority of individuals will require further investigations, which the authors discuss with confidence born from experience. They consider T_1 sequence gadolinium-enhanced magnetic resonance imaging (MRI) as the single most useful test to rule out lesions of the cerebellopontine angle. This is a test that may not be always accessible; nevertheless, it is important to know the contemporary standards.

Hain and Zee's cautions are as valuable as their assertions. They warn against ruling out benign paroxysmal positional vertigo on the basis of a single examination for positional nystagmus; they advocate long-term vigilance rather than labeling of patients with vertigo of uncertain origin, and they caution against the "microvascular compression syndrome," characterized by vague definitions and heroic surgery.

The authors do not discuss two conditions that are common in the offices of the general physician: hyperventilation and hypotension. Strictly speaking, they are not disorders of the vestibular system, which the authors emphasize, but they frequently present as problems of "dizziness."

Involuntary and unnoticed hyperventilation tends to occur in the anxious, the troubled, and the depressed. The patient will often complain of lightheadedness, unsteadiness, and buzzing in the ears.

When patients are asked to hyperventilate for 3 minutes, they often will stop after 1 or 2 minutes, complaining of the symptoms. This usually means that they are "prehyperventilated," and it takes a shorter time to reach symptomatic hypocarbic levels. It is important to ask patients whether they have ever felt like that before, rather than ask leading questions, because some patients distressed by vestibular disorder will also hyperventilate, compounding the symptoms.

Hypotension often occurs in the elderly, especially those on many medications. A close inquiry and determination of the blood pressure lying and standing may identify the nature of the "dizziness" that many individuals have so much difficulty describing.

VCH

The term "dizziness" carries a heavy load, being commonly used to describe anxiety, disorientation, and impending syncope, as well as the violent sense of bodily rotation that follows vestibular nerve section. Here we will discuss dizziness and imbalance due to disorders of the vestibular system. We will emphasize principles of pathophysiology that are often forgotten in the approach to the dizzy patient, certain controversial or ill-defined causes of vertigo, and the role of medications and physical therapy in management.

PATHOPHYSIOLOGY OF DIZZINESS

The symptoms and signs of vestibular disease cannot be understood unless the clinician has an explicit understanding of the function of the vestibular apparatus. The purpose of the vestibular system is to register angular (rotational) and linear (translational) motion. This information is used to help us to move and see at the same time (the vestibulo-ocular reflex [VOR]), and to assist vision and proprioception in maintaining postural stability (the vestibulo-spinal reflex [VSR]). In a three-dimensional world, there are three potential axes about which rotation and translation can occur. Our vestibular system needs to track a total of six motion coordinates, three of which are related to translation and three to rotation.

Not surprisingly, then, the peripheral vestibular apparatus is organized in such a way as to separate linear from angular movement and to analyze motion according to its axis. The three semicircular canals each respond to angular acceleration in their own plane, producing a complete set of orthogonal information encoding the direction and amplitude of head velocity. Two otolith organs, the utricle and the saccule, respond to linear acceleration in their planes by encoding the direction and amplitude of head translation as well as the orientation to gravity.

This sensory information is reflected by firing patterns in the vestibular nerve and vestibular nucleus that are characterized by two parameters, namely, tone and gain.

Tone is the baseline firing rate in the vestibular nerve or nucleus in the absence of head movement. Tone is normally equal on both sides. *Gain* is the ratio of output to input when the head is moved. *Most disorders of vestibular function can be related to abnormalities of tone or gain.*

The rate and pattern with which vestibular lesions recover determines the prognosis of a patient with a vertiginous episode. Recovery of tone and gain occur at different rates. Let us consider the case of an acute vestibular nerve section of the right side. Immediately after the section, there exists both a tone imbalance and a gain inadequacy. Loss of the resting firing of one side of the vestibular system amounts to the equivalent of rotation at 90° per second to the left. Furthermore, because the vestibular afferents from one labyrinth are gone, the gain acutely drops to 0.5. Most of the recovery from the imbalance in tone occurs in a few days and appears to be "automatic," not requiring visual input. Compensation for reduced gain depends on visual inputs and occurs more slowly, taking months to years to complete.[9] For high speeds and high accelerations, compensation may never be complete. The clinical implication of these observations is that nystagmus usually is a transient sign of a vestibular lesion, whereas movement-induced symptoms are often chronic.

HISTORY AND EXAMINATION OF THE DIZZY PATIENT

Considerable useful information can be gained from a careful description of symptoms. Patients with vestibular tone imbalance complain of *vertigo* (a spinning sensation), *impulsion* (a sensation of linear movement), or a sensation of *tilt*. Although textbooks often emphasize that one should determine direction of vertigo, this procedure is rarely useful. Remember that with the eyes open, spontaneous nystagmus causes retinal images to move on the retina, which gives rise to a directional sense of rotation that is *opposite* to the direction of rotation perceived when the eyes are closed. In other words, vestibular-induced sensation indicates head rotation in the opposite direction as motion inferred from the visual consequence of nystagmus.

More important is to distinguish between horizontal turning, tumbling, and cartwheeling and between rotatory motion and sensations of impulsion, tilt, or floating, as thereby one may be able to separate horizontal from vertical canal imbalance and otolith-induced from canal-induced vertigo. Sensations of tilting or impulsion are rare in peripheral vestibular disorders, perhaps because the hair cells of the otolithic maculae are oriented in multiple directions and a lesion may not produce a pattern of firing resembling natural stimulation.

Patients with normal vestibular tone but inappropriate vestibular gain complain of *movement-induced vertigo*. It is more common and less specific than vertigo due to tone imbalance. Patients with movement-induced vertigo should be questioned about the situations in which their symptoms occur. In particular, is it stimulated by a change in the attitude of the head with respect to gravity (positional vertigo) or by a sudden head rotation in the horizontal plane (when the orientation to gravity does not change).

The objective of the clinical examination is to establish the location and severity of the lesion, with severity expressed in terms of imbalance of tone and abnormalities of gain. Not infrequently an etiology can be established from the examination alone. The essential equipment necessary for an examination of vestibular function includes a set of Frenzel glasses, an ophthalmoscope and otoscope, a visual acuity chart, and a syringe of ice water.

Spontaneous nystagmus indicates imbalance of tone. To see spontaneous nystagmus it is often necessary to remove fixation and magnify the eyes. Frenzel glasses, which are magnifying lenses (+20 diopter) mounted in goggles that occlude the rest of vision, are ideal for this purpose. The ophthalmoscope also works well as long as one remembers that the back of the eye moves oppositely to the front of the eye. The direction of nystagmus indicates which canal(s) or central projections of canals are involved.

Postural instability can arise from both abnormal tone and gain. Patients who persistently fall in one direction may have abnormalities of vestibulospinal tone. Such abnormalities of postural stability are nonspecific, because proprioceptive loss and cerebellar, basal ganglia, and motor disorders can all contribute to poorer performance for difficult balancing tasks.

VOR gain can be evaluated with the ophthalmoscope.[38] If the head is gently oscillated, the optic disc should not move, because a functioning VOR keeps the eye still in space. Another method of assessing VOR gain is by comparing visual acuity with the head moving gently back and forth, against acuity to head still. This has been called the "dynamic illegible E test." It is important that the examiner does not let the patient "cheat" by stopping at turnaround points. A drop in acuity of two lines or more is significant.[19]

The *head-shaking test* can detect *compensated* unilateral vestibular lesions, which is to say that it can detect vestibular lesions that have been present long enough for the spontaneous nystagmus and gain decrease that occurs acutely to be repaired by central adaptations.[14] Here one moves the patient's head (or asks the patient to do so) back and forth as fast as is reasonably tolerated (about 2 Hz) for a total of 20 cycles. Then one stops the head and observes for nystagmus using Frenzel glasses. Normal subjects have no head-shaking nystagmus. Patients with unilateral vestibular paresis or loss may have nystagmus, usually directed so that it beats toward the nonparetic ear. The presence of head-shaking nystagmus in peripheral lesions depends on central storage of asymmetrical activity coming from labyrinthine activation induced by each half-cycle of head rotation. Because central storage is often decreased by vestibular lesions, not all patients with unilateral lesions have head-shaking nystagmus; accordingly, this test can be used to infer the presence of a vestibular gain imbalance but cannot be used to exclude one.

Rapid Rolls. Recently a new clinical test for compensated lesions has been proposed that also depends on rapid head motion. In this test one instructs the subject to fixate a point. One then suddenly and unpredictably rotates the head to one side, looking for "catch-up" saccades at the end of the movement. These indicate that the VOR is not adequate to keep the eyes on the target during the rapid rotation.[15] The utility of this test in a large series of patients with known lesions remains to be established.

The *minimal ice-water caloric* test is a valuable method of detecting a vestibular loss.[24] In this test one uses only 0.2–0.5 mL of ice water as opposed to the 50 mL needed in the testing of the comatose patient.[27] Nystagmus is detected with Frenzel glasses. This is a "yes or no" test — subtle amounts of vestibular paresis will not be detected. We usually use this test to confirm an impression of vestibular loss already gained from the history and other examination procedures.

Hearing should be tested routinely at the bedside because peripheral dizziness is often accompanied by hearing loss. As high-frequency and conductive deficits can be easily appreciated on clinical examination, the main question is: who needs audiometry? Certainly patients with nonvestibular causes of dizziness do not need audiometry, but this may not be apparent early in the evaluation process. Most patients younger than 50 with hearing complaints should be sent for audiometry. However, because of the high prevalence of hearing loss in the elderly, one should screen for severity and asymmetry in older patients. In certain disorders such as benign paroxysmal positional vertigo, hearing assessment is not needed. However, if one is considering Ménière's syndrome or when hearing loss is asymmetrical, audiometry is essential. Of course, the ear should *always* be examined for signs of otitis, tumor, or deformity.

Several ancillary maneuvers are performed to detect for specific vertigo syndromes. One should always attempt to elicit *pressure sensitivity*, which occurs in dizziness due to perilymph fistula. Pressure sensitivity is best assessed with a Politzer bag with an olive tip, but tragal compression can sometimes be enough to cause visible ocular torsion or a subjective sensation of motion. *Positional nystagmus* should be assessed using the Barany and Hallpike maneuvers. Positional testing is most helpful for detecting the upbeat/torsional nystagmus of benign paroxysmal positional vertigo (BPPV). *Hyperventilation-induced nystagmus* is an occasional sign of acoustic neurinomas or other lesions within the petrous bone.

THE ROLE OF VESTIBULAR FUNCTION TESTS

Conventional vestibular function tests are unable to detect lesions of the vertical canals or otoliths and only provide information regarding lateral semicircular canal function. Accordingly, *vestibular function tests can establish that a patient has a peripheral vestibular lesion but cannot exclude one.* *Caloric tests*, also called electronystagmography (ENG), are commonly available in the community, and rotatory tests are available in many university hospitals. Often these tests are accompanied by an evaluation of oculomotor function.

Caloric tests provide only one useful piece of information, called "canal paresis." A canal paresis greater than 25% is abnormal in the statistical sense and implies that there is a decrease in the response of the lateral canal on the side of paresis relative to the other side. Caloric tests are insensitive to moderate degrees of bilateral vestibular paresis because of the large range of responses found in the normal population.[4] While information regarding spontaneous and positional nystagmus is usually provided with the caloric result, these signs are more easily and accurately identified at the bedside with the ophthalmoscope and Frenzel glasses. Positional nystagmus in particular is poorly registered by ENG because (1) the recordings cannot detect torsional nystagmus, (2) without a specific fixation point spontaneous nystagmus can easily be confused with gaze-evoked nystagmus, and (3) the usual eyes-closed recording technique is fraught with artifact. *Reports of positional nystagmus on ENG should always be confirmed by direct observation.*

Rotatory tests provide two useful pieces of information — gain and time constant. The *time constant*, a measure of the duration of response to a constant velocity rotation, is a nonspecific but sensitive measure of vestibular dysfunction indicating that a structural vestibular lesion is present. When the time constant is normal, the search for central or nonvestibular causes of dizziness should be intensified. A significant decrease in rotatory test *gain* indicates a bilateral vestibular weakness. Rotatory testing only rarely separates peripheral from central disorders and as conventionally performed cannot indicate the site of lesion. The central versus peripheral distinction must be made from history and examination and the side of lesion localization from examination and caloric test result.

From the perspective of the neurologist, only access to a rotatory testing facility is necessary as the caloric test and oculomotor evaluation are best done at the time of examination, as described previously. While results of formal caloric testing are valuable if you are familiar with reliability of the testing laboratory, many caloric tests are performed in physicians' offices in which the quality control is not high. When in doubt, always perform your own bedside caloric test. There is, however, no substitute for rotational testing, since the VOR time constant cannot be measured using bedside testing techniques.

Other tests commonly used in evaluating dizziness include brainstem audio evoked responses (BAER), MRI, and petrous tomograms. A T_1 sequence gadolinium MRI, with cuts through the cerebellopontine angle, is the most useful single test. Although acoustic neuromas can be detected by BAERs, an MRI with gadolinium contrast enhancement is equally sensitive and also serves to exclude other causes of dizziness. Petrous tomograms have been supplanted by MRI except when certain bony lesions are suspected.

Electrocochleography (ECochG) is a newer test of vestibular function that is advocated as a method of diagnosing Ménière's disease.[33] The test is positive when there is pathologic enlargement of the cochlear summating potential. There are two difficulties with this test. First, although the test was originally developed using needle electrodes inserted into the middle ear through the tympanic membrane, the test as usually performed in the clinical setting uses electrodes placed on the external auditory meatus. This technique makes it possible for technicians to perform it safely, but the signal quality is degraded. Second, unless a patient has some hearing at high frequencies, ECochG is unreliable. It is too early to say how useful ECochG will become.

Moving-platform posturography has recently been made available commercially and has been advocated as a method of screening for vestibular dysfunction.[5,35] Posturography is less sensitive to vestibular paresis than is a simple clinical examination. We find the main uses of posturography are to document psychogenic disorders of equilibrium and to follow objectively the progress of patients over time.

DIFFERENTIAL DIAGNOSIS OF DIZZINESS

Figure 1–1 illustrates the most common causes of dizziness, according to location. This organization is useful in generating a differential diagnosis once a general category of disease (e.g., central vascular) is known. Often, however, little information is available concerning location of lesion. In this case, it is more useful to use an approach that considers the relative power of the various examination maneuvers and historical features. For example, characteristic findings on positional testing in patients with BPPV are quite specific for this common and treatable syndrome.

Figure 1–2 illustrates the logic used to assign diagnoses to dizzy patients. First one tries to assign a diagnosis using any physical findings that are usually pathognomonic for a specific condition. Generally, about half of the patients referred to a typical "dizzy" clinic will have either BPPV, orthostasis, hyperventilation syndrome, or multiple sensory deficits. Carotid sinus hypersensitivity and perilymphatic fistula also may be diagnosable at the time of the physical examination.

Next, one considers whether or not enough evidence is available to assign the patient to the peripheral or central category. Peripheral disorders typically are accompanied by nausea, hearing disturbance, mild disequilibrium, and quick recovery. Patients with central disorders may be without nausea; usually do not have hearing disturbance; and usually also have paresthesia, weakness, or other signs of central disturbance. Peripheral disorders commonly last hours to days. Central disorders, especially ischemic ones, are more variable, often lasting only minutes, but unlike peripheral disorders, central conditions can cause permanent vertigo. A complete neurologic examination and careful inquiry into risk

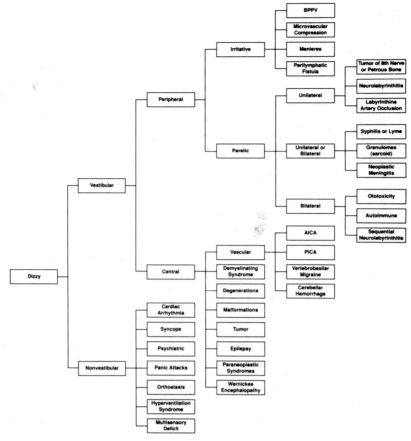

FIGURE 1-1. Causes of dizziness.

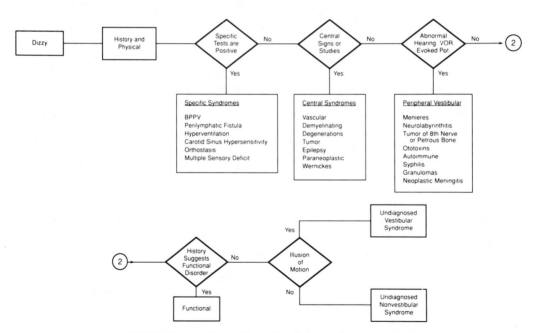

FIGURE 1-2. Logic used to assign diagnoses to dizzy patients.

factors for vascular disease is mandatory when the question of a central origin arises. Findings peculiar to central disorders include purely vertical or torsional spontaneous nystagmus and cross-coupled head-shaking nystagmus (vertical nystagmus after horizontal head shaking). While these particular findings are clues to localization, there are still many patients in whom a clear-cut localization is impossible. The clinical picture of lesions in the labyrinth, vestibular nuclei, and vestibular cerebellum may be identical. MRI scanning is the key in these cases.

In the peripheral cases it is important to make a distinction between unilateral and bilateral disorders. Results from the head-shaking, caloric, and rotatory chair tests are usually helpful. A caloric asymmetry, positive head-shaking test, and decrease in the VOR time constant all suggest a unilateral lesion. Symmetrical or diminished calorics, accompanied by decreased amplitude and by a low time constant of the VOR and decreased visual acuity whenever the head is in motion, support the diagnosis of bilateral paresis or loss. In peripheral disorders, if one can establish that the condition is unilateral, one may be able to treat disorders such as acoustic neuroma, perilymph fistula, or unilateral Ménière's syndrome. On the other hand, bilateral vestibular disorders should prompt a search for ototoxins and for inflammatory and granulomatous disorders.

The remaining patients (entry point 2, Fig. 1 – 2) are essentially undiagnosed and include patients with dizziness due to various nonvestibular causes and patients in whom their vestibular disease produces no abnormalities on clinical or laboratory testing. A functional disorder is suggested by dizziness accompanied by bizarre symptoms, or a previous psychiatric history, and a normal workup including an audiogram and a caloric or rotatory test. However, the diagnosis of a functional syndrome must always be tentative, with an ongoing willingness to reconsider alternatives. Remember that currently available diagnostic tests are unable to detect lesions of the otoliths or vertical semicircular canals.

Specific diagnoses are usually made by recognizing a pattern incorporating history, examination, and test results. We will next discuss the pattern (or lack of pattern) of the most common vertigo syndromes.

Benign Paroxysmal Positional Vertigo

BPPV is the most common cause of vertigo in the elderly.[7] The diagnosis is easily made through a history of positional vertigo and a typical torsional/upbeat nystagmus that appears on the Hallpike maneuver. *The diagnosis of BPPV can definitely be established only through direct observation of a mixed upbeat/torsional nystagmus that appears in a burst.* ENG recordings are inadequate to refute or establish the diagnosis of BPPV because one has no method of ascertaining that the maneuver was done properly and because ENG does not register torsional nystagmus. Remember also that the absence of positional nystagmus on a single examination does not exclude BPPV, especially if the head is not brought quickly to the dependent position.

Ménière's Syndrome

Ménière's syndrome is often the catchall diagnosis for patients with intermittent vertigo and hearing complaints because the criteria for its diagnosis are nonspecific. The diagnosis should be considered in any patient who has both intermittent dizziness combined with a static or fluctuating hearing deficit or dizziness and an abnormal sensation of pressure or fullness in one ear. Ménière's syndrome is probable when (1) a spontaneous nystagmus is observed on at least one occasion, (2) hearing can be documented to be fluctuating on audiometry, and (3) studies necessary to exclude structural lesions of the labyrinth have been performed. In this case, the hearing loss should be of a "cochlear pattern." Most of these patients will also state that ear pain, pressure, fullness, or tinnitus accompanies their vertigo. The clinical picture in Ménière's syndrome does not differ greatly from that of perilymph fistula and from some disorders of the eighth nerve, which will be discussed subsequently. The diagnosis of "vestibular Ménière's" is often made in patients with recurrent vertigo without hearing abnormalities; most of these patients have another cause for their vestibular symptoms.

Microvascular Compression Syndrome

The diagnostic criteria for vestibular symptoms due to a blood vessel compressing the eighth nerve vary markedly. Janetta and coworkers[17] suggest that the syndrome consists of positional vertigo, normal hearing except for tinnitus, and an abnormal BAER. McCabe and Gantz[21] feel that the syndrome is easily confused with "vestibular Ménière's disease" and consists of brief spells of vertigo, disabling motion intolerance, normal hearing, and abnormal peripheral vestibular function. Ryu and associates[29] suggest instead that the typical pattern is to have tinnitus, sensorineural hearing loss, and decreased caloric responses on the affected side. They also found that BAERs are not useful for the diagnosis. Applebaum and Valvassori[1] reported patients who presented with unilateral hearing loss, episodic vertigo, and vascular anomalies on air cisternogram–computed tomography. Since most normal persons have blood vessels crossing the cerebellopontine cistern,[28] having a vessel in the internal auditory canal does not establish that symptoms are due to the vessel and, accordingly, the diagnosis cannot be confirmed at surgery. There is no typical clinical picture for this syndrome,[23] and how important this syndrome is in the overall context of all vestibular disorders is unknown.

Migraine and Vascular Disease

Patients with vertebrobasilar migraine often have recurrent vestibular symptoms, either together with or apart from their headaches. This diagnosis should be considered in patients with typical migraine histories, and particularly in children or young adults with a previous migraine history and unexplained recurrent vertigo.

Vestibular symptoms commonly accompany the lateral medullary syndrome and ischemia in the distribution of the anterior inferior cerebellar artery.[10] The problem arises in separating central from peripheral

causes in otherwise normal patients with recurrent dizziness and vascular risk factors. Grad and Baloh[13] have recently suggested that sudden onset of vertigo lasting minutes in a patient with known cerebrovascular disease suggests an ischemic cause. However, this conclusion was based on their experience with 84 patients with vertigo "presumed" to be of cerebrovascular origin.

Anxiety/Phobic Disorder

As with Ménière's syndrome, the diagnosis of an anxiety/phobic disorder can be applied to patients in a catchall fashion. There are many patients whose test results are entirely normal, but as we have tests only for the lateral canals, it is unclear how to interpret this fact. Some clinicians label these persons as having "anxiety/phobic disorders" and refer them to psychiatrists. *There is no infallible method of recognizing a psychogenic vertigo patient.* Many symptoms that sound bizarre to physicians are actually quite common and presumably have a physiologic substrate. For example, some patients are disturbed by riding in elevators or navigating curves on the highway.[26] Presumably, these symptoms are related to abnormal processing of otolithic signals.

Cervical Vertigo

Cervical vertigo is rare. Theoretically, cervical vertigo might arise from (1) impingement of the vertebral arteries in the neck, (2) compression of the brainstem by a craniocervical junction abnormality such as the Chiari malformation, or (3) an abnormal pattern of inputs from neck proprioceptors.[25] Vertigo is almost never due to occlusion of the vertebral arteries in the neck.[10] Support for the mechanism of vertigo due to abnormal neck proprioception is derived from the experiments of DeJong and associates,[8] in which nystagmus and ataxia were elicited by injection of local anesthetics into the necks of cats and monkeys. In a single human trial, an injection caused ataxia but no nystagmus.

Only craniocervical junction abnormalities are an important cause of cervical vertigo. These patients complain of positional vertigo elicited by either prolonged unusual positioning of the head or neck or repeated flexion/extension movements of the neck.

The usual mistake is to assign vertigo elicited by hyperextension of the head to a cervical origin. In most cases, symptoms are not provoked by having the patient bend forward at the waist and then hyperextending the neck, thus positioning the head upright with respect to gravity but extended with respect to the body. This maneuver usually produces no nystagmus, proving that the symptoms require reorientation of the head with respect to gravity rather than being solely due to the position of the head on the body.

Perilymph Fistula

A perilymph fistula is an abnormal communication between the inner and middle ear due to an otic capsule or labyrinthine window defect. Patients with fistula classically complain of episodic vertigo that worsens with activity; sensitivity to pressure or noise (Tulio's phenomenon); and hearing loss. The symptoms of perilymph fistula closely resemble those of Ménière's syndrome, with the added precipitants of activity, pressure, or noise. The treatment of this condition is surgical exploration and plugging of the defect, but the indications for exploration are highly controversial.[22]

The problem is that exploratory tympanotomy is required to confirm a diagnosis of perilymph fistula, but then the diagnosis still rests on a subjective assessment by the surgeon. Usually about half of such explorations are "dry taps."[31] We feel that exploration should be confined to patients with pressure sensitivity; typical symptoms combined with a history of barotrauma, unusual exertion, or head trauma; or with congenital malformation of the inner ear such as the Mondini deformity. Patients with spontaneous fistulas are exceedingly rare.

Autoimmune Vestibulopathy

Patients with autoantibodies to mesenchymal structures of the inner ear have been well documented,[2] and a syndrome of autoimmune sensorineural hearing loss has been proposed. Many of these patients also complain of gait ataxia resembling that of bilateral vestibular paresis or loss.[20] Little attention has been directed toward this entity. It may account for some cases of "idiopathic bilateral vestibulopathy,"[3] as well as disequilibrium in patients with autoimmune disorders such as Cogan's syndrome, lupus erythematosus, Sjögren's syndrome, and other connective tissue disorders. Whether an autoimmune vestibulopathy occurs without concomitant hearing loss is unknown.

All patients with bilateral vestibular paresis should have serum drawn for antinuclear antibody and sedimentation rate tests. Although a variety of autoimmune tests have been advocated as being sensitive to this disorder,[2,16,36] which of these are appropriate is uncertain. In patients with hearing loss, one may consider immunosuppression, but it is unclear whether or not immunosuppressive treatment should be used in patients who have vestibular complaints alone.

Vestibular Syndromes caused by Syphilis and Lyme Disease

Syphilis is still an important cause of deafness and vestibular paresis. Recently, another spirochete, *Borrelia burgdorferi*, which causes Lyme disease, has come to the attention of the medical community. Lyme disease, like syphilis, can cause a variety of distinct neurologic syndromes, but unlike syphilis, it often affects the cranial nerves; vestibular loss can be associated with positive Lyme serology.[18] As both syphilis and Lyme disease are amenable to antibiotic treatment, patients with undiagnosed vestibular syndromes should always have a fluorescein treponemal antibody test, and if they are from an area endemic for Lyme disease, also a Lyme titer. It is important to remember that the Lyme titer may be negative even in the presence of active disease.

TREATMENT OF VERTIGO

General Considerations in Treatment

There are two sources of symptoms in patients with vertigo: vegetative symptoms, such as nausea, vomiting, and malaise, and distress due to the abnormal sensory function that accompanies a loss of vestibular function, such as movement-induced vertigo, ataxia, and oscillopsia. The problem in treatment is that measures aimed at alleviating the vegetative symptoms, such as bed rest and medication, may harm the patient by denying the nervous system the ability to compensate for a vestibular lesion. Our strategy is to use as few medications as possible and to encourage early ambulation.

When there appears to be no alternative to medication, the question then becomes, which medication is appropriate? Drugs in common use include anticholinergics such as scopolamine (Transderm); antiemetic phenothiazines such as prochlorperazine (Compazine) and promethazine (Phenergan); minor tranquilizers such as diazepam (Valium) and lorazepam (Ativan); and drugs with a mixture of anticholinergic and antihistamine properties such as meclizine (Antivert) and dimenhydrinate (Dramamine). Because of side effects, all of these medications are useful only for short-term management.

Many clinicians fail to distinguish between anticholinergic drugs that are intended to prevent motion sickness, such as scopolamine; drugs that are intended to suppress emesis, such as promethazine or prochlorperazine; and drugs that aim to "sedate" the vestibular system (and usually the patient), such as diazepam. Although scopolamine is useful for prevention of motion sickness, scopolamine and oral meclizine are ineffective in treating acute vestibular imbalance.[37] Antiemetics may reduce nausea and vomiting, but they do not alter the sensation of vertigo per se.

Similarly, a number of other drugs are used commonly to treat dizziness but have no proven efficacy. These include intravenous histamine, carbon dioxide inhalation, nicotinic acid, papaverine, and zinc sulfate.[34] Because most peripheral vestibular disorders resolve spontaneously, any medication that is harmless can be used for its placebo effect. Meclizine in small, ineffective doses (12.5 mg/d) is probably the most useful because of its fortunate brand name ("Antivert").

Management of the *abnormal sensory*

situation that accompanies permanent vestibular paresis or loss is more difficult. This problem arises as the vegetative symptoms abate. Drug treatment is not useful — inasmuch as these symptoms are due to loss of function, suppression of more function does not help matters. Instead, patients should be warned about sudden head movements but be encouraged to attempt as much normal activity as is possible without triggering emesis. A formal vestibular rehabilitation program is a useful method of ensuring activity.

Treatment of Benign Paroxysmal Positional Vertigo

Drugs are not useful in BPPV because while the vertigo is severe, an episode lasts only seconds. There are two approaches to treatment: exercises and surgery. Exercises are effective in 75% of cases.[6] These consist of the process of repeatedly bringing on symptoms until either the disorder remits or the patient learns to tolerate the symptoms. Recently, a new single-step exercise treatment, the "liberatory maneuver," has been proposed by Semont and associates[32] and is claimed to be effective in about 84% of cases. The concept behind this maneuver is that the "stones" that are causing positional nystagmus can be moved out of the posterior canal into the vestibule. Controlled studies comparing this maneuver with the conventional exercises and with no treatment at all are indicated.

The other treatment option is to cut the nerve to the posterior semicircular canal, that is, to perform a singular neurectomy. According to Gacek,[11] this procedure fails in about 10% of cases because of failure to properly diagnose BPPV as well as failure to recognize the singular nerve in the middle ear. There is also a risk of hearing loss of 3% to 7%.

Treatment of Ménière's Disease

Both medical and surgical treatments exist for Ménière's disease. Medical treatment of Ménière's disease includes salt restriction, diuretics, and antiemetics. Surgical treatment is considered only in extremely symptomatic patients in whom medical management fails, if the symptoms can be localized to one side, and if the patient is a good surgical candidate.

Surgical options include several types of labyrinthectomy, as well as specific procedures that aim to decompress the endolymphatic system, such as cochleo-sacculotomy and tacks.[12] These operations attempt to create a permanent fistula between the endolymph and perilymph and to ameliorate symptoms. They relieve vertigo in about 60% of cases, but hearing may deteriorate. Endolymphatic shunts attempt to release excess pressure developed within the endolymphatic space by draining the space into the mastoid.[30] Hearing is improved in some cases and vertigo is usually controlled, although the relapse rate is high.

The results of surgery must be viewed with some skepticism, as a variety of procedures including traction on the spinal column as well as inflating the middle ear through the eustachian tube have also claimed equivalent rates of success in the treatment of Ménière's disease.[34] Presumably, this relates to the self-limited nature of the condition. In extremely intractable cases, a destructive procedure such as labyrinthectomy or vestibular nerve section is employed.

RESEARCH QUESTIONS

It is clear from the preceding discussion that there are many aspects of vestibular disorders needing to be investigated. We are still ignorant about the causes and the treatment of dizziness in most of our patients.

The first step to a neurologic diagnosis is to localize the site of lesion. We need methods of detecting lesions in the vertical semicircular canals and in the otolith organs before we can tell our patients why they feel dizzy. The technology to stimulate a single vertical canal or a single otolith organ is not yet available, and efforts should be made to develop it.

Until we can accurately diagnose patients, only general forms of treatment are likely to succeed. Physical therapy approaches that attempt to promote recalibration of the ves-

tibular system and to encourage new sensory or motor strategies are promising, but it is unclear how important the various types of recovery strategies are in individuals or what the optimum approach might be. Prospective trials of physical therapy using objective and functional methods of assessing improvement are needed.

Finally, as our goal is to optimize the *long-term* well-being of our patients, the question arises whether there are drugs that might promote adaptation. Unfortunately, the drugs we prescribe for the short-term comfort of our patients may actually slow or impede optimal compensation. Research aimed at quantifying the effect of commonly used agents such as meclizine on compensation and identifying drugs that speed adaptation to structural vestibular lesions is indicated.

SUMMARY

The bedside examination is the most important part of the evaluation of the dizzy patient. Armed with an ophthalmoscope, otoscope, Frenzel glasses, a syringe of ice water, and an understanding of vestibular physiology, the neurologist can usually separate central from peripheral lesions and identify a reasonable approach to treatment. Numerous causes of dizziness are often poorly documented or defined and should be viewed with some skepticism. These include vestibular Ménière's syndrome, microvascular compression syndrome, psychogenic vertigo, and perilymph fistula. Treatment must consider that the sources of symptoms in vertigo include not only vegetative responses to tone imbalance but also sensory loss or distortion (e.g., ataxia and oscillopsia) and that measures that abate vegetative symptoms may slow down the rate of compensation and eventual recovery.

REFERENCES

1. Applebaum, EL and Valvasorri, G: Internal auditory canal vascular loops: Audiometric and vestibular system findings. J Otol (Suppl)6:110–113, 1985.
2. Arnold, W, Pfaltz, R, and Altermatt, HJ: Evidence of serum antibodies against inner ear tissues in

the blood of patients with certain sensorineural hearing disorders. Acta Otolaryngol (Stockh) 99:437–444, 1985.

3. Baloh, RW, Jacobson, K, and Honrubia, V: Idiopathic bilateral vestibulopathy. Neurology 39:272–275, 1989.

4. Barber, HO and Stockwell, CW: Manual of Electronystagmography. CV Mosby, St. Louis, 1980.

5. Black FO: Vestibular function assessment in patients with Ménière's disease: The vestibulospinal system. Laryngoscope 92:1419–1436, 1982.

6. Brandt, T and Daroff, RB: Physical therapy for benign paroxysmal positional vertigo. Arch Otolaryngol 106:484–485, 1980.

7. Buchele, W and Brandt, T: Benign paroxysmal positional vertigo and posture. In Bles, W and Brandt, T (eds): Disorders of Posture and Gait. Elsevier, Amsterdam, 1986.

8. DeJong, PTVM, DeJong, JMBV, Cohen, B, and Jongkees, LBW: Ataxia and nystagmus induced by injection of local anesthetics in the neck. Ann Neurol 1:240–246, 1977.

9. Fetter, M and Zee, DS: Recovery from unilateral labyrinthectomy in rhesus monkey. J Neurophysiol 59:370–393, 1988.

10. Fisher, CM: Vertigo in cerebrovascular disease. Arch Otolaryngol 85:85–90, 1967.

11. Gacek, RR: Singular neurectomy update. Ann Otol Rhinol Laryngol 91:469–473, 1982.

12. Glasscock, ME, Kveton, JF, and Christiansen, SG: Current status of surgery of Ménière's disease. Otolaryngol Head Neck Surg 92:67–72, 1984.

13. Grad, A and Baloh, RW: Vertigo of vascular origin: Clinical and electronystagmographic features in 84 cases. Arch Neurol 46:281–284, 1989.

14. Hain, TC, Fetter, M, and Zee, DS: Head shaking nystagmus in unilateral peripheral vestibular lesions. Am J Otol 8:36–47, 1987.

15. Halmagyi, GM and Curthoys, IS: A clinical sign of canal paresis. Arch Neurol 45:737–740, 1988.

16. Hughes, GB, Barna, BP, Calabrese, LH, Kinney, SE, and Nalepa, NJ: Clinical diagnosis of immune inner-ear disease. Laryngoscope 98:2251–2253, 1988.

17. Janetta, PJ, Moller, MB, and Moller, AR: Disabling positional vertigo. N Engl J Med 310:1700–1705, 1984.

18. Krejcova, H, Bojar, M, Jerabek, J, Tomas, J, and Jirous, J: Otoneurological symptomatology in Lyme disease. Adv Otorhinolaryngol 42:410–212, 1988.

19. Longridge, NS and Mallinson, AI: The dynamic illegible E-test. Acta Otolaryngol (Stockh) 103: 273–279, 1987.

20. McCabe, BF: Autoimmune sensorineural hearing loss. Ann Otol Rhinol Laryngol 88:585–589, 1979.

21. McCabe, BF and Gantz, BJ: Vascular loop as a cause of incapacitating dizziness. Am J Otol 10:117–120, 1989.

22. Meyer, H: Peer review's limits visible once again. Am Med News, May 5, 1989, pp. 1–11.

23. Nadol, JB: Disabling positional vertigo. N Engl J Med 311:1053–1054, 1984.

24. Nelson, JR: The minimal ice water caloric test. Neurology 19:577, 1969.

25. Norre, ME: Neurophysiology of vertigo with special reference to cervical vertigo: A review. Medica Physica 29:183–194, 1986.

26. Page, NGR and Gresty, MA: Motorist's vestibular disorientation syndrome. J Neurol Neurosurg Psychiatry 48:729–734, 1985.

27. Plum, F and Posner, JB: The Diagnosis of Stupor and Coma, ed 3. FA Davis, Philadelphia, 1980.

28. Quaking, GE: Microsurgical anatomy of the arterial loops in the ponto-cerebellar angle and the internal auditory Meatus. In Samii, M, Janetta, PJ (eds): The Cranial Nerves. Springer-Verlag, Berlin, 1981, pp 388–390.

29. Ryu, H, Uemura, K, Yokayama, T, and Nozue, M: Indications and results of neurovascular decompression of the eighth cranial nerve for vertigo, tinnitus and hearing disturbances. Adv Otorhinolaryngol 42:280–283, 1988.

30. Schuknecht, HF and Bartley, M: Cochlear endolymphatic shunt for Ménière's disease. Am J Otol (Suppl) 20–22, 1985.

31. Seltzer, S and McCabe, BF: Perilymph fistula: The Iowa experience. Laryngoscope 96:37–49, 1986.

32. Semont, A, Freyss, G, and Vitte, E: Curing the BPPV with a liberatory maneuver. Adv Otorhinolaryngol 42:290–293, 1988.

33. Shea, JL and Orchik, DJ: Electrocochleography and low-frequency harmonic acceleration in Ménière's disease. Arch Otorhinolaryngol Head Neck Surg 112:929–933, 1986.

34. Torok, N: Old and new in Ménière's disease. Laryngoscope 11:1870–1877, 1977.

35. Wall, C and Black, FO: Postural stability and rotational tests: Their effectiveness for screening dizzy patients. Acta Otolaryngol (Stockh) 95: 235–236, 1983.

36. Wei, NR and Giebel, W: Optimierung des immunofluoreszenztest für antikorper im serum von patienen mit innenohrerkrankungen. Laryngorhinootologie (Stuttgart) 66:6–10, 1987.

37. Wennmo, C, Bergenius, J, Henriksson, NG, Hyden, D, Enbom, H, Magnusson, M, Odkvist, LM, Pyykko, I, Rosenhall, U, Schalen, L, and Siegborn, J: Transdermal scopolamine and vertigo of peripheral vestibular origin. In Grahm, MD and Kemink, JL (eds): The Vestibular System: Neurophysiologic and Clinical Research. Raven Press, New York, 1987, pp 607–611.

38. Zee, DS: Opthalmoscopy in examination of patients with vestibular disorders. Ann Neurol 3:373, 1978.

CHAPTER 2

• •

THE DIZZY PATIENT: TREATMENT OPTIONS

Robert W. Baloh, M.D.

If "normality" is to be defined statistically, then after the age of 65 years being dizzy is normal and not being dizzy is abnormal. Baloh quotes evidence that as many as 70% of the elderly living at home complain of dizziness.

"Dizziness" is like an overcoat, ample but unrevealing. As Baloh points out, spinning is one of the few sensations described as dizziness that has diagnostic significance, nearly always implying a vestibular disorder.

The author provides a balanced and reasoned account of diagnosis and management of the common disorders afflicting the dizzy patient.

VCH

EXTENT OF THE PROBLEM

Dizziness is a common symptom in patients of all ages. As many as 5% of all patients seen by general practitioners and 10% to 15% of patients seen by otolaryngologists and neurologists present with the complaint of dizziness.[42] According to the 1980–1981 national ambulatory medical care survey, dizziness was the single most common presenting complaint among aged patients 70 years and older in office practice.[35] Among adults age 65 years and older living at home as many as 70% complain of dizziness, with the incidence rising with advancing age and generally being higher in women than in men.[27] Dizziness is a difficult symptom to assess for several reasons: (1) it is a subjective sensation, that is, it cannot be measured; (2) it represents several different overlapping sensations; and (3) it is caused by many different pathophysiologic mechanisms and a variety of diagnoses.

TYPES OF DIZZINESS

"Dizziness" is a nonspecific term that describes a sensation of altered orientation in space.[4] Since visual, proprioceptive, and vestibular signals provide the main source of information about the position of the head and body in space, damage to any of these afferent systems can lead to a complaint of dizziness. Furthermore, changes in the brain centers that integrate these orienting signals can also lead to the sensation of dizziness. Inasmuch as the evaluation and management differ markedly depending on the category of dizziness, it is critical that the examining physician determine the type of dizziness before proceeding with diagnostic studies (Table 2–1).

Vertigo. The afferent nerves from the otoliths and semicircular canals of each labyrinth maintain a balanced tonic rate of firing to the vestibular nuclei. Asymmetric involvement of this baseline activity anywhere

15

TABLE 2–1. **MECHANISM AND COMMON CAUSES OF DIFFERENT TYPES OF DIZZINESS**

Type	Mechanism	Common Causes
Vertigo	Imbalance of tonic vestibular signals	Benign positional vertigo, Ménière's syndrome, neurolabyrinthitis, vertebrobasilar insufficiency
Presyncopal lightheadedness	Diffuse cerebral ischemia	Orthostatic hypotension, vasovagal episode, cardiac arrhythmia, hyperventilation
Psychophysiologic dizziness	Impaired central integration of sensory signals	Anxiety, panic attacks, phobias
Dysequilibrium	Loss of vestibulospinal, proprioceptive, cerebellar function	Ototoxicity, peripheral neuropathy, stroke, cerebellar atrophy
Ocular dizziness	Visual-vestibular mismatch due to impaired vision	Change in magnification, oculomotor paresis
Multisensory dizziness	Partial loss of multiple sensory systems	Diabetes mellitus, aging
Physiologic dizziness	Sensory conflict due to unusual combination of sensory signals	Motion sickness, height vertigo, mal de debarquement

in the peripheral and central vestibular pathways can lead to an illusion of movement, vertigo. The same sensation can result from lesions in such diverse locations as the inner ear, the deep paravertebral stretch receptors of the neck, the visual-vestibular interaction centers in the brainstem and cerebellum, or the subjective sensation pathways of the thalamus or cortex. Furthermore, well-documented lesions within the vestibular pathways sometimes produce only a nonspecific sensation of disorientation without a clearly defined illusion of movement.

Vestibular versus Nonvestibular Dizziness. Although the description alone does not distinguish between vestibular and nonvestibular causes of dizziness, certain words are commonly used to describe each type of dizziness. A sensation of spinning nearly always indicates a vestibular disorder. Patients with nonvestibular dizziness occasionally will report a sensation of spinning inside the head but the environment remains still and they do not have nystagmus. Patients with vestibular lesions often liken the sensation to that of being drunk or motion sick. They describe feelings of imbalance as though they are falling or tilting to one side. Patients with nonvestibular dizziness use terms such as "light-headed," "floating," "giddy," or "swimming." The sensation that one has left one's body is

characteristic of psychophysiologic dizziness.

Vertigo is an episodic phenomenon, whereas nonvestibular dizziness is often continuous. An exception would be presyncopal lightheadedness caused by postural hypotension or cardiac arrhythmia. Patients with psychophysiologic dizziness often report being dizzy from morning to night without change for months to years at a time. Vertigo is typically aggravated by head movements, while nonvestibular dizziness is often aggravated by movements of visual targets. Episodes of dizziness induced by position change suggest a vestibular lesion if postural hypotension has been ruled out. Although stress can aggravate both vestibular and nonvestibular dizziness, dizziness that is reliably precipitated by stress suggests a nonvestibular cause. Finally, episodes of dizziness occurring only in specific situations (e.g., driving on the freeway, entering a crowded room, or shopping in a busy supermarket) suggests a nonvestibular cause.

The presence of associated symptoms can also help one distinguish between vestibular and nonvestibular causes of dizziness. Nausea and vomiting are usual with vertigo but uncommon with other types of dizziness. Associated auditory or neurologic symptoms suggest a vestibular disorder, presyncopal symptoms and syncope a nonvestibular disorder. Multiple symptoms of acute and chronic anxiety commonly accompany psychophysiologic dizziness.

PATHOPHYSIOLOGY AND MANAGEMENT OF COMMON VESTIBULAR DISORDERS

Benign Positional Vertigo

Benign positional vertigo is not a disease but rather a syndrome that can be the sequelae of several different inner ear diseases; in about half the cases no cause can be found.[5,33] Patients with the disorder develop brief episodes of vertigo (<30 second) with position change typically when turning over in bed, getting in and out of bed, bending over and straightening up, or extending the neck to look up. Diagnosis rests on finding a characteristic fatigable paroxysmal positional nystagmus after the patient is rapidly moved from the sitting to the head-hanging position (the so-called Hallpike maneuver). Studies of the temporal bone in patients with typical benign positional vertigo have revealed basophilic deposits on the cupulae of the posterior semicircular canals.[54] These deposits were prominent only on one side, the side that was undermost when paroxysmal positional nystagmus and vertigo were induced. The deposits are probably otoconia released from a degenerating utricular macule. The octonia settle on the cupula of the posterior canal (situated directly under the utricular macule), causing it to become heavier than the surrounding endolymph and thus sensitive to changes in the direction of gravity. When the patient moves from the sitting to head-hanging position, the posterior canal moves from an inferior to a superior position, a utriculofugal displacement of the cupula occurs, and a burst of nystagmus is produced. The latency before nystagmus onset could be due to the period of time required for the otoconial mass to be displaced, and fatigability may be caused by the dispersing of particles in the endolymph. Consistent with this theory, the burst of paroxysmal positional nystagmus is in the plane of the posterior canal of the "down ear" with the fast component directed upward, as would be predicted from ampullofugal stimulation of

the posterior canal.[7,26] Additional support for this concept has come from reports showing disappearance of fatigable paroxysmal positional nystagmus after the ampullary nerve has been sectioned from the posterior canal on the diseased side.[22]

Management

Once the diagnosis is made, a simple explanation of the nature of the disorder and its favorable prognosis can help relieve the patients' anxiety. It is important to be aware, however, that although it is a benign disorder, the course is often protracted and most patients will have recurrences at some time. Positional exercises can accelerate remissions in most cases of benign positional vertigo. The patient is instructed to sit on the edge of a bed and rapidly assume the lateral position to induce positional vertigo.[11] After the vertigo subsides, the patient returns to the upright position, usually experiencing a lesser episode of vertigo. These positional changes are repeated in each session until the vertigo fatigues; the sessions are repeated three times a day until the vertigo no longer occurs. In our experience patients who show the most prominent fatigue on the standard diagnostic positional tests will derive the most benefit from positional exercises. It has been hypothesized that these positional maneuvers work by dislodging the calcium carbonate material from the cupula of the posterior semicircular canals. Central adaptation is another possible explanation for their benefit.

Viral Neural Labyrinthitis

Of the thousands of infants born deaf every year, about 20% of cases are thought to be the result of congenital viral infections.[45] More than 4000 persons are stricken each year with "sudden deafness," a sensorineural hearing loss of acute onset, presumed to be of viral origin in most cases.[65] A like number of individuals are stricken with the acute onset of intense vertigo (so-called vestibular neuronitis or neuritis) unaccompanied by any neurologic or audiologic symptoms and also presumed to be of viral origin.[53] Despite the strong suspicion of a viral origin for these common disorders, proof of a viral pathophysiology in a given case is difficult to obtain. Serologic studies demonstrate that a virus infected the patient but do not prove that the infectious agent caused inner ear damage. Furthermore, isolation of a virus from the nasopharynx or any tissue other than the membranous labyrinth does not prove a causal relationship between the virus and the inner ear disease.

Probably the most convincing data supporting a viral cause for these common neurotologic syndromes are the temporal bone studies of Schuknecht and his colleagues in Boston.[51,52,53] These investigators found lesions consistent with viral involvement of the cochlea and auditory nerve in patients with a history of sudden deafness and of the vestibular end organ and vestibular nerve in patients with a history of an acute vestibulopathy. The atrophy of the nerves and end organs was identical to that associated with well-documented viral syndromes (such as mumps or measles). Furthermore, experimental studies in animals have shown that several viruses will selectively infect the labyrinth and/or eighth nerve.[17,43]

Viral neurolabyrinthitis can present with sudden deafness, acute vertigo, or with some combination of auditory and vestibular symptoms. Although the term "sudden deafness" is commonly used, the hearing loss due to viral infection usually comes on over several hours and may even extend over several days.[51,65] The loss is often profound and may be permanent, although it reverses at least partially in most cases. Normal function returns in more than 50% of patients (with or without treatment).[37] Vestibular neurolabyrinthitis (vestibular neuronitis, vestibular neuritis) is typically manifested by a gradual onset of vertigo, nausea, and vomiting over several hours.[52] The symptoms usually reach a peak within 24 hours and then gradually resolve over several weeks. During the first day there is severe truncal unsteadiness and imbalance and the patient has difficulty focusing because of spontaneous nystagmus. Most patients have a benign course with complete recovery within 3 months. There are important exceptions to this rule, however. Occasional patients, particularly the elderly, will have

intractible dizziness that persists for months to years. Twenty to 30% of patients will have at least one recurrent bout of vertigo (this is usually less severe than the initial episode).[15] This may represent reactivation of a latent virus, since it is often associated with a systemic viral illness. A small percentage of these patients will have multiple recurrent episodes of vertigo leading to a profound bilateral vestibulopathy (so-called bilateral sequential vestibular neuritis).[55] The episodic vertigo is eventually replaced by persistent disequilibrium and oscillopsia.[6]

Management

Management of patients who present with isolated episodes of auditory and/or vestibular loss is controversial because the pathophysiology is often uncertain. As suggested earlier, unless there is convincing evidence to support a vascular or nonviral infectious cause, the patient should be managed as a presumed case of viral neurolabyrinthitis, that is, with symptomatic treatment. Although steroids have been recommended for their anti-inflammatory effect,[1] there have been no controlled studies to assess the risk-benefit ratio for these drugs. Numerous so-called vasodilating regimens have been proposed, but they would have little effect on the presumed viral pathophysiology. Although about one third of patients with vestibular neurolabyrinthitis are left with permanent loss of vestibular function (as documented by serial caloric examinations), the central nervous system (CNS) is able to adapt to the vestibular loss, and residual symptoms are usually minimal once the compensation has occurred. Vestibular exercises (Table 2–2) should be started immediately after the acute nausea and vomiting subside and should be continued until dizziness and imbalance are minimal.[8] Although antiviral agents such as cytosine arabinase and acyclovir have been used for treating systemic viral illnesses in children, it is unclear whether the hearing loss that is often associated with disorders such as cytomegalovirus and rubella infections is altered by such treatment. There have been no reports on the efficacy of antiviral agents in adults with viral neurolabyrinthitis.

TABLE 2-2. VESTIBULAR EXERCISES

In Bed

Eye movements at first slow, then quick
  Gazing up and down
  Gazing from side to side
  Focusing on finger moving from 30-10 cm away
    from face
Head movements at first slow, then quick, later with
    eyes closed
  Bending forward and backward
  Turning from side to side

Sitting

Head movements as above
Shoulder shrugging and circling
Bending forward and picking up objects from ground

Standing

Eye and head movements, shoulder shrugging and
    circling as above
Changing from sitting to standing position with eyes
    open and closed
Throwing small ball from hand to hand (above eye level)
Throwing ball from hand to hand under knee
Changing from sitting to standing position, turning
    around in between

Moving About

Circling around center person who will throw large
    ball and to whom it will be returned
Walking across room with eyes open and then closed
Walking up and down slope with eyes open and then
    closed
Walking up and down steps with eyes open and then
    closed
Performing any game involving stooping and
    stretching and aiming, such as skittles, bowling,
    or basketball

Ménière's Syndrome

Ménière's syndrome is characterized by episodes of hearing loss, tinnitus, vertigo, and a sensation of fullness or pressure in the ear. In the early stages the hearing loss is completely reversible, but in later stages a residual hearing loss remains between attacks. The main pathologic finding in patients with Ménière's syndrome is distention of the endolymphatic system.[25,44] The membranous labyrinth progressively dilates until the saccular wall makes contact with the stapes footplate and the cochlear duct occupies the entire vestibular scala. The cochlear and vestibular end-organs and nerves show minimal pathologic changes. Membranous labyrinth herniations and ruptures are common, the latter frequently involving Reissner's membrane and the walls of the saccule, utricle, and ampullae. Occasionally, a rupture is followed by complete collapse of the membranous labyrinth.

Although the pathologic changes have been well described, the mechanism for the fluctuating symptoms and signs of Ménière's syndrome are not well understood. A leading theory is that the episodes of hearing loss and vertigo are caused by ruptures in the membrane, separating endolymph from perilymph, producing a sudden increase in potassium concentration in the latter.[57] As the potassium is slowly cleared over several hours, symptoms and signs subside. Another possible explanation is mechanical deformation of the end-organ, which is reversible as the endolymphatic pressure decreases. The infrequent but dramatic sudden falling attacks seen in patients with Ménière's syndrome are most likely due to a sudden deformation or displacement of one of the vestibular sense organs.[61]

Management

Since the cause of Ménière's syndrome is usually unknown, treatment is empiric. Medical management consists of symptomatic treatment of the acute spells of vertigo (see below) and long-term prophylaxis with salt restriction and diuretics.[9,31] The mechanism by which a low-salt diet decreases the frequency and severity of attacks with Ménière's syndrome is unclear, but there is strong empiric evidence for its efficacy. We recommend salt restriction in the range of 1 to 2 g of sodium per day with a minimum therapeutic trial of 2 to 3 months. Fluid and food intake should be regularly distributed throughout the day. Binges (particularly foods with high sugar or salt content) should be avoided. Occasionally, patients will notice that certain foods (e.g., alcohol, coffee, chocolate) may precipitate attacks. Diuretics (acetazolamide, 250 mg bid, or hydrochlorathiazide, 50 mg bid) provide additional benefit in some patients, although they cannot replace a salt restriction diet.

Two different types of surgery have been used for treating Ménière's syndrome: endolymphatic shunts and destructive procedures. While shunts are logical based on the presumed pathophysiology of Ménière's syndrome, several factors limit the probability of achieving a functional shunt.[50] Furthermore, recent clinical studies question their efficacy.[56,59] The rationale for ablative surgery in treating Ménière's syndrome is that the nervous system is better able to compensate for complete loss of vestibular function than for partial loss that is fluctuating in degree. Ablative procedures are most effective in patients with unilateral involvement who have no functional hearing on the damaged side. Obviously, ablative surgery should not be considered if the abnormal side is not well defined or if the nature of the underlying disorder is not absolutely clear. Severe vertigo is expected during the immediate postoperative period, but most patients who follow a structured vestibular exercise program (Table 2–2) can return to normal activity within 1 to 3 months. Ablative surgical procedures generally should be avoided in elderly patients, since the elderly have greater difficulty adjusting to vestibular imbalance.

Perilymph Fistula

Perilymph fistulae result from the disruption of the limiting membranes of the labyrinth, usually at the oval or round windows. The symptoms and signs are remarkably variable; fistula must be considered in the differential diagnosis of sudden hearing loss, recurrent vestibulopathy, Ménière's syndrome, congenital sensorineural hearing loss, posttraumatic hearing loss and vertigo, and stapedectomy failure.[40] The cause is obvious when there is a disruption of the otic capsule or a tear in the membranous labyrinth associated with trauma, surgery, or infection, but spontaneous fistulae are more difficult to explain. A sudden negative or positive pressure change in the middle ear from violent nose blowing, sneezing, or barotrauma or a sudden increase in cerebrospinal fluid (CSF) pressure associated with lifting, straining, coughing, or vigorous activity may lead to rupture of the round window.[23] In the last case, the change in CSF pressure is transmitted to the inner ear via the cochlear aqueduct and/or internal auditory canal. Perilymph fistulae may also be associated with developmental abnormalities of the middle ear and otic capsule. The classical presentation of an acute perilymph fistula is a sudden audible pop in the ear immediately followed by hearing loss, vertigo, and tinnitus. The key to the diagnosis is to identify the characteristic precipitating factors mentioned previously.

Management

The great majority of perilymph fistulae spontaneously heal without intervention. For this reason, most authors advocate conservative management with an initial period of bed rest, sedation, and head elevation and measures to decrease straining.[40] The one exception to this conservative approach is acute barotrauma, in which immediate exploration has been advocated.[47] Persistent fluctuating auditory and vestibular symptoms are indications for exploration of the middle ear after an initial trial of conservative management. Even in these cases, however, only about half to two thirds of ears are found to have fistulae.

Acoustic Neuroma

Acoustic neuroma (vestibular schwannoma) usually begins in the internal auditory canal, producing symptoms by compressing the nerves in the narrow confines of the canal. As the tumor enlarges, it protrudes through the internal auditory meatus, producing a funnel-shaped erosion of the bone surrounding the canal, stretching adjacent nerves over the surface of the mass, and deforming the brainstem and cerebellum. Acoustic neuromas account for about 5% of intracranial tumors and over 90% of cerebellopontine (CP) angle tumors.[10] By far the most common symptoms associated with acoustic neuromas are slowly progressive hearing loss and tinnitus from compression of the cochlear nerve.[20,41] Rarely, an acute hearing loss occurs, apparently from compression of the labyrinthine vasculature. Vertigo occurs in fewer than 20% of patients, but approximately 50% complain of imbalance or disequilibrium. Next to the auditory nerve, the most commonly involved cranial nerves (by compression) are the seventh and fifth, producing facial weakness and numbness, respectively. Involvement of the sixth, ninth, tenth, eleventh, and twelfth nerves occurs only in the late stages of disease with massive tumors. Large acoustic neuromas may also produce increased intracranial pressure from obstruction of CSF outflow.

Management

With few exceptions, the management of tumors in the internal auditory canal and CP angle is surgical. Occasionally, one might follow the case of a patient with a small acoustic neuroma, particularly if the patient is elderly or has underlying medical problems.[63] These tumors can remain confined to the internal auditory canal for years; symptoms may be restricted to those of the eighth nerve.

Vertibrobasilar Insufficiency

Vertibrobasilar insufficiency (VBI) is a common cause of vertigo in patients over the age of 50.[21,64] Whether the vertigo originates from ischemia of the labyrinth, brainstem, or both structures is not always clear, since the circulation to both the labyrinth and vestibular nuclei originates from the vertebrobasilar system. Isolated episodes of vertigo, however, are almost certainly due to selective ischemia in the end-artery circulation of the vestibular labyrinth.[24] Vertigo with VBI is abrupt in onset, usually lasts several minutes, and is frequently associated with nausea and vomiting. The key to the diagnosis is to find associated symptoms resulting from ischemia in the remaining territories supplied by the posterior circulation. Common associated symptoms include formed and unformed visual hallucinations, diplopia, drop attacks, dysarthria, numbness, and weakness. These symptoms occur in episodes (lasting minutes) either in combination with the vertigo or in isolation. Vertigo may be an isolated initial symptom of VBI, but repeated episodes of vertigo without other symptoms suggests a disorder other than VBI.[21,24]

The cause of VBI is usually atherosclerosis of the subclavian, vertebral, and basilar arteries.[13] Other, less common, causes of arterial occlusion include dissecting aneurysms, arteritis, emboli, polycythemia, thromboangitis obliterans, and hypercoagulation syndromes. In rare cases, occlusion or stenosis of the subclavian or innominate arteries just proximal to the origin of the vertebral artery results in the so-called subclavian steal syndrome. In this syndrome, VBI results from siphoning blood down the vertebral artery from the basilar system to supply the upper extremity. Also, rarely, episodes are precipitated by postural hypotension, Stokes-Adams attacks, or mechanical compression from cervical spondylosis.

Management

Knowledge of the natural history of VBI is obviously critical in assessing any treatment regimen.[12] It has been our impression that patients with episodes of vertigo of typical vascular onset and duration, with or without associated symptoms, have the most benign course of the VBI syndromes. More worrisome are patients who present with episodes of quadraparesis, perioral numbness, bilateral blindness, or loss of consciousness. These last symptoms are often prodroma of basilar artery thrombosis. Treatment of VBI usually consists of controlling risk factors (diabetes, hypertension, hyperlipidemia) and the use of antiplatelet drugs (aspirin).[34] Anticoagulation is reserved for patients with frequent incapacitating episodes or for patients with symptoms and signs suggesting a stroke in evolution, particularly basilar artery thrombosis. Although surgical reconstruction and revascularization procedures have been performed successfully in the vertebrobasilar system, their specific indications have yet to be defined. Controlled studies with modern angiographic and surgical techniques are needed to assess the risk-benefit ratio.

SYMPTOMATIC TREATMENT OF VERTIGO

Vertigo is a frightening symptom. Regardless of its cause, the physician can provide support and reassurance to the patient. If the patient's fear and anxiety can be alleviated, the symptom is less distressing. Patients with acute vertigo prefer to lie still in bed in a dark and quiet room. Fortunately, the CNS has a remarkable ability to compensate for most types of vestibular imbalance and therefore, regardless of cause, acute vertigo usually resolves over several days.

As the acute vertiginous episode subsides, rehabilitation should begin promptly. Because vertigo is aggravated by head movements, patients typically hold themselves stiffly when turning and moving about. They also tire easily with physical activity. Patients beginning rehabilitation should realize that a gradual return to normal physical activity is vital to recovery. For the nervous system to recalibrate the relationship between visual, proprioceptive, and vestibular signals, repeated head, eye, and body movements are essential. Patients may drift into a state of chronic invalidism if they are unaware of this requirement.

Antivertiginous Medications

The commonly used antivertiginous medications and their dosages are listed in Table 2–3. It is often difficult to predict which drug or combinations of drugs will be most effective in a given patient; some respond to one drug but not to others in the same class. The mechanism of action of these drugs is not completely known, although most have been shown either to decrease the efficacy of transmission from primary to secondary vestibular neurons or to decrease the overall excitability of neurons in the vestibular nucleus.

The choice of a drug or combination of drugs is based on the known effects of each drug (see Table 2–1) and on the severity and time course of symptoms. In patients with acute severe vertigo, sedation is desirable and drugs such as promethazine and diazepam are particularly useful. If nausea and vomiting are severe, the antiemetic prochlorperazine can be combined with another antivertiginous medication. The patient with chronic recurrent vertigo usually is attempting to carry on normal activities and therefore sedation is undesirable. In this setting, meclizine, dimenhydrinate, and scopolamine are often useful. Of the antihistamines, promethazine has the most sedating effect and is therefore useful only when moderate sedation is desired. A com-

TABLE 2–3. DOSAGE AND EFFECTS OF COMMONLY USED ANTIVERTIGINOUS MEDICATIONS

Class	Drug	Dosage	Sedation	Antiemetic Actions	Dryness of Mucous Membranes	Extra-pyramidal Symptoms
Anticholinergic	Scopolamine	0.6 mg orally q4–6h or 0.5 mg transdermally q3d	+	+	+++	−
Monoaminergic	Amphetamine	5 or 10 mg orally q4–6h	−	+	+	+
	Ephedrine	25 mg orally q4–6h	−	+	+	−
Antihistamine	Meclizine (Antivert)	25 mg orally q4–6h	+	+	+	−
	Dimenhydrinate (Dramamine)	50 mg orally or intramuscularly q4–6h or 100-mg suppository q8h	+	+	+	−
	Promethazine (Phenergan)	25 or 50 mg orally, intramuscularly, or as suppository q4–6h	++	++	+	−
Phenothiazine	Prochlorperazine Compazine)	5 or 10 mg orally or intramuscularly q6h or 25-mg suppository q12h	+	+++	+	+++
Benzodiazepine	Diazepam (Valium)	5 or 10 mg orally, intramuscularly, or intravenously q4–6h	+++	+	−	−

bination of promethazine and the sympatho-
mimetic ephedrine (25 mg of each) produces less sedation than promethazine
alone and is more effective in relieving associated autonomic symptoms.

Vestibular Exercises

In 1945, Cooksey[16] and Cawthorne[14] reported that vestibular compensation occurred more rapidly and was more complete
if patients began exercising as soon as possible after a labyrinthine injury or ablation.
Subsequent controlled studies in primates
have supported this clinical observation.
Baboons whose hind limbs are restrained by
a plaster cast after a unilateral vestibular
neurectomy show markedly delayed compensation for ataxia compared with control
animals that are allowed normal motor exploration after an identical neurectomy.[36]
Squirrel monkeys given daily exercises in a
motor-driven rotating cage compensate for a
unilateral labyrinthectomy faster than control animals given no exercise.[30]

Vestibular exercises are designed to gradually retrain the eye and body musculature
to use visual and proprioceptive signals to
compensate for the lost vestibular signals
(see Table 2–2). The eye and head movements are performed in bed as soon as possible after acute vertigo, nausea, and vomiting
have subsided. The remaining exercises are
then gradually introduced as the patient recovers. Three exercise sessions per day for at
least 5 minutes are recommended. The patient should be encouraged to seek out the
head positions and movements that cause
dizziness as far as can be tolerated, since the
more frequently dizziness is induced the
more quickly compensation occurs. Antivertiginous medications can be used during
the course of the exercises to make the dizziness more tolerable.

Grouping patients together for their vestibular exercises is ideal, since they can encourage each other and beginners can wit-
ness the progress of long-term members.
The purpose of the exercises should be explained to each patient and each should receive written instructions outlining the exercise regimen. The exercises are usually
continued for 1 to 3 months. During this
time, the patient is encouraged to return to a
normal schedule of work and leisure activities as soon as possible.

IMPORTANT RESEARCH AREAS

New Diagnostic Techniques

Vestibular Function Tests

As with other sensory systems, there are
two general categories of tests of vestibular
function: those relying on the subjective response of the patient and those relying on
objective measurements of the reflex activity. Unlike tests of the auditory and visual
systems, however, quantifying the sensation
of movement derived from excitation of the
vestibular receptors has been a difficult task.
It is often impossible for a patient to differentiate those sensations that are strictly vestibular from visual and proprioceptive sensations. Equally important, awareness of
vestibular stimulation depends on a patient's general state of alertness and degree
of cooperation. For these reasons, modern
vestibular function testing has focused on
objective measurements of vestibular reflex activity.[3] The horizontal semicircular
canal–ocular reflex has received the most
attention to date because there are several
relatively simple techniques for stimulating
(caloric and rotational) and recording
(electronystagmography). Tests of the other
vestibulo-ocular reflexes (vertical semicircular canal and otolith) and of the vestibulo-
spinal reflexes (posturography) have yet to
be shown useful in the clinical setting.[3]

Vestibular Evoked Potentials

A vestibular evoked potential would provide an objective measure of peripheral vestibular function that would be independent
of either the oculomotor or postural control
systems. Despite the fact that sensory
evoked potentials using auditory, visual,
and somatosensory signals have been developed and are in routine clinical use, short-
latency vestibular evoked potentials have
been recorded successfully only in small
laboratory animals.[18,19] This lack of development is related to the difficulty in delivering a vestibular stimulus that is capable of

triggering a coordinated volley of neural activity, a requirement for eliciting a measurable evoked potential. The vestibular equivalent of an auditory click, visual flash, or somatosensory prick is a brief, abrupt, high-intensity movement equivalent to that encountered during a blow to the face, that is, an angular acceleration in the range of 7000 deg/s^2. Prior research regrading human vestibular evoked potentials has focused on recording long-latency cortical potentials rather than brainstem evoked potentials.[28,29,46,49] The results of these studies are conflicting; it is unclear whether the recorded potentials are specific for the vestibular system. Considering their possible clinical usefulness, research on vestibular evoked potentials continues in several centers.

Neuroimaging

Computed tomography (CT) and magnetic resonance imaging (MRI) have markedly improved the diagnosis of lesions involving the temporal bone and posterior fossa.[2,60,62] The relative merit of these two imaging techniques is still being defined, although MRI is clearly superior to CT for imaging soft-tissue lesions. MRI can identify small acoustic neuromas confined to the internal auditory canal, tumors that are missed with CT (Fig. 2–1A). MRI can also reliably identify gliomas of the brainstem and cerebellum, tumors that may be isodense on CT (Figure 2–1B). CT is most useful for identifying bony erosion, hemorrhage, and/or calcification within tumors. In some cases CT can compliment MRI by differentiating between tumor and associated edema.

Pharmacology of Vestibular Neurotransmitters

The pharmacology of the peripheral and central vestibular pathways is poorly understood. Animal studies suggest that drugs with anticholinergic activity diminish the excitability of vestibular nucleus neurons.[32,39,48] Such drugs suppress both the spontaneous firing rate and the response to vestibular nerve stimulation, indicating a cholinergic transmission from primary to secondary vestibular neurons. The antivertiginous properties of the antihistamines (e.g., meclizine and dimenhydrinate) may be due, at least in part, to the anticholinergic activities. Both the anticholinergic and antihistaminic drugs also have parasympatholytic activity, which may account for their effectiveness in relieving the autonomic symptoms associated with vertigo.

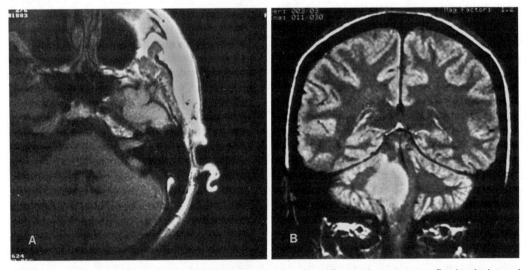

FIGURE 2–1. Magnetic resonance imaging (MRI) scans showing: A, small acoustic neuroma confined to the internal auditory canal (transverse section, T_1 weighted) and B, glioma involving root entry zone of eighth nerve (coronal section, T_2 weighted). Neither tumor was seen on computed tomography (CT) scans.

Several tranquilizers are effective in suppressing vertigo. Diazepam decreases the resting activity of vestibular nucleus neurons, possibly by decreasing the reticular facilitory influence or by increased crossed vestibular and/or cerebellovestibular inhibitory transmission.[38,58] The phenothiazines, in addition to their well-known dopaminergic blocking effects, have weak antihistaminic and anticholinergic effects. Prochlorperazine is particularly effective in suppressing nausea and vomiting, presumably through direct action on the chemoreceptive trigger zone in the brainstem. As our understanding of the pharmacology of the vestibular system improves, more rational therapy should evolve.

SUMMARY

Treatment of vertigo can be divided into two general categories: specific and symptomatic. Specific therapies discussed in this article include positional exercises for benign positional vertigo, salt restriction for Ménière's syndrome, surgery for perilymph fistula and acoustic neuroma, and anticoagulation for vertebrobasilar insufficiency. The key is to make a correct diagnosis so that specific therapies can be applied. As a general rule, the usefulness of the different antivertiginous drugs has been determined by empiric observation. The strategy for deciding which drug or combination of drugs to use is based on the known effects of each drug (outlined in Table 2–2) and on the severity and time course of symptoms. A major change in treatment strategy that has evolved over the past few years is to encourage patients to return to normal physical activity as rapidly as possible after an acute vertiginous attack. Repeated head, eye, and body movements (vestibular exercises) allow the brain to recalibrate the relationship between visual, proprioceptive, and vestibular signals.

REFERENCES

1. Adour, KK, Sprague, MA, and Hilsinger, RL: Vestibular vertigo: A form of polyneuritis. JAMA 246:1564, 1981.

2. Baker, HL: The application of magnetic resonance imaging in otolaryngology. Laryngoscope 96:19, 1986.

3. Baloh, RW and Furman, JM: Modern vestibular function testing. West J Med 150:59, 1989.

4. Baloh, RW and Honrubia, V: Clinical Neurophysiology of the Vestibular System, ed 2. FA Davis, Philadelphia, 1990.

5. Baloh, RW, Honrubia, V, and Jacobson, K: Benign positional vertigo: Clinical and oculographic features in 240 cases. Neurology 37:371, 1987.

6. Baloh, RW, Jacobson, K, and Honrubia, V: Idiopathic bilateral vestibulopathy. Neurology 39:272, 1989.

7. Baloh, RW, Sakala, SM, and Honrubia, V: Benign paroxysmal positional nystagmus. Am J Otolaryngol 1:1, 1979.

8. Baloh, RW: The dizzy patient: Symptomatic treatment of vertigo. Postgrad Med 73:317, 1983.

9. Boles, R, Rice, DH, Hybels, R, and Work, WP: Conservative management of Ménière's disease: Furstenberg regimen revisited. Ann Otol Rhinol Laryngol 84:513, 1975.

10. Brackman, DE and Bartels, LJ: Rare tumors of the cerebellopontine angle. Arch Otolaryngol Head Neck Surg 88:555, 1980.

11. Brandt, T and Daroff, RB: Physical therapy for benign paroxysmal positional vertigo. Arch Otolaryngol Head Neck Surg 106:484, 1980.

12. Caplan, LR: Treatment of patients with vertebrobasilar occlusive disease. Compr Therapy 12:23, 1986.

13. Caplan, LR: Vertebrobasilar disease. In Barnett, HJM, Mohr, JP, Stein, BM, Yatsu, FM (eds): Stroke: Pathophysiology, Diagnosis and Management. Churchill Livingstone, New York, 1986, pp 549–620.

14. Cawthorne, T: Vestibular injuries. Proc Roy Soc Med 39:270, 1945.

15. Coats, AC: Vestibular neuronitis. Acta Otolaryngol (Stockh) (Suppl)251:1, 1969.

16. Cooksey, FS: Rehabilitation in vestibular injuries. Proc Roy Soc Med 39:220, 1945.

17. Davis, LE and Johnsson, LG: Viral infections of the inner ear: Clinical, virologic and pathologic studies in humans and animals. Am J Otolaryngol 4:347, 1983.

18. Elidan, J, Lanhofer, L, and Honrubia, V: Recording of short-latency vestibular evoked potentials induced by acceleration impulses in experimental animals: Current status of the method and its application. Electroencephalogr Clin Neurophysiol 68:58, 1987.

19. Elidan, J, Sohmer, H, and Nizan, M: Recording of short-latency vestibular evoked potentials to acceleration in rats by means of skin electrodes. Electroencephalogr Clin Neurophysiol 53:501, 1982.

20. Erickson, L., Sorenson, G, and McGavran, M: A review of 140 acoustic neurinomas (neurilemmomas). Laryngoscope 75:601, 1965.

21. Fisher, CM: Vertigo in cerebrovascular disease. Arch Otolaryngol Head Neck Surg 85:855, 1967.

22. Gacek, RR: Further observations on posterior am-

pullary nerve transection for positional vertigo. Ann Otol Rhinol Laryngol 87:30, 1978.

23. Goodhill, V: Leaking labyrinth lesions, deafness, tinnitus and dizziness. Ann Otol Rhinol Laryngol 90:99, 1981.

24. Grad, A, and Baloh, RW: Vertigo of vascular origin: Clinical and ENG features in 84 cases. Arch Neurol 46:281, 1989.

25. Hallpike, C and Cairns, H: Observations on the pathology of Ménière's syndrome. J Laryngol Otol 53:625, 1938.

26. Harbert, F: Benign paroxysmal positional nystagmus. Arch Ophthalmol 84:298, 1970.

27. Hinchcliffe, R: Epidemiology of balance disorders in the elderly. In Hinchcliffe, R (ed): Hearing and Balance in the Elderly. Churchill Livingstone, New York, 1983, p 227.

28. Hofferberth, B: Evoked potentials to rotatory stimulation. Acta Otolaryngol (Stockh) (Suppl) 406:134, 1984.

29. Hood, JD and Kayan, A: Observations upon the evoked responses to natural vestibular stimulation. Electroencephalogr Clin Neurophysiol 62:266, 1985.

30. Igarashi, M, Levy, JK, O-Uchi, T, Reschker, MF: Further study of physical exercise and locomotor balance compensation after unilateral labyrinthectomy in squirrel monkeys. Acta Otolaryngol (Stockh) 92(1–2):101, 1981.

31. Jackson, CG, Glasscock, ME, Davis, WE, Hughes, GB, and Sismanis, A: Medical management of Ménière's disease. Ann Otol Rhinol Laryngol 90:142, 1981.

32. Jaju, BP and Wang, SC: Effects of diphenhydramine and dimenhydrinate on vestibular neuronal activity of cat: A search for the locus of their antimotion sickness action. J Pharmacol Exp Ther 76:718, 1971.

33. Katsarkas, A and Kirkham, TH: Paroxysmal positional vertigo: A study of 255 cases. J Otolaryngol 7:320, 1978.

34. Kistler, JP, Ropper, AH, and Heros, RC: Therapy of ischemic cerebral vascular disease due to atherothrombosis. N Engl J Med 311:27, 1984.

35. Koch, H, and Smith, MC: Office-based ambulatory care for patients 75 years old and over: National Ambulatory Medical Care Survey, 1980 and 1981. National Center for Health Statistics, Public Health Advance Data No. 110. US Government Printing Office, Hyattsville, MD, 1985.

36. Lacour, M, Roll, JP, and Appaix, M: Modifications and development of spinal reflexes in the alert baboon (Papio papio) following a unilateral vestibular neurotomy. Brain Res 113(2):255, 1976.

37. Laird, N and Wilson, WR: Predicting recovery from idiopathic sudden hearing loss. Am J Otolaryngol 4:161, 1983.

38. Matsuoka, I, Chikamori, Y, Takaori, S, Morimoto, M: Effects of chlorpromazine and diazepam on neuronal activites of the lateral vestibular nucleus in cats. Arch Otorhinolaryngol Suppl 209:89, 1975.

39. Matsouka, I, Domino, EF, and Morimoto, M: Adrenergic and cholinergic mechanisms of single vestibular neurons in the cat. Adv Otorhinolaryngol 19:163, 1973.

40. Mattox, DE: Perilymph fistulas. In Cummings, CW, Fredrickson, JM, Harker, LA, Krause, CJ, Schuller, DE (eds): Otolaryngology: Head and Neck Surgery. CV Mosby, St Louis, 1986, p 3113.

41. Mattox, DE: Vestibular schwannomas. Otolaryngol Clin North Am 20:149, 1987.

42. National Hearing Association: Dizziness: If, Where, and Why. NHA, 1981.

43. Nomura, Y, Kurata, T and Saito, K: Sudden deafness: Human temporal bone studies and an animal model. In Nomura, Y (ed): Hearing Loss and Dizziness. Igaku-Shoin, Tokyo, 1985, p 58.

44. Paparella, MM: Pathology of Ménière's disease. Ann Otol Rhinol Laryngol (Suppl 112)93:31, 1984.

45. Pappas, DG: Hearing impairments and vestibular abnormalities among children with subclinical cytomegalovirus. Ann Otol Rhinol Laryngol 92:552, 1983.

46. Pirodda, E, Ghedini, S, and Zanetti, MA: Investigation into vestibular evoked responses. Acta Otolaryngol (Stockh) 104:77, 1987.

47. Pullen, FW, Rosenberg, GH, and Cabeza, CH: Sudden hearing loss in divers and fliers. Laryngoscope 84:1373, 1979.

48. Ryu, JH, and McCabe, BF: Effects of diazepam and dimenhydrinate on the resting activity of the vestibular neuron. Aerospace Med 45 (10):1177, 1974.

49. Salamy, J, Potvin, A, Jones, K, Landreth, J: Cortical evoked responses to labyrinthine stimulation in man. Psychophysiology 12:55, 1975.

50. Schuknecht, HF: Endolymphatic hydrops: Can it be controlled? Ann Otol Rhinol Laryngol 95:36, 1986.

51. Schuknecht, HF, Kimura, RR, and Nanfal, PM: The pathology of idiopathic sensorineural hearing loss. Arch Otorhinolaryngol Suppl 243:1, 1986.

52. Schuknecht, FH, and Kitamura, K: Vestibular neuritis. Ann Otol Rhinol Laryngol (Suppl)90:1, 1981.

53. Schuknecht, HF: Neurolabyrinthitis: Viral infections of the peripheral auditory and vestibular systems. In Nomura, Y (ed): Hearing Loss and Dizziness. Igaku-Shoin, Tokyo, 1985, p 1.

54. Schuknecht, H and Ruby, R: Cupulolithiasis. Adv Otorhinolaryngol 20:434, 1973.

55. Schuknecht, HF and Witt, RL: Acute bilateral sequential vestibular neuritis. Am J Otolaryngol 6:255, 1985.

56. Silverstein, H, Smouha, E, and Jones, R: Natural history vs surgery for Ménière's disease. Arch Otolaryngol Head Neck Surg 100:6, 1989.

57. Silverstein, H: The effects of perfusing the perilymphatic space with artificial endolymph. Ann Otol Rhinol Laryngol 79:754, 1970.

58. Steiner, FA and Felix, D: Antagonistic effects of GABA and benzodiazepines on vestibular and cerebellar neurons. Nature (Lond) 260 (5549):346, 1976.

59. Thomsen, J, Brettan, P, Tos, M, and Johnsen, NJ:

Placebo effect of surgery for Ménière's disease. Arch Otolaryngol Head Neck Surg 107:271, 1981.

60. Thomsen, J, Gyldensted, C, and Lester, J: Computer tomography of cerebellopontine angle lesions. Arch Otolaryngol Head Neck Surgery 103:65, 1977.

61. Tumarkin, I: Otolithic catastrophe: A new syndrome. Br Med J 2:175, 1936.

62. Valvassori, GE: Diagnosis of retrocochlear and central vestibular disease by magnetic resonance imaging. Ann Otol Rhinol Laryngol 97:19, 1988.

63. Wazen, J, Silverstein, NH, and Besse, B: Preoperative and postoperative growth rates in acoustic neuromas documented with CT scanning. Otolaryngol Head Neck Surg 93:151, 1985.

64. Williams D and Wilson, TG: The diagnosis of the major and minor syndromes of basilar insufficiency. Brain 85:741, 1962.

65. Wilson, WR, Veltri, RW, Laird, N: Viral and epidemiologic studies of idiopathic sudden hearing loss. Otolaryngol Head Neck Surg 91:653,1983.

CHAPTER 3

• •

THE WHIPLASH PATIENT:
A SYMPATHETIC APPROACH

Robert W. Teasell, B.Sc., M.D., F.R.C.P(C)

Soft neck collars have become the formal dress of too many claimants to allow a dispassionate examination of the whiplash patient.

Teasell argues convincingly about how the acute injury is real. What remains difficult is the assessment of chronic suffering, since it is often distorted by emotion, frustration, and hope of financial gain.

The author decries the lack of scientific rigor in the field, but unavoidably, at times he has to anchor his own views on anecdotage, since whiplash injury is so often enmeshed in litigation and hence difficult to study. Teasell's own province of Ontario has recently introduced no-fault car insurance. This will provide an excellent opportunity for studying whiplash injury devoid of legal entanglements. Let us hope that the opportunity is grasped.

VCH

Whiplash injuries are a controversial clinical entity and represent a perplexing problem for both patient and physician. "Whiplash" is an ominous and misleading term that has nevertheless become firmly established in the medical literature, in litigation procedures, and in laypersons' vocabulary. Whiplash generally refers to *a sudden forced hyperextension-flexion injury of the cervical region following a motor vehicle accident, which results in soft tissue injuries* and is also known as cervical musculoligamentous sprain, flexion-extension injury, and acceleration-deceleration injury. Patients with chronic whiplash injuries present with subjective symptoms often out of proportion to physical findings; this disproportion, combined with the psychologic consequences of chronic pain, pending litigation, and a poor response to conventional therapeutic interventions, often leads to doubts about the reality of their complaints.[68] Experimental and clinical evidence, however, clearly points to a physiologic origin for the persistent symptoms following whiplash injuries. Alternative explanations such as "compensation neurosis" and malingering may account for a small minority of patients but should not be generalized to include all chronic whiplash patients.

THE WHIPLASH INJURY

A Historical Perspective

Whiplash injuries are a modern-day disease without a natural parallel. They were first recorded as a clinical entity with the diagnosis of "railway spine" injuries following train accidents. Erichsen[31] wrote about these injuries in 1886 and even then noted that individuals struck from behind suffered more serious injuries.

> *I have often remarked that in railway accidents those passengers suffer most seriously from concussion of the nervous system who sit with their backs turned towards the end of the train which is struck. Thus when a train runs into an obstruction on the line, those who are sitting with their backs to the engine will probably suffer most; whilst if a train is run into from behind, those who are facing the engine will most frequently be the greatest sufferers.*[31]

"Railway spine" was regarded back then as a medicolegal problem[58] much as whiplash is today. The term "whiplash" is thought to have originated with Crowe[23] in 1928 and was later popularized by a number of authors.[40,42]

The last four decades have seen a growing epidemic of whiplash injuries as a result of motor vehicle accidents, most commonly rear-end collisions. In 1971, the Insurance Institute for Highway Safety noted a 24% incidence of these injuries following rear-end collisions. Another study[60] estimated that neck injury occurred in one fifth of all accidents involving rear-end collisions. In 1971 the National Safety Council estimated that there were approximately 4 million rear-end collisions in the United States, resulting in as many as 1 million reported injuries per year.[21,73]

Biomechanics of Injury

Typically the injured individual is the occupant of a stationary vehicle that is struck from behind with little or no warning.[8,19,39,57,60-64] Injury results because the neck is in a vulnerable position and is physically unable to compensate adequately for the rapidity of neck movements and the magnitude of the acceleration forces generated at the time of impact.

The Mechanism of Injury

Neck injury most frequently follows an acceleration impact from a rear-end collision, which produces a sudden hyperextension followed by rapid forward flexion of the neck. Soft-tissue injuries after head-on deceleration accidents or side-on collisions are less common and less persistent than those following rear-end acceleration accidents.[19,40] MacNab[60-64] studied three groups of patients: those who suffered lateral flexion injuries in side-on collisions, those who suffered flexion injuries because they were facing backwards at the time of a rear-end collision, and those who sustained hyperextension injuries in typical rear-end collisions. Patients in the first two groups recovered, while those in the typical rear-end collision group[8] went on to develop the chronic symptoms characteristic of whiplash.

Experiments have demonstrated that the struck vehicle acquires a peak acceleration almost equal to that of the striking vehicle, followed by acceleration of the head, neck, and shoulders of the occupant more than twice as great as that of the vehicle.[85] For instance, one study[85] found that a low-velocity, 15 km/h (8 mph) rear-end collision produced a 2-g acceleration force of the vehicle and a 5-g acceleration force of the head, all within 300 milliseconds. The cervical spine extended up to 120 degrees following impact, well beyond the normal physiologic maximum of 70 degrees.

After a delay of 100 milliseconds following impact, the torso is accelerated forward by the back of the seat or is forced backward into the seat back.[21] The head, because of its inertia and lack of support, lags behind. In other words, the head initially remains in its original position while the thorax accelerates forward beneath it, causing the head to fall back and forcing the neck into hyperextension (Fig. 3–1). The neck is also subjected to very high tensile forces, which equates to axial stretching.[22] Following neck extension, the inertia of the head is overcome and the head accelerates forward at a faster rate than that of the torso, forcing the neck into flexion.[8] One study[85] observed acceleration forces up to 11 g in anthropometric dummies, whereas a mathematical model[65] demonstrated that relative to the trunk, the head acceleration could be as high as 12 g in the extension phase and 16 g in the flexion phase. The entire sequence

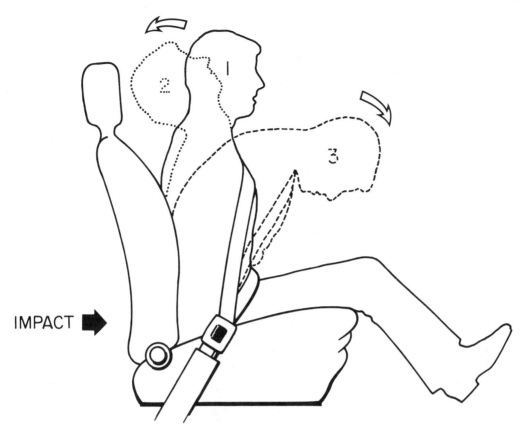

FIGURE 3–1. The sequence of movements of the car occupant following a rear-end collision. The head and neck extend backward as the torso is accelerated forward (2). Next, the head and neck are catapulted into forward flexion as the inertia of the head is overcome (3).

was completed within less than 500 milliseconds. Thus, low-speed rear-end collisions can generate substantial forces and result in significant injuries.

Head Restraints and Seat Belts

In 1968, the US Department of Transportation recognized whiplash injuries as a major public health problem when it required all passenger cars manufactured after December 31, 1968 to be equipped with head restraints for front seat occupants. Overall, however, installing head restraints has not prevented cervical soft-tissue injuries. In 1971, the Insurance Institute noted no difference in the incidence of neck injuries for cars equipped with head restraints when compared with those without head restraints. However, head restraints have been reported to reduce the incidence of neck extension injuries by 18% to 24%.[76,90] Because of improper usage and inadequate design, head restraints often are ineffective in countering the acceleration forces generated in motor vehicle accidents. Many head restraints are kept too low by the occupant to be of any benefit. Also, in most automobiles the seat is inclined backwards, whereas most motorists tend to sit upright or forward, so that the headrest is rarely near the occiput but is generally some distance behind[8] (Fig. 3–2). Under these circumstances the back of the seat strikes the torso, accelerating it forward before the headrest contacts the occiput. The neck may then go into hyperextension before the head restraint can prevent it. Thus, the head should be as close as possible to the restraint before impact; 2.5 cm may be a suitable distance.[36]

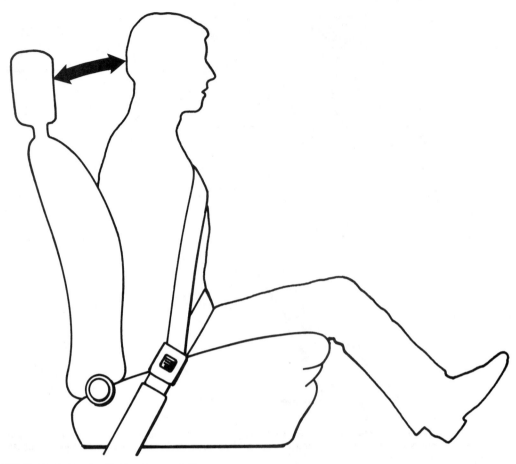

FIGURE 3–2. Head restraints often are ineffective because, whereas car seats often are inclined backward at a slight angle for maximum comfort, most occupants, particularly drivers, do not incline backward into the seat but tend to lean forward while driving. Thus, the headrest-to-occiput distance may be too great to allow the headrest to function properly.

Underestimation of the importance of the subsequent flexion as a mechanism of injury may also explain the ineffectiveness of head restraints.[98] If injury occurs when the neck is catapulted into flexion at high g forces, the head restraint would be ineffective in preventing soft-tissue injuries.

Despite the obvious benefits of lap and shoulder restraints in preventing serious injuries and death, a slightly higher incidence of neck sprains has been reported in individuals involved in rear-end collisions wearing seat belts[24,46,47] when compared with those not wearing them. A possible explanation is that the torso restrained by the shoulder belt cannot dampen the rate of head accelera-

tion, causing the neck to experience increased flexion movements relative to the trunk.[24] It is also possible that because unbelted individuals suffer more serious (i.e., traumatic brain or spinal cord) injuries, neck sprains are accorded a lower priority.

Pathophysiology of Injury

Physiologic Restraints to Injury

Exceeding the physiologic range of motion of the cervical spine will injure soft tissues of the neck (i.e., muscles, ligaments, and joint capsules). There are natural restraints to hyperflexion as the chin strikes the chest, and to lateral flexion as the head strikes the shoulder. Neck extension, however, is restrained only by the upper thorax, so that angulation of up to 120 degrees may be attained, far beyond the physiologic maximum of 70 degrees. If the head is rotated to the right or left at the time of impact, the physiologic limit of extension is even less and injury is theoretically more likely to occur. Although the consensus view is that hyperextension is the etiology of most injuries, it is important to remember that there are also significant flexion forces that may be potentially more injurious.[98]

Much of the initial neck movement following impact occurs before the neuromuscular system can adequately react to control it. The motor response is often delayed relative to neck movements and in some cases may actually aggravate the impact forces and the degree of soft-tissue injuries. For instance, sudden neck hyperextension results in reflex contraction of neck flexors, which may paradoxically add to the forces driving the neck into subsequent forward flexion.

Women are reported to experience whiplash injuries more often and more severely than men. Women generally have slimmer, less muscular necks, which may place them at greater risk of cervical soft-tissue injuries following acceleration forces generated at the time of impact.

Hypothetical Model of Injury

When a vehicle is struck from behind, the occupant's torso is accelerated forward, causing the unrestrained head and neck to fall back into hyperextension (see Fig. 3–1). Rapid and forceful hyperextension of the neck stretches the anterior cervical muscles. If rapid and forceful enough, the stretch will overcome muscle tone and elasticity and result in rupture of individual muscle fibers. Once muscle resistance is overcome, the brunt of the remaining force would be taken up by the anterior longitudinal ligament and anterior fibers of the annulus fibrosus,[21] which in turn may become stretched or undergo some localized tearing.[62] McKenzie and Williams[66] claimed that maximum injurious forces occur in hyperextension and are found mainly in the re-

gion of C-6 and C-7. Following acceleration and hyperextension, deceleration and flexion of the neck occurs. This later deceleration-flexion may be more injurious than the initial acceleration-hyperextension,[98] with the upper cervical spine or region sustaining the greatest injury because of its position as the pivot point.[94] Croft[21] suggests that the muscles in the upper cervical region (i.e., suboccipital and occipitofrontalis muscles) are smaller and more specialized and hence more susceptible to trauma than the larger paraspinal muscles. The posterior joint capsules, interspinous ligament, and ligamentum flavum would be susceptible to injury during forward flexion.

Pathology of Whiplash Injuries

The pathologic lesions accounting for the whiplash syndrome remain poorly defined. Attempts have been made to determine the pathologic lesions of whiplash injuries using theoretical constructs as well as animal and human cadaver experiments.[8] Animal experiments in which whiplash injuries are produced in a laboratory setting have proved to be the most informative regarding the pathology of such injuries. This approach has obvious drawbacks, since animals differ from humans both anatomically and physiologically and their pathologic lesions may not correlate well with human injuries. Human cadaver studies offer an anatomically better model, but cadavers differ in their response to injury since they lack the reflex responses and tissue quality seen in live subjects. Experimental and clinical experiences have demonstrated a wide variety of possible pathologic lesions[8,60–64,99] (Table 3–1).

Chronic pain may arise from a variety of sources. Musculoligamentous injuries often take a long time to heal, and the repair process may be incomplete, particularly in ligaments that possess a relatively poor blood supply. Damaged ligaments, tendons, joint capsules, and muscles may allow abnormal movements at intervertebral joints and may not get an opportunity to heal properly because full immobilization of the neck is impossible. Pain may then result in increased muscle tension or spasm in an effort to splint or protect injured tissues.[22]

TABLE 3–1. **POSSIBLE PATHOLOGIC LESIONS IN WHIPLASH INJURIES**

Anterior longitudinal ligament sprain or tear[19,40,60–64]
Intraspinous ligament sprain or tear[51]
Intervertebral disc herniation[40]
Vertebral body fracture[19]
Zygapophysial joint sprain or fracture[38,57]
Muscle strain, or rupture tear[38,39,57,58,60–64]
Retropharyngeal hematoma[57,60–64]
Esophageal hemorrhage[60–64]
Sympathetic trunk injury[35,60–64,75,91,100,102]
Vertebral artery ischemia
Concussion or minor head injury[35,40,91,102]
Thoracic outlet syndrome[15]
Temporomandibular joint dysfunction[37,39,56,80,96]

TABLE 3–2. **TRIGGER POINT CHARACTERISTICS**

Localized tender point, often in a firm band of muscle or fascia
Locally painful to palpation
Referred pain pattern characteristic of that specific trigger point (see Figs. 3–3, 3–4)
Muscle may be shortened (by 10%–20%), subjectively weaker, and more easily fatigued

Pain arising from structures below the deep fascia (ligament, tendon, capsule, bone) often presents as an aching discomfort made worse with stretching or activating the involved structures.[22] Experimental mechanical irritation[22,33,34,50] of deep tissues (i.e., muscles, ligaments, tendons, and joint capsules) in humans results in a poorly localized aching or burning pain often associated with muscle soreness and tenderness over bony prominences.[50] This referred pain, although often delayed in onset, is surprisingly consistent and may be accompanied by autonomic phenomena. In one study sympathetic blockade failed to reduce the pain. Furthermore, this pain is referred to areas that are anaesthetic, suggesting the peripheral nervous system is not responsible for referred pain.[33] This has obvious relevance in whiplash injuries, where pain is often delayed, referred in nonanatomical patterns, and unresponsive even to nerve blocks.

Myofascial pain syndrome is a controversial clinical entity regarded by some as a "wastebasket" diagnosis, but it does have characteristic clinical features, in particular the presence of a trigger point, which allow the diagnosis to be made with a certain degree of consistency (Table 3–2) (Fig. 3–3). Myofascial pain is thought to occur as a result of an acute strain or "overload" that occurs at the time of impact. One hypothesis is that a small area of muscle contraction develops and becomes self-sustaining (Fig. 3–4), followed by development of a tender

point in this localized band of contracted muscle.

THE CLINICAL PICTURE

The Whiplash Syndrome

Although whiplash remains poorly defined in pathologic terms, it is a common clinical phenomenon with a consistent constellation of symptoms.[8] The whiplash syndrome is generally dominated by neck and head pain and may be associated with a variety of poorly explained neurologic symptoms. The clinical picture may be complicated by psychologic reactions to chronic pain as well as by pending litigation. Potential complications are listed in Table 3–3.

A delay in symptoms ranging from several hours up to 48 hours is characteristic of whiplash injuries. Some symptoms may actually be delayed for several weeks. This history of delayed symptoms is similar to ligamentous sports injuries, in which a history may be given of continued athletic play after an injury is sustained. This delay may be due to the time required for the onset of traumatic edema and hemorrhage in damaged soft tissues.[58] As discussed earlier, experimental mechanical irritation of deep tissues results in the delayed onset of pain.[50] For the first few hours following injury, physical findings on examination are generally minimal.[49] With time, however, limitation of neck motion, tightness, muscle spasm and/or swelling, and tenderness of both anterior and posterior cervical structures become apparent.[49,51]

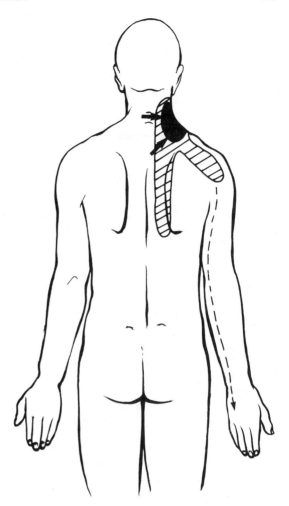

FIGURE 3–3. Trigger points within the right levator scapulae muscle are indicated with arrows. The main area of referred pain is shown as the consolidated area; some pain also may refer down the medial border of the scapula and out into the posterior shoulder. Referral of pain also may occur down the medial aspect of the arm and into the fourth and fifth fingers. (Adapted from Travell and Simons.[92])

Neck Pain

Neck pain is the most commonly reported symptom and is described as a deep, aching, posterior cervical discomfort, often associated with burning and stiffness, radiating out over the trapezius ridge, down into the interscapular region, up into the occiput, or down the arms. Many patients describe a disturbing "cracking" or crepitus when they move the neck, which they often associate with ongoing bony or articular damage. Range of motion of the cervical spine is often restricted, and tenderness is often present over the spinous posterior prominence of the 6th cervical vertebra and the posterior cervical paraspinal musculature.

Radiologic studies of the cervical spine are generally unremarkable or reveal evidence of preexisting degenerative changes. The most commonly reported abnormal x-ray finding in the acute phase is straightening of the normal cervical lordotic curve.[48] Computed tomographic scanning and magnetic resonance imaging should be reserved for those cases where cervical disk protrusion or spinal cord injury is suspected. Radionucleotide bone scanning has proved to be a sensitive test for detecting occult fractures or active inflammation of facet joints.

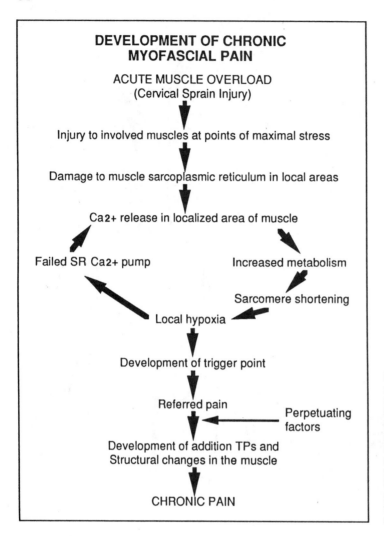

DEVELOPMENT OF CHRONIC MYOFASCIAL PAIN

ACUTE MUSCLE OVERLOAD
(Cervical Sprain Injury)

Injury to involved muscles at points of maximal stress

Damage to muscle sarcoplasmic reticulum in local areas

$Ca2+$ release in localized area of muscle

Failed SR $Ca2+$ pump

Increased metabolism

Sarcomere shortening

Local hypoxia

Development of trigger point

Referred pain

Perpetuating factors

Development of addition TPs and Structural changes in the muscle

CHRONIC PAIN

FIGURE 3–4. Proposed mechanism for development of chronic myofascial pain following whiplash injury. An acute muscle overload at the time of impact results in damage to muscle fibers, which develop localized, self-sustaining areas of muscle contraction. Within these localized bands of muscles, typical trigger points develop with the characteristic referred pain. (SR = sarcoplasmic reticulum).

Headache

Headache is a very common and often disabling symptom. Within 24 hours of the accident, many patients complain of diffuse neck and head pain. The head pain may be limited to the occipital area or may spread to involve the vertex, temporal, frontal, and retroorbital areas.[89] The pain is most often described as a dull ache or a pressurelike, squeezing sensation, although some individuals describe it as pounding or throbbing.[3,89] Muscle contraction and common migraine headaches are often present simultaneously (posttraumatic mixed headache) with associated nausea, vomiting, and photophobia. Headaches have been reported in

up to 97% of cases,[101] and in some patients it is the predominant symptom.

Common migraine or tension-vascular headaches are frequently seen following whiplash injuries and often occur in individuals with no prior history of migraine or vascular headaches. Traditionally, tension and migraine headaches have been regarded as entirely separate entities, with differing characteristics, mechanisms, and treatment. However, the distinction may not be so apparent in clinical practice, and overlapping features between tension and migraine headaches are often present. The clinical spectrum of benign, recurrent headache appears to include classic migraine at one end, the variations of common migraine and ten-

TABLE 3-3. FACTORS INFLUENCING MYOFASCIAL PAIN FOLLOWING WHIPLASH INJURIES

Aggravating Factors

Strenuous use of involved muscles, especially in the shortened position (e.g., heavy lifting, strenuous exercise)

Excessive rapid stretching of the involved muscles

Sustained or repeated contraction of the muscle (e.g., working with arms above shoulder level, repetitive arm work)

Placing the involved muscle in one position for prolonged periods of time (e.g., long car rides, reading, typing, sleeping)

Applying pressure to trigger point

Cold drafts or dampness (changes with weather)

Periods of muscle tension (anxiety, anger)

Alleviating Factors

Short period of rest following activity

Slow, steady, passive stretch of the involved muscles

Ice (for less than 5 min) or moist heat applied over the trigger point

Short periods of light activity following prolonged posturing or rest

Specific myofascial therapy (spray and stretch, local injections)

---

sion-vascular headache occupying the vast middle ground, and tension headache at the other end.[78]

Dysphagia

Dysphagia occurring early after whiplash injury may be the result of esophageal and/or pharyngeal injury or a retropharyngeal hematoma. The early occurrence of dysphagia suggests a more serious injury, with a large hematoma, and is an important prognostic sign.[62] Hoarseness may also be reported and may be the result of laryngeal stretch or hyperemia.[99] Dysphagia and hoarseness tend to be short-lived and rarely persist beyond 1 week.

Visual Disturbances

Whiplash patients commonly complain of intermittent blurring of vision; eyeglass wearers may even obtain a change in their prescriptions, but without improvement. One explanation put forward for blurred vision[8] is based on cervical pain evoking an efferent sympathetic discharge to the eye, resulting in abnormal accommodation. Blurring of vision by itself is not thought to be of prognostic significance. Photophobia commonly accompanies migrainous headaches.

Dizziness

Symptoms of dizziness or vertigo are frequently reported following whiplash injuries. Many patients complain of suddenly "veering" to one side or feeling dizzy if they move their neck or change their posture too quickly. A variety of theories have been proposed to explain these features, including vertebral artery insufficiency, inner ear damage, injury to the cervical sympathetic chain, and an impaired neck-righting reflex. One theory, known as the "reflex" or "neuromuscular" theory, proposes that interference with normal signals coming from the upper cervical joints, muscles, or nerves to the inner ear induces a feeling of ataxia.[25,62] This could explain the posture-related vertigo experienced by many of these patients.

Tinnitus

Tinnitus is another frequent complaint and may be due to vertebral artery insufficiency, injury to the cervical sympathetic chain, or inner ear damage. Tinnitus itself does not appear to have any prognostic value.[62] Many patients complain that their ear(s) feels plugged; additional auditory complaints include decreased hearing and difficulty with loud noises. Electronystagmographic abnormalities have been reported in a large number of whiplash victims.[20]

Arm Pain and Thoracic Outlet Syndrome

Arm pain and paresthesiae are reported frequently following whiplash injuries. The source of these arm symptoms remains obscure. As mentioned previously, nonneurogenic radiation of pain may result from chronic irritation of deep musculoligamentous, joint, and intervertebral disk structures. The arm ipsilateral to the most symptomatic side often becomes subjectively weaker, owing in part to lack of use as a result of habitual and instinctive avoidance of activities or movements that cause pain. Travell and Simons[92] feel that the muscle itself tends to limit the force of its contraction below the pain threshold, resulting in clinical weakness. Nerve conduction, F-wave, and needle electromyographic studies are usually normal.

Numbness or parasthesiae are commonly noted along the ulnar side of the forearm and hand or felt diffusely throughout the entire arm. MacNab[62] speculated that numbness along the ulnar aspect of the distal upper extremity may be secondary to spasm of the scalene muscles compressing the brachial plexus and resulting in a transient thoracic outlet syndrome. Alternatively, Bogduk[8] speculated that acute injury to the zygapophysial or facet joint, with subsequent edema or hemorrhage, may compromise the adjacent nerve roots posteriorly.[19,39] In the chronic stage, organization of pericapsular exudates may result in nerve root fibrosis or scarring. Objective data supporting these theoretical explanations are lacking, however.

Low Back Pain

The lumbar and thoracolumbar spine may suddenly be forced into extension or flexed forward as the torso moves in an arc over a fixed pelvis. One study of 320 uncomplicated whiplash victims[101] reported a 60% incidence of low back pain. This was thought to be the result of a sprain or mechanical injury to the supporting ligaments of the lumbar spine occurring during sudden flexion-extension of the lower back. Others[9] reported low back pain in 42% of whiplash patients, with sciaticlike symptoms in 15%. Another group[21] reported low back pain in 57% of individuals with moderate to severe whiplash injuries arising from rear-end collisions. Side-on collisions, however, were associated with a 71% incidence of low back pain, causing the authors to speculate that the lumbar spine was more vulnerable to injury during lateral flexion trauma than during forward flexion or extension. A soft seat back and a lap seat belt with no shoulder strap would be expected to increase the risk of low back pain.

Low back pain is typically described as an aching, often burning discomfort located in the lumbosacral region and/or the buttock(s). Prolonged sitting, standing, and lying down all tend to worsen the low back pain. It is common for patients to experience paresthesiae and referred pain down the leg, which may be mistaken for sciatica. A particularly confusing group of patients are those with low back pain appearing several weeks following the accident. Ameis[2] states, "back ache occurring for the first time several weeks post trauma probably reflects the effect of spasm and the chronic alteration of posture, anxiety, increased body weight and reduced fitness brought on by the indolence of a prolonged illness."[2]

Miscellaneous Symptoms

Anterior chest pain is sometimes seen and may be mistaken for angina. It is generally an achy pain, made worse with exercise, often associated with neck pain, and presenting with anterior chest wall tenderness. Fatigue and irritability are very common complaints, and many patients have evidence of sleep disturbance. Often they are restless sleepers, waking many times during the night, and feeling tired and unrefreshed on awakening. Memory and concentration problems are common complaints.

Psychologic Problems

Psychologic problems brought on by chronic pain and the subsequent disability are extremely common following chronic whiplash injuries and only serve to complicate an already difficult situation. Personality changes, depression, difficulty coping with everyday activities, anxiety, anger, frustration, and a preoccupation with somatic complaints are common. Many clinicians find it difficult to determine whether the patient's psychologic response to his or her symptoms is appropriate. Often the psychologic response varies significantly between individuals and is influenced by a variety of factors (Fig. 3–5). Unfortunately, the emotional and behavioral problems that frequently accompany persistent whiplash injuries are often misinterpreted as the

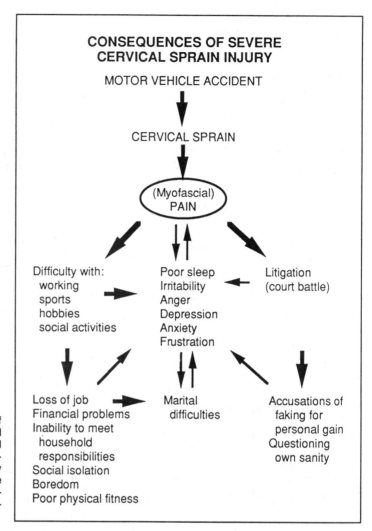

FIGURE 3–5. Consequences of whiplash injuries may go beyond the pain and affect the individual psychosocially. After severe injuries, chronic pain can completely dominate the patient's life. These psychosocial consequences interact with each other and may eventually influence the pain itself.

source of, rather than the result of, pain. This belief has enjoyed significant popularity in the past and has been reinforced by the particular selection bias of patients attending specialty practices and by the absence of hard, objective evidence of injury.

Poor Premorbid Coping Skills

Patients bring to any stressful situation an array of differing coping skills and strategies. Some patients cope with persistent pain and disability better than others with similar symptoms and disability. "Poor" copers often are individuals with a history of premorbid psychologic problems, poor self-esteem, and nonsupportive environments. Often their symptoms and subsequent disability are out of proportion to physical signs. These individuals may have maladaptive coping styles that adversely affect how well they deal with their symptoms. Similar maladaptive coping strategies are often seen in other patients with chronic, disabling diseases. Poor copers account for a disproportionately large number of referrals to chronic pain specialists and neurologists. Some characteristic features of poor copers are listed in Table 3–4.

TABLE 3-4. **CLUES TO DIAGNOSING INDIVIDUALS WITH POOR COPING SKILLS**

Premorbid psychologic problems (e.g., depression, suicide attempt)
Premorbid personality disorder
History of childhood abuse (physical, sexual, or psychologic)
Comes from a broken home
Difficulty establishing interpersonal relationships
Marital problems
Dramatic presentation
History of alcohol and drug abuse
Women more likely than men
Immigrant with poor communication skills
Limited education and/or skills
Dependent and demanding behavior

Posttraumatic Stress Syndrome

This syndrome is a form of anxiety neurosis that is seen in up to one third of accident victims and that is most prevalent in the first few weeks or months after the accident. Essentially the patient experiences panic attacks, often repetitively reliving the accident or manifesting an unreasonable fear of riding in a car. This is thought to be a learned response and is closely related to trauma or "assaults" of a deeply personal nature.[2] Over time this response disappears, but in more severe cases patients may benefit from a gradual exposure to the anxiety-provoking activity or stimulus.

Compensation Neurosis

The role of compensation in prolonging pain and disability after motor vehicle accidents has served as the focus of much of the controversy surrounding whiplash injuries. Among many clinicians there has been a suspicion bordering on conviction that the availability of compensatory awards prejudices the outcome after injury. MacNab[62] notes that,

Although there is general agreement about the types of symptoms to be expected, widely divergent views are held regarding their significance. These viewpoints, rigidly held and hotly contested, are usually based on impressions only. . . . Many

physicians believe that those with the "whiplash" syndrome are a group of hysterical, neurotic, if not frankly dishonest people.[62]

"Compensation neurosis" is a concept used to describe the persistence of symptoms attributable to compensable accidental injuries that linger long after their expected recovery and that fail to respond adequately to treatment and rehabilitation. The accident victim is felt to be preoccupied with the amount of the award, and symptoms are thought to resolve promptly on resolution of litigation. In 1946, Kennedy[53] wrote, "compensation neurosis is a state of mind born out of fear, kept alive by avarice, stimulated by lawyers and cured by a verdict."[53] The term was made popular by the influential writings of Miller[72] in 1961, and the concept has persisted.

The symptoms following a whiplash injury are accompanied by a paucity of clinical (especially neurologic) signs and objective radiographic evidence. Patients complain of pain and a variety of associated symptoms that often appear to be neurologically non-anatomical and are often confined to regions (regional pain syndromes) as opposed to dermatomes. Psychologic reactions to chronic pain are often interpreted as abnormal or as evidence of a "neurotic" predisposition.

The predominance of plaintiffs among whiplash patients seeking medical attention is a well-known phenomenon and lends support to the concept that symptoms are generated out of a desire for monetary gain. The litigation process and/or compensation system may work against the patient's optimal recovery and prolong chronic pain and disability. To receive compensation, victims must prove that they are suffering from pain and disability as a result of the accident. As the case drags on in court, fiscal rehabilitation to compensate for lost wages is often delayed or inadequate, creating financial stresses and anxiety. The litigation process is itself necessarily adversarial, which creates stress. The popular notion of dramatic cures following financial compensation is based on anecdotal experiences in the absence of adequate follow-up and is not supported by outcome studies.

The notorious reputation often attributed to whiplash injuries can be explained in part by conflicts that develop between whiplash patients and their physicians. The interaction between needy, often demanding patients with chronic disabling pain and ill-prepared physicians who are uncertain how to deal with them inevitably leads to an unsatisfactory encounter for both parties. Many chronic whiplash patients are less-than-ideal patients whose expectations of the medical system are often unrealistic. Current medical training often places the physician at a disadvantage because of its emphasis on the "acute medical model" or reductionistic approach to disease (Fig. 3-6). Chronic whiplash, with its persistent symptoms, paucity of clinical neurologic signs, and intractability to treatment may make the clinician feel inept and challenge his or her need to feel competent. The problem is further complicated by the fact that many physicians still think in terms of a *mind-body dualism* which views patients' complaints as either physical or psychologic rather than a combination of both. Faced with clinical uncertainty and a feeling of ineptness, some physicians attribute symptoms to a psychologic origin so that in one sense the patient is held to be responsible, either consciously or subconsciously, for his or her continuing complaints. As a result, these patients are often labeled as neurotic, hysterical, malingering, or as seeking some form of "secondary gain." Diamond and Grauer[27] state,

> *The major reactions of physicians to patients with the chronic pain syndrome are frustration, disapproval, anger, uncertainty and rejection. The physician must understand that although these reactions are normal, they may interfere with optimal rapport and management. Understanding these reactions can help guide the physician in the management of patients with chronic pain.[27]*

Compelling evidence points to a physiologic origin for the whiplash symptom complex, as opposed to a psychologic basis. Attributing symptoms to compensation neurosis does not explain the impressive consistency of symptoms reported by whiplash patients, the predominance of rear-end collisions in those with persistent symptoms, or the failure of symptoms to resolve with compensation settlement. The most compelling evidence for a physiologic cause of the whiplash syndrome is the impressive consistency of the clinical picture. Bogduk[8] speaks to this issue when he states, "It is unbelievable that were there not a common organic syndrome, there exists among patients a deliberate, international, translingual conspiracy that enables them all to consistently report the same symp-

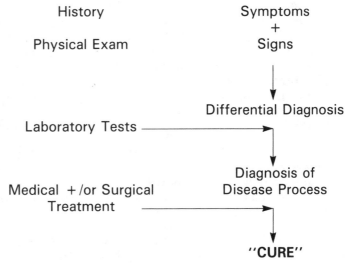

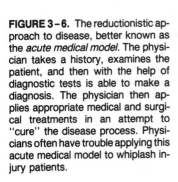

FIGURE 3-6. The reductionistic approach to disease, better known as the *acute medical model.* The physician takes a history, examines the patient, and then with the help of diagnostic tests is able to make a diagnosis. The physician then applies appropriate medical and surgical treatments in an attempt to "cure" the disease process. Physicians often have trouble applying this acute medical model to whiplash injury patients.

toms.'' More than 80% of patients with the most persistent symptoms were involved in collisions where they were the occupant of a car hit from behind.[24,60,62] Rear-end collisions account for only 20% of motor vehicle accidents. This discrepancy suggests a physiologic origin. If the whiplash patient's persistent symptoms were generated solely out of a desire for compensation, one would expect that symptoms would continue unabated until the time of the compensation settlement and disappear sometime afterwards. In clinical practice, however, many patients experience a marked improvement or resolution of their symptoms prior to resolution of litigation, whereas a substantial number still have significant symptoms and disability years after settlement.

Recovery from Whiplash Injuries

Soft-tissue injuries following motor vehicle accidents demonstrate a slow, steady resolution of symptoms in the majority of cases. A minority of patients (more than 10%) go on to develop chronic disabling pain generally centered in the neck or interscapular region. During the acute stage, the patient presents with pain, muscle spasm, and restriction of neck movement. Symptoms generally develop over several hours after the accident and peak the following morning or during the following few days. Dysphagia may be present initially, and the patient may complain of dizziness, tinnitus, or blurred vision. Within the first few days or weeks there is an easing of muscle spasm, allowing more neck movement to occur. This may be prolonged by injudicious collar use or excessive guarding and overprotection by the patient. Dizziness gradually disappears over the ensuing weeks or even months; however, new symptoms, in particular, arm or low back pain, may appear.

Eventually patients regain full neck range of motion and strength, paralleled by the resumption of normal activities. However, there are generally upper limits to the intensity and duration of activities these individuals can perform without suffering from neck pain and headaches. Difficulty with prolonged positioning in one posture is very common. Vigorous return to sport or work is often painful and frequently results in intolerable pain. Patient motivation and pain tolerance are important in determining return to regular activities. This stage may be very prolonged, and symptoms often persist indefinitely even in the best-motivated patients.

Outcome Studies

Outcome studies of whiplash injuries suffer from a variety of problems including lack of prospective design, selection bias in the group of patients selected, and a lack of measurable, objective data. The studies that do exist provide some interesting insights.

Gotten[42] surveyed 100 patients who were referred for neurosurgical consultation after cervical whiplash injury. After several years, 12% were still sufficiently symptomatic to be wearing cervical collars, sleeping in traction, receiving physiotherapy, and periodically seeing their physicians for help. Another 34% suffered "minor" residual symptoms. MacNab[60,62] reviewed 266 patients who had suffered cervical whiplash injuries and had had court settlements 2 or more years previously. A minimum of 45% were still symptomatic. The symptomatic group was comprised primarily of patients who had suffered hyperextension injuries, whereas most asymptomatic patients had lateral flexion or forward flexion injuries. Virtually all other injuries (e.g., sprained ankles, broken wrists) had healed within the normal healing times, but the neck injuries had not. In most patients the residual symptoms constituted a continuing nuisance rather than a significant disability. DePalma and Subin[26] found that among 386 of their patients with cervical pain syndromes, only 25% were involved in litigation. The outcome after therapy was the same in both the litigation and nonlitigation groups, suggesting that litigation did not have a significant influence on outcome. Schutt and Dohan[84] found that at 6 months, 50 of 67 women (75%) continued to experience neck pain. No difference was apparent between those patients who had pending litigation and those whose litigation had been resolved. Hohl[48] observed 146 patients with neck injuries following car accidents for 5 years. Within the first month following injury, virtually all patients experienced aching and stiffness in the neck, two thirds had headaches, and one third complained of shoulder pain. The duration of symptoms ranged from a few days to more than 5 years, with an average of about 24 months. At 5-year follow-up, 57% of these patients had made a "symptomatic recovery;" that is, the patient felt there were no residual problems related to the original injury. Forty-three percent were still symptomatic. Mendelson[70] reported on 101 unselected consecutive patients involved in litigation and referred for psychiatric assessment after motor vehicle or industrial accidents. Thirty-five of the patients resumed work before settlement. An average of 15.7 months after settlement, 9 of the remaining 66 patients had returned to work, 49 were not working, and 13 were lost to follow-up. Thus one third of patients resumed work before settlement of their litigation, whereas half failed to resume work when reviewed more than a year after settlement. Norris and Watt[74] reviewed 61 patients who were occupants of cars struck in rear-end collisions. They found residual neck pain at 6 months in 40% of patients with milder injuries and 90% of those with severe injuries. More recently, Deans[24] reported the findings of a retrospective study of 137 car occupants seen in the emergency room following injuries suffered during motor vehicle accidents during a 6-month period and consequently contacted after 2 years with follow-up questionnaires. Sixty-two percent of the 137 reported neck pain after their accident; of those, the pain lasted only 1 week in 17%, longer than 6 months in 56%, and longer than 1 full year in 42%. In this later group, 36% had occasional pain and only 6% had continuous pain.

Determining the Prognosis

Providing an accurate prognosis is often difficult following cervical "whiplash" soft-tissue injuries. Factors that indicate a poorer prognosis are listed in Table 3–5. Some conclusions can be drawn from outcome studies and clinical experiences. The patient with a cervical soft-tissue injury persisting several weeks after a motor vehicle accident has an 85% to 90% chance of achieving a functional recovery,[2] but 40% to

TABLE 3–5. FACTORS INDICATING A POORER PROGNOSIS FOLLOWING CERVICAL WHIPLASH INJURY

Rear-end collision
Wearing seat belt (especially shoulder strap)
Female sex
Increasing age
Preexisting cervical degenerative disk disease
Initial dysphagia, Horner's syndrome, or loss of consciousness
Previous whiplash or neck injury
Arm numbness and pain
Persisting sleep disturbance
Prolonged collar use
Generalized pain syndrome (i.e., fibromyalgia)
Evidence of poor coping skills (see Table 3–4)
Vocation requiring manual labor
?Litigation

70% retain some degree of intermittent discomfort or nuisance symptoms.[42,62] The symptoms are distracting and may be occasionally disabling, but the individual can still perform his or her job and enjoy most leisure activities and in that sense has achieved a "functional recovery." A functional recovery occurs when the patient is able to carry out a full spectrum of normal activities with a frequency, duration, and level of intensity reasonable for his or her age, skills, and needs. The chances of achieving a functional recovery decrease with the duration of disabling symptoms following injury.[2] If at the end of 6 weeks the patient still has continuous and significant pain, he or she can be expected to have intermittent symptoms for a minimum of 6 to 12 months.[62] Of those who have suffered significant whiplash injuries, at least 50% will have made a functional recovery at the end of the first year; a further 25% recover during the next 6 months.[2] Patients still symptomatic enough after 18 months that they cannot return to work or engage in regular leisure activities have a poor prognosis.

What is often not appreciated is that the level of activities required for a functional recovery varies significantly from patient to patient and is largely dependent on the external physical demands placed on the individual. For example, an office worker or a professional may eventually achieve a functional recovery, whereas a manual laborer may not, despite similar injuries. More than 10% of patients with cervical soft-tissue injuries following motor vehicle accidents fail to achieve a functional recovery even after the passage of 2 to 3 years.[2] This means that the patient is left with sufficient pain and discomfort to seriously interfere with his or her ability to perform work and engage in leisure activities. Much of this difficulty is related to the individual's type of work and is much more common in persons engaging in known pain-aggravating activities.

MANAGEMENT OF WHIPLASH INJURIES

Practical management of whiplash patients begins with a recognition that the pain and subsequent disability associated with these soft-tissue injuries may be prolonged and that "quick cures" often sought by patients are not available. The treating clinician should develop a rational, progressive program geared to the individual patient, taking into account not only the injury but the individual's peculiar reaction to the pain and impairment; the impact it has on family, vocational, and avocational activities; and the influence of outside environmental factors.

The Treatment Program

Any treatment program should consider a wide variety of available therapeutic interventions outlined in Table 3–6. The con-

TABLE 3–6. ELEMENTS OF TREATMENT

Rule out treatable radiologic abnormalities
Patient education
Avoidance of prolonged cervical collar use
Attention to good posture
Graduated stretching exercise program
General aerobic fitness
Changing maladaptive coping patterns
Relaxation techniques and stress management
Avoidance of aggravating environmental factors
Limited use of medications
Work modification and retraining
Emphasis on return to function and pain control

cept that some injuries resulting in pain may be inaccessible to physical and pharmacologic treatments is among the most difficult for many patients (and some clinicians) to grasp and accept. Patients hope and often expect that treatment will result in a "cure" for their pain, whereas the primary goals of any treatment program should be pain control and subsequent recovery of function.

Education

Education of the patient (and family) is the most crucial component of any treatment program, and yet clinicians consistently fail to provide adequate information. Education and reassurance should be provided as soon as possible after the accident, with the patient being made aware of treatment goals (i.e., return of function versus complete relief of pain) and the likely prognosis (i.e., gradual improvement). The clinician should warn the patient that recovery may be slow but should remain optimistic, stressing that the majority of individuals eventually make a functional recovery and return to employment. This helps patients to plan realistically for the future, reduces anxiety, increases confidence and a sense of control, helps reduce psychologic complications, builds confidence in the physician, and improves compliance with the treatment program. Education of the family helps to reduce family and marital conflicts and overprotectiveness by family members.

After the acute stage is over, a very important concept for the patient to understand is that "*hurt is not harm.*" Most patients feel that when they experience neck and shoulder pain they must be redamaging the involved area. As a result they may limit their activities and movement of the neck in a logical attempt to avoid pain and, by inference, further tissue damage. Complete avoidance of pain-aggravating activities must be actively discouraged to prevent subsequent loss of range of motion and overall physical deconditioning. Advice against specific aggravating activities such as prolonged desk work, typing, lifting heavy loads, or prolonged reading with the neck in a flexed position and advice on proper pacing of activities may help to prevent significant exacerbations of pain.

Cervical Collar

Neck splinting with a soft cervical collar is controversial, but it is often recommended initially for all but the mildest injuries. A recent controlled double-blind study demonstrated that patients mobilized early without a cervical collar did better, with greater reduction of pain and improved cervical range of motion.[67] Continuous use of the cervical collar for more than 2 weeks after the accident should be discouraged. Prolonged collar use leads to disuse atrophy of the neck muscles, contractures, increased dependency, and enhancement of feelings of disability. Collar use should not be abruptly withdrawn; the patient should be weaned from it gradually in conjunction with a neck exercise program. Failure to use a collar weaning/exercise program may only perpetuate pain complaints and collar use[58] (Fig. 3–7). A cervical collar may occasionally still be recommended at night and may also be useful during long car rides or periods of reading or studying.

Posture

Careful attention to posture is another important but often overlooked element of pain management. Proper sitting posture is of particular importance to individuals who must sit at their place of work for long pe-

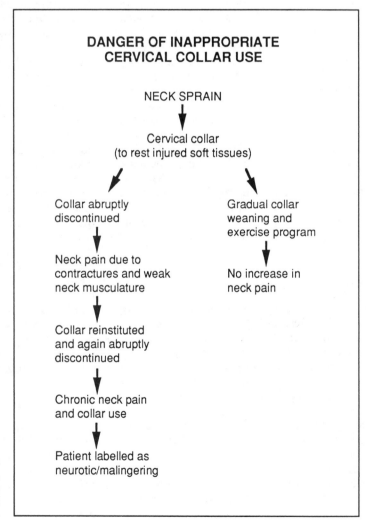

FIGURE 3–7. Excessive collar wearing and the lack of a collar-weaning program may result in iatrogenic dependency on the collar.

riods of time. Sitting for prolonged periods with the neck in forward flexion generally exacerbates neck pain and headache. This commonly occurs during long car rides; while studying for examinations; and in clerical/typing/computer jobs, which whiplash patients invariably find difficult. One way to reduce discomfort is to have patients take a regular break every 30 or 40 minutes, during which they should move the neck around and change their position. Whiplash patients should be taught that the ideal posture when sitting or standing is to keep the neck straight with the shoulders pulled back. One of the most painful positions for whiplash patients is working with their arms above the level of the shoulders. Washing windows, painting, haircutting, filing, or reaching for objects in a high cupboard all can result in an increase in neck and trapezius pain, so that this position should be avoided whenever possible.

Poor sleeping postures can result in an intensification and prolongation of symptoms. Ideally the patient should be supine with adequate support of the cervical lordosis. Side lying is an acceptable sleeping position, provided that the neck can be kept in a neutral position and not laterally flexed. Lying prone is contraindicated as it keeps the neck laterally rotated and under strain. The patient should be encouraged to sleep with one small pillow or a special cervical pillow designed to support the cervical lordosis while preventing lateral flexion and rotation.

Physical Therapies

Physical therapy should be directed along rational lines, and its use should be time-limited. Local heat and cold, ultrasound, traction, manipulation, and massage therapy may provide temporary relief of pain but do not appear to provide any significant long-term benefits. Therefore, use of these physical therapeutic techniques should not take away from time at work and must lead to some improvement in functional abilities if their long-term use is to be justified. In the early acute phase of whiplash, icing may be helpful to limit muscle swelling. After the acute phase (3 to 10 days after the accident), local hot packs, ultrasound, and in-

terferential or transcutaneous electrical stimulation (TENS) may be helpful in temporarily reducing pain. Moist heat tends to be more effective than dry heat. Many patients find it useful to apply ice to involved areas 3 to 5 minutes before stretching the involved muscles.

Exercises and Cervical Traction

Exercises with an emphasis on stretching and increasing overall physical activity form the cornerstone of any treatment program. Exercises are best taught to the patient initially by a physiotherapist to ensure that they are being performed properly. After that, the emphasis is on a daily home exercise program that encourages the patient to take an active role in his or her recovery. *Early mobilization* of the neck should be gentle and graduated to avoid excessive exacerbations of pain. One or 2 days after the injury, most patients can be started on gentle, progressive stretching exercises. The stretching of muscles to their normal length is a necessary step toward restoration of normal function and minimization of pain. Isometric strengthening exercises of the cervical musculature should be left until later in the program. If strengthening exercises are introduced too early or too aggressively in the early phases, they often result in intolerable exacerbations of pain, and the patient may discontinue all exercises.

In our experience, mechanical cervical *traction* often aggravates symptoms in both the acute and later stages. In the acute phase, mechanical traction is contraindicated, as distractive forces may increase pain and further damage healing tissues. Manual traction provided by a physiotherapist may be useful in providing temporary relief of pain but is not a substitute for a proper stretching program.

Manipulation

Of all therapeutic techniques available to treat whiplash victims, cervical manipulation is the most controversial. The best-known form of manipulation is the *high-velocity, low-amplitude thrust*. It begins with the patient positioned in such a way that muscles or joints are placed at maximum stretch, so that the stretched muscle cannot effectively resist the manipulating thrust. At this point the manipulator applies additional stretch; consequently, movement is increased slightly beyond the physiologic limit into the paraphysiologic range. A second, final barrier may then be met, formed by the stretched ligaments and capsule. This is the limit of anatomic integrity, and forcing movement beyond this point will damage ligaments and the joint capsule. The additional abrupt stretch on the maximally extended muscles likely stimulates muscle spindles and connective tissue proprioceptive organs, resulting in relaxation of the muscles and a transient relief of pain that can sometimes last for several days, followed by a gradual return of pain. There are a variety of postulated mechanisms of pain relief following manipulation, including an alteration of sensory input from joints and soft tissues through mechanoreceptor stimulation, reflex effects on increased muscle tone, restoration of extensibility to soft tissues, and the psychologic effects of being carefully assessed and sympathetically treated.

Forceful cervical manipulation procedures may result in very rare but serious complications such as vertebral artery dissection and cervical spinal cord injury. Disease processes that damage bone, joints, and ligaments, making them especially vulnerable to sudden stresses, are contraindications to forceful manipulation (Table 3–7). A transient worsening of pain and discomfort is common. The greatest drawback of manipulation is that its effects are transient and the procedure needs to be performed repeatedly, fostering passivity and dependency in patients. Practitioners of manipulation often use it in isolation and not as a component of a more comprehensive pain management program. From a pragmatic standpoint, however, it does relieve pain in some patients, albeit temporarily, allowing them to function better and improving overall life quality.

Massage

Massage therapy is a time-honored treatment for pain of musculoligamentous origin, although there is no evidence that it

TABLE 3–7.
CONTRAINDICATIONS TO CERVICAL MANIPULATION

Malignant disease of bone or soft tissues
Osteomyelitis
Osteoporosis of cervical vertebrae
Spinal cord compression
Recent fracture of cervical vertebrae
Vertebrobasilar insufficiency
Inflammatory arthritis, in particular, rheumatoid arthritis
Bony or ligamentous instability of cervical spine
Severe nerve root irritation or compression
Pain of unknown origin
Acute whiplash injury of the neck (first several weeks)
Anticoagulant therapy
Recent steroid therapy
Severe pain made worse with manipulation
Worsening of signs and symptoms while being manipulated
Developing psychologic dependence on cervical manipulation

produces any long-lasting benefits. Like manipulation, massage therapy can play a role in keeping the patient functional by providing some temporary relief or lessening of pain. It is particularly effective in situations where muscle tension and pain gradually build (e.g., an office worker or a student studying for examinations). Massage therapy should be gentle, since aggressive or deep friction massage techniques often result in an increase in pain.

Medications

Medications have a limited role in the management of whiplash injuries and carry with them the potential for misuse and side effects. Many whiplash victims take substantial quantities of *analgesics*, often narcotics, even though they may be only minimally effective in relieving pain. Too often the side effects of the drug outweigh the benefits of pain reduction and control or of improvement in function. Analgesic medications have their greatest application in the acute stage. Nonsteroidal anti-inflammatory drugs are more likely to benefit patients through their analgesic properties than through their anti-inflammatory properties. Narcotic analgesics may be needed in the first few weeks, but their use must be carefully monitored and limited because of the risk of addiction. Analgesics are best given on a regular schedule and not on an "as needed" or demand basis.

Tricyclic antidepressants such as amitriptyline, administered in small doses before bedtime, are often helpful in reducing the pain experienced by whiplash patients. The mechanism of action is unclear but may be related to the ability of tricyclic antidepressants to block the reuptake of serotonin in neurons in selected regions of the central nervous system. Tricyclics may then work by enhancing endogenous pain control pathways or alternatively by reducing alpha-wave intrusion into the normal delta-wave pattern of non-REM stage 4 sleep and helping to restore a more normal sleep pattern. The major side effects of amitriptyline are dry mouth and morning drowsiness. Most patients who benefit from this medication need only 10 to 50 mg at bedtime. *Cyclobenzaprine* also is a tricyclic compound similar to amitriptyline in its chemical structure but marketed as a muscle relaxant. Cyclobenzaprine is prescribed in doses of 10 mg given one to three times per day and may serve as an alternative medication for individuals unable to tolerate amitriptyline.

Psychology

The psychologist's role is to identify emotional problems common to chronic pain (e.g., anger, depression, and anxiety); poor coping strategies; and aggravating environmental factors. The psychologist may then provide emotional support, help the patient develop better coping strategies, teach methods to reduce muscle tension, and encourage proper pacing of activities. Family or marital therapy is used where appropriate.

Muscular tension contributes to pain throughout axial regions of the body (i.e., head, neck, and back), most commonly around the injured neck and upper thorax. Anxiety, anger, and emotional stress can increase muscle tension, resulting in increased pain and discomfort, which in turn may lead to further muscle tension, anxiety, and emotional stress until a self-perpetuating cycle develops (Fig. 3–8). The psychologist can teach the patient to consciously reduce muscle tension before the pain reaches

intolerable levels. Learning to relax, perhaps aided by the use of relaxation tapes, may prevent the development of intolerable pain. Electromyographic biofeedback techniques may help a patient learn to control muscle tension either through auditory or visual feedback. Self-hypnosis and imagery techniques are methods of mental manipulation of the experience of pain designed to limit the experience of pain. Proper pacing of activities and avoiding situations of emotional stress further aid in reducing muscle tension and subsequent pain.

Vocational Adjustments and Retraining

A crucial element of management involves returning the patient to work. Certain postures, heavy manual labor, and repetitive arm movements are frequent aggravators of symptoms. Often pain builds to the point where the injured person is no longer able to work. The inability to work often leads to loss of self-esteem, financial stresses, depression, and accusations of malingering or secondary gain. The most important prognostic factor in determining whether a patient with chronic whiplash symptoms will return to work is the type of work itself. Failure to recognize the importance of vocational type to symptoms often results in failure to return the patient to employment.

Heavy lifting tends to aggravate pain in the neck and upper thoracic regions. Repetitive arm work also is difficult, particularly when the arms are held above the level of the shoulders. With both heavy lifting and repetitive arm work, the volume and the intensity of work is crucial. Putting the patient on light duties with frequent breaks may allow the patient to keep pain within tolerable limits. Prolonged sitting and standing postures (sometimes for less than 20 minutes) are also well-known aggravators of neck, upper thoracic, and low back pain after whiplash injuries. Some special adaptations, such as using a drafting style of desk that can be tilted up to reduce neck flexion or standing on a platform to limit shoulder abduction, are often helpful.

Return to work should be encouraged as soon as possible following the accident. Initially, part-time work with avoidance of

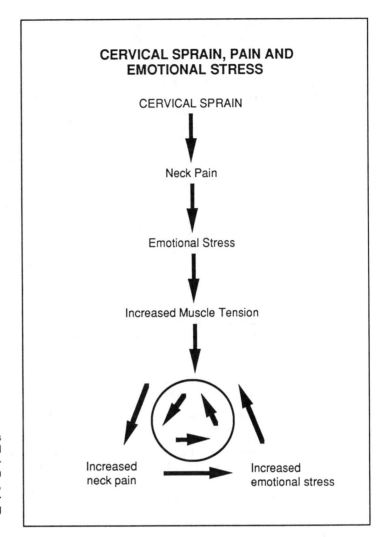

CERVICAL SPRAIN, PAIN AND EMOTIONAL STRESS

CERVICAL SPRAIN

Neck Pain

Emotional Stress

Increased Muscle Tension

Increased neck pain

Increased emotional stress

FIGURE 3-8. Emotional stress can influence pain from a cervical sprain by increasing muscle tension. The resulting increase in pain leads to further emotional stress, further muscle tension, and a self-perpetuating cycle of increasing pain, stress, and tension.

pain-aggravating activities will be more successful than a sudden return to regular duties. In those cases where the patient cannot return to previous employment, vocational counseling and retraining for a suitable job may become necessary. It must be made clear to the patient that return to some form of work is an essential part of rehabilitation.

CONCLUSION

Whiplash injuries remain a controversial clinical entity, and whiplash patients are among the most frustrating and difficult patients that neurologists must deal with. Symptoms following whiplash injuries ap-

pear to have a physiologic origin and do improve, albeit at different rates and to different degrees. Morbidity may persist for years. The majority of these patients are left with residual "nuisance" symptoms that are not disabling, while a small minority continue to have unremitting, disabling symptoms. Management of these patients should emphasize education, pain control, and recovery of function. Traditional medical training combined with a difficult chronic-pain patient provides fertile ground for patient-physician conflicts that compromise objective assessment and optimal management. Too often this has resulted in an overestimation of the role of litigation in prolongation of symptoms.

Possible solutions to the problem of

whiplash include prevention through improved car safety features and design, helping patients develop better adaptive coping skills and alternative vocational options, training physicians to deal better with chronic whiplash patients, and providing adequate and rapid financial compensation. More research is required into the pathophysiology, management, and outcome of whiplash injuries.

REFERENCES

1. Alves, WM, Colohan, ART, O'Leary, TJ, Rimel, RW, and Jane, JA: Understanding post-traumatic symptoms after minor head injury. J Head Trauma Rehabil 1(2):1–12, 1986.
2. Ameis, A: Cervical whiplash: Considerations in the rehabilitation of cervical myofascial injury. Can Fam Physician 32:1871–1876, 1986.
3. Balla, JI and Moraitis, S: Knights in armour: A follow-up study of injuries after legal settlement. Med J Aust 2:355–361, 1970.
4. Balla, JI: The late whiplash syndrome. Aust N Z J Surg 50(6):601–614, 1980.
5. Becker, H: The motor vehicle accident in family practice. Can Fam Physician 34:589–593, 1988.
6. Bland, JH: Disorders of the Cervical Spine. WB Saunders, Philadelphia, 1987.
7. Blumer, D and Heillbronn, H: Chronic pain as a variant of depressive disease: The pain prone disorder. J Nerv Ment Dis 170(7):381–406, 1982.
8. Bogduk, N: The anatomy and pathophysiology of whiplash. Clin Biomechanics 1:92–101, 1986.
9. Braaf, MM and Rosner, S: Symptomatology and treatment of injuries of the neck. NY J Med 55:237, 1955.
10. Braaf, MM and Rosner, S: Whiplash injury of neck: Fact or fancy? Int Surg 46:176, 1966.
11. Braaf, MM and Rosner, S: Trauma of cervical spine as a cause of chronic headache. J Trauma 15(5):441–446, 1975.
12. Brena, SF and Chapman, SL: The "learned pain syndrome." Postgrad Med 69:53–62, 1981.
13. Brena, SF and Chapman, SL: Chronic pain: Physiology, diagnosis, management. In Lelek, JC, Gershwin, ME, Fowler, WM (eds): Principles of Physical Medicine and Rehabilitation in the Musculoskeletal Diseases. Grune & Stratton, Orlando, FL, 1986, pp 189–216.
14. Cailliet, R: Neck and Arm Pain, ed 2. FA Davis, Philadelphia, 1981.
15. Campbell, SM, Gatter, RA, Clark, S, and Bennett, RM: A double-blind study of cyclobenzaprine versus placebo in patients with fibrositis (abstr). Arthritis Rheum 27:576, 1984.
16. Capistrant, TD: Thoracic outlet syndrome in whiplash injury. Ann Surg 185:175–178, 1977.
17. Carette, S, McCain, GA, Bell, DA and Fam, AG: Evaluation of amitriptyline in primary fibrositis: A double-blind, placebo-controlled study. Arthritis Rheum 29:655–659, 1986.
18. Colachis, SC: Diagnosis and management of whiplash injuries. Current concepts on pain. Analgesia 4(4):1–2, 1977.
19. Commack, KV: Whiplash injuries to the neck. Am J Surg 93:663–666, 1957.
20. Compere, WE: Electronystagmographic findings in patients with "whiplash" injuries. Laryngoscope 78:1226–1232, 1968.
21. Croft, AC: Biomechanics. In Foreman, SM and Croft, AC: Whiplash Injuries: The Cervical Acceleration Deceleration syndrome. Williams & Wilkins, Baltimore, 1988.
22. Croft, AC: Developmental anatomy. In Foreman, SM and Croft, AC: Whiplash Injuries: The Cervical Acceleration Deceleration Syndrome. William & Wilkins, Baltimore, 1988.
23. Crowe, ME: Injuries to the cervical spine. Presented at the meeting of the Western Orthopedic Association, San Francisco, 1928.
24. Deans, GT: Incidence and duration of neck pain among patients injured in car accidents. Br Med J 292:94–95, 1986.
25. deJong, PTVM, deJong, JMBV, Cohen, B, and Jongkees, LBW: Ataxia and nystagmus induced by injection of local anaesthetics in the neck. Ann Neurol 1:240–246, 1977.
26. De Palma, A and Subin, D: Study of the cervical syndrome. Clin Orthop 38:135–142, 1965.
27. Diamond, EL and Grauer, K: The physician's reactions to patients with chronic pain. Am Fam Physician 34(3):117–122, 1986.
28. Dunn, EJ and Blazlar, LS: Soft-tissue injuries of the lower cervical spine. In The Cervical Spine Research Society Editorial Committee (eds): The Cervical Spine. J. B. Lippincott, Philadelphia, 1983, pp 499–512.
29. Dunsker, SB: Hyperextension and hyperflexion injuries of the cervical spine. In Youmans, JR (ed): Neurological Surgery, ed 2. WB Saunders, Philadelphia, 1982, pp 2338–2343.
30. Elton, D, Stanley, and Burrows, G: Psychological Control of Pain. Grune & Stratton, North Ryde, Australia, 1983.
31. Erichson, JE: Concussion of the spine: Nervous shock and other obscure injuries to the nervous system: Clinical and medicolegal aspects. William Wood & Co, New York, 1886, p 57.
32. Farbmann, AA: Neck sprain, associated factors. JAMA 223:101–1015, 1973.
33. Feinstein, B, Langton, JNK, Jameson, RM, and Schiller, F: Experiments of pain referred from deep somatic tissues. J Bone Joint Surg 36A(5):981–997, 1954.
34. Feinstein, B: Referred pain from paravertebral structures. In Buerger, AA and Tobis, JS (eds): Approaches to the Validation of Manipulation Therapy. Charles C Thomas, Springfield, IL, 1977, pp 139–174.
35. Fisher, CM: Whiplash amnesia. Neurology (NY) 32:667–668, 1982.
36. Fox, JC and Williams, JF: Mathematical model for

investigating combined seatback–head restraint during rear end impact. Med Biol Eng Comput 14:263, 1976.

37. Frankel, VH: Temporomandibular joint pain syndrome following deceleration injury to the cervical spine. Bull Hosp Joint Dis Orthop Inst 26:47, 1969.

38. Frankel, VH: Whiplash injuries to the neck. In Hirsch, C and Zotterman, Y (eds): Cervical Pain. Pergamon, Oxford, 1972, pp 97–112.

39. Frankel, VH: Pathomechanics of whiplash injuries to the neck. In Morley, TP (ed): Current Controversies in Neurosurgery. WB Saunders, Philadelphia, 1976, pp 39–50.

40. Gay, JR and Abbott, KH: Common whiplash injuries of the neck. JAMA 152:1698–1704, 1953.

41. Gorlin, R and Zucker, HD: Physician's reactions to patients: A key to teaching humanistic medicine. N Engl J Med 308:1059–1063, 1983.

42. Gotten, N: Survey of 100 cases of whiplash injury after settlement of litigation. JAMA 162:865–867, 1956.

43. Greenfield, J, and Ilfeld, FW: Acute cervical strain: Evaluation and short term prognostic factors. Clin Orthop 122:196–200, 1977.

44. Hass, DC: Whiplash amnesia. Neurology (NY) 33:525, 1983.

45. Hendler, N: Chronic pain patient versus the malingering patient. In Foly, KM and Payne, RM: Current Therapy of Pain. Philadelphia BC Decker, 1985, pp 14–22.

46. Hobbs, CA: The effectiveness of seat belts in reducing injuries to car occupants. Transport and Road Research Laboratory Report No. 811, 1978.

47. Hobbs, CA: Car occupant injury patterns and mechanisms. Transport and Road Research Laboratory Supplementary Report No. 648, 1981.

48. Hohl, M: Soft tissue injuries of the neck in automobile accidents: Factors influencing prognosis. J Bone Joint Surg 56A:1675–1682, 1974.

49. Hohl, M: Soft tissue injuries of the neck. Clin Orthop 109:42–49, 1975.

50. Inman, VH and Saunders, JBdeCM: Referred pain from skeletal structures. J Nerv Ment Dis 99:660–667, 1944.

51. Janes, J and Hooshmand, H: Severe extension-flexion injuries of the cervical spine. Mayo Clinic Proc 40(5):353–369, 1965.

52. Kenna, C and Murtagh, J: Whiplash. Aust Fam Physician 16(6):727–736, 1987.

53. Kennedy, F: The mind of the injured worker: Its effect on disability periods. Compens Med 1:19–24, 1946.

54. Kirkaldy-Willis, WH (ed): Managing low back pain, ed 2. Churchill Livingstone, New York, 1988.

55. Kuch, K, Swinson, RP, and Kirby, M: Post-traumatic stress disorder after car accidents. Can J Psychiatry 30:426–427, 1985.

56. Lader, E: Cervical trauma as a factor in the development of TMJ dysfunction and facial pain. Craniomandibular Pract 1:85, 1983.

57. LaRocca, H: Acceleration injuries of the neck. Clin Neurosurg 25:205–217, 1978.

58. Lieberman, JS: Cervical soft tissue injuries and cervical disc disease. In Principles of Physical Medicine and Rehabilitation in the Musculoskeletal Diseases. Grune & Stratton, Orlando, FL, 1986, pp 263–286.

59. Lloyd, JH: Compensation neurosis. Aust Fam Physician 9:84–87, 1980.

60. MacNab, I: Acceleration injuries of the cervical spine. J Bone Joint Surg 46A:1797–1799, 1964.

61. MacNab, I: Acceleration extension injuries of the cervical spine. In AAOS Symposium of the Spine. CV Mosby, St Louis, 1969, pp 10–17.

62. MacNab, I: The "whiplash syndrome." Orthop Clin North Am 2:389–403, 1971.

63. MacNab, I: The whiplash syndrome. Clin Neurosurg 20:232–241, 1973.

64. MacNab, I: Acceleration extension injuries of the cervical spine. In Rothman, RH and Simeone, FA (eds): The Spine, ed 2. WB Saunders, Philadelphia, 1982, pp 647–660.

65. Martinez, JL and García DJ: A model for whiplash. J Biomechanics 1:23–32, 1968.

66. McKenzie, JA and Williams, JF: The dynamic behavior of the head and cervical spine during "whiplash." J Biomechanics 4:474–490, 1971.

67. Mealy, K, Brennan, H, and Fenelon, GCC: Early mobilization of acute whiplash injuries. Br Med J 292:656–657, 1986.

68. Meffan, P and Welsh, P: The whiplash syndrome: A problem for doctor and patient. Mod Med Can 38(6):743–745, 1983.

69. Mendelson, G: Persistent work disability following settlement of compensation claims. Law Institute Journal (Melbourne) 55:342–345, 1981.

70. Mendelson, G: Not "cured by a verdict": Effect of a legal settlement on compensation claimants. Med J Aust 2:132–134, 1982.

71. Merskey, H: Psychiatry and the cervical sprain syndrome. Can Med Assoc J 130:1119–1121, 1984.

72. Miller, H: Accident neurosis: Lecture II. Br Med J 1:992–998, 1961.

73. National Safety Council: Accident Facts, 47. Chicago, 1971.

74. Norris, SH and Watt, F: The prognosis of neck injuries resulting from rear-end vehicle collisions. J Bone Joint Surg 65B:608–611, 1983.

75. Ommaya, AK, Faas, F, and Yarnell, P: Whiplash and brain damage. JAMA 204(4):285, 1968.

76. O'Neill, BL, Haddon, W Jr, Kelley, AB, and Sorenson, WW: Automobile head restraints: Frequency of neck injury claims in relation to the presence of head restraints. Am J Public Health 62:399, 1972.

77. Parker, N: Accident litigants with neurotic symptoms. Med J Aust 2:318–322, 1977.

78. Raskin, NH: Headache, ed 2. Churchill Livingstone, New York, 1988.

79. Roca, PD: Ocular manifestations of whiplash injuries. Ann Ophthalmol 4:63–73, 1972.

80. Roydhouse, RH: Whiplash and temporomandibular dysfunction. Lancet 1:1394, 1973.

81. Rubin, W: Whiplash with vestibular involvement. Arch Otolaryngol Head Neck Surg 97:85–87, 1973.

82. Sandoz, R: Some physical mechanisms and effects of spinal adjustments. Annals of the Swiss Chiropractic Association 6:91, 1976.

83. Sandoz, R: Some reflex phenomena associated with spinal derangements and adjustments. Annals of the Swiss Chiropractic Association, 7:45, 1981.

84. Schutt, CH and Dohan, FCS: Neck injuries to women in auto accidents. A metropolitan plague. JAMA 206:2689–2692, 1968.

85. Severy, DM, Mathewson, JH, and Bechtol, CO: Controlled automobile rear-end collisions: An investigation of related engineering and medical phenomena. Can Sev Med J 11:717–759, 1955.

86. Simons, DG: Myofascial pain syndromes: Where are we? Where are we going? Arch Phys Med Rehabil 69:207–212, 1988.

87. Slater, E: Diagnosis of "hysteria." Br Med J 1:1395–1399, 1965.

88. Slater, EO and Glithero, E: A follow-up of patients diagnosed as suffering from "hysteria." J Psychosom Res 9:9–13, 1965.

89. Speed, WG: Psychiatric aspects of posttraumatic headaches. In Adler, CS, et al. (eds): Psychiatric Aspects of Headache. Williams & Wilkins, Baltimore, 1987, pp 201–206.

90. States, JD, Balcerak, JC, Williams, JS, et al.: Injury frequency and head restraint effectiveness in rear-end impact accidents. Proceedings of the 16th STAPP Car Crash Conference, Detroit, MI 1972, p 228.

91. Torres, F and Shapiro SK: Electroencephalograms in whiplash injury. Arch Neurol 5:40, 1961.

92. Travell, J and Simons, DG: Myofascial pain and dysfunction: The trigger point manual. Williams & Wilkins, Baltimore, 1983.

93. Tyler, GSI, McNeely, HE, and Dick, ML. Treatment of post-traumatic headache with amitriptyline. Headache 20:213–216, 1980.

94. Unterharnscheidt, F: Traumatic alterations in the Rhesus monkey undergoing GX impact accelerations. Neurotraumatology 6:151–167, 1983.

95. Vasudevan, SV: Clinical perspectives on the relationships between pain and disability. Neurol Clinics 7(2):429–439, 1989.

96. Weinberg, S and LaPointe, H: Cervical extension-flexion injury (whiplash) and internal derangement of the temporomandibular joint. J Oral Maxillofac Surg 45:653–656, 1987.

97. White, AA, Johnson, RM, Panjabi, MM, et al.: Biomechanical analysis of clinical stability in the cervical spine. Clin Orthop 109:85–95, 1975.

98. Wickstrom, JK, Rodriguez, RP Jr, and Martinez, JL: Experimental production of acceleration injuries of the head and neck. Highway Safety Research Institute, Washington, DC, 181, 1967.

99. Wickstrom, JK, Martinez, JL, Rodriguez, R, et al.: Hyperextension and hyperflexion injuries to the head and neck of primates. In Gurdjian, ES and Thomas, LM (eds): Neckache and Backache. Charles C Thomas, Springfield, IL, 1970, pp 108–119.

100. Wickstrom, J and LaRocca, H: Management of patients with cervical spine and head injuries from acceleration forces. Curr Pract Orthop Surg 6:83, 1975.

101. Wiley, AM et al.: Musculoskeletal sequelae of whiplash injuries. Advocates Q 7:65–73, 1986.

102. Yarnell, PR and Rossie, GV: Minor whiplash head injury with major debilitation. Brain Inj 2(3):255–258, 1988.

SECTION TWO

. . . .

INTENSIVE CARE NEUROLOGY

Editor's Commentary

Neurologic care is becoming more intense, complex, and costly. Cardiac disease, brain trauma, and neurologic complications associated with prolonged management in an intensive care unit represent but three areas of expanded activity within the realm of diseases of the nervous system.

Salazar deals with the epidemiology, pathogenesis, management, and rehabilitation of patients with traumatic brain injury. The frequency and seriousness of head injury are so high and the difficulties of dealing with the consequences are so great that one wonders whether physicians would have a greater impact as educators in prevention than as therapists. Both roles are important but appear puny when compared to the dimensions of the problem.

A poor outcome is always unwelcome, particularly if unexpected. Samuels reviews the close link between the nervous system and cardiopulmonary function and offers a unifying hypothesis to explain sudden death in neurologic patients. Overactivity of the sympathetic limb of the autonomic nervous system may explain the all-too-common deaths in subarachnoid hemorrhage, status epilepticus, and head trauma.

VCH

CHAPTER 4

. . . .

TRAUMATIC BRAIN INJURY: THE CONTINUING EPIDEMIC

Andres M. Salazar, M.D., COL, M.C., USA

More death and disability from brain injury is sustained in the homes and on the highways of North America than have ever been inflicted on its battlefields. Salazar appreciates the dimensions of the problem both as a neurologist and as a military man. He rightly emphasizes the relative neglect of this important field and the persistence of practices based more on habit than proof, such as the use of corticosteroids in head-injured patients.

The author also deals with the sequelae of "minor" head injury. Headache, fatigue, and dizziness lead the list. "Dizziness" reemerges yet again as a nonspecific but troubling symptom.

VCH

Traumatic brain injury (TBI) is the leading cause of death and disability in young adults today; every 5 minutes one American dies and another is permanently disabled from TBI.[12] Largely because it affects the young, the total economic cost of TBI has been estimated at over $25 billion per year. The incidence of TBI requiring hospitalization is about 200 per 100,000; from a neurologic point of view it is a much larger problem than HIV infection. Yet it has been generally ignored by neurologists, perhaps as no other subject in the specialty relative to its incidence. So little is known about TBI that the entire field is a challenge and fertile ground for basic, pharmacologic, acute clinical, behavioral, and neurorehabilitation research. While basic laboratory, acute clinical, and prevention research may be more likely to lead to long-term solutions, the need for immediately practical clinical research into the behavioral and rehabilitation problems of TBI patients is particularly pressing at this time, for both economic and humanitarian reasons. Additionally, certain kinds of head-injured patients with focal lesions (such as gunshot or fragment wounds) continue to offer unique opportunities for studying specific aspects of brain function.

This chapter will briefly review our current understanding of the pathogenesis of TBI, with an emphasis on certain areas of active research, and then outline a practical management approach to the TBI patient based on that knowledge.

PATHOPHYSIOLOGY OF TBI

The most important challenges in the TBI field today relate to expanding our understanding of the basic pathophysiology. A brief review is warranted, since recognition of the various pathologic components of this condition is particularly important to the present day management of the head-injured patient. In the first place, we must recognize that TBI is a dynamic process. Not only does

55

the pathologic picture continue to evolve over the first few hours and days after trauma, often with devastating secondary injury, but the physiologic and clinical aspects of the recovery process itself can continue for a period of years. Thus, the notion of a "dynamic prognosis" requiring intermittent revision is especially relevant to the head-injured patient, both because of the long period of recovery and because the multiple poorly understood variables involved still make outcome prediction as much of an art as a science.

In addition, we should remember that the TBI victim often manifests a multitude of systemic abnormalities, not only as a consequence of concomitant trauma elsewhere in the body but secondary to the brain injury itself. Changes in nutrition,[21] cardiopulmonary status,[8,26] circulating catecholamines,[63] and coagulation[35] are among those described.

Pathology

Over the past decades we have moved from conceptualizing the pathology of closed head injury (CHI) in terms of hematomas and "coup-contrecoup" contusions to a four-component classification.[31] Three parallel components were initially identified: (1) focal injury, (2) diffuse axonal injury (DAI), and (3) superimposed hypoxia-ischemia. More recently, (4) diffuse microvascular injury with loss of autoregulation has been implicated as playing an important role in the acute stage of moderate and severe head injury. All of these pathologic features have been reproduced in animal models of angular acceleration without impact.[23]

Focal injury. Focal contusions often occur under the site of impact and thus result in focal neurologic deficits referable to that area (e.g., aphasia, hemiparesis), but by far the most common location for contusions after acceleration-deceleration injury is in the orbitofrontal and anterior temporal lobes, where brain lies next to bony edges. Thus, a relatively typical pathologic picture is often seen in CHI, and the most troubling clinical sequelae are behavioral and cognitive abnormalities that may be referable to

the frontal and temporal lobe injury. Subdural hematomas are most common with rapid decelerations such as occur with impact after a fall, especially in the aged, and are often due to rupture of bridging veins. Recent studies suggest that delays longer than 4 hours in the surgical management of hematomas significantly worsens prognosis. Delayed hematomas, as well as bleeding into contusions, are particularly important in the so-called "talk and die" patient, who may initially appear to be at low risk but then deteriorates unexpectedly.[41]

Diffuse axonal injury is one of the most important causes of persistent severe neurologic deficit in CHI. Originally described as a "shearing" injury of axons, it was characterized microscopically by axonal "retraction" balls in the hemispheric white matter, corpus callosum, and brainstem.[56,24] Recent work with mild to moderate fluid-percussion injury in animal models, however, shows that the typical light microscopic histopathology of DAI may not emerge until 12 to 24 hours postinjury. The only early abnormality is a relatively subtle focal intra-axonal disruption seen on electron microscopy, with an intact axon sheath. This leads to a disturbance of axonal flow, accumulation of transport material with axonal ballooning proximal to the injury, and then eventual severing of axons several hours later.[50,51] The role of alterations in calcium metabolism at the injured site on the axon may be particularly important. One obvious clinical implication of these findings is that there may be a potential 12- to 24-hour window of therapeutic opportunity postinjury during which future treatments may prevent total axonal disruption. Another important conclusion from these studies is that DAI can be demonstrated even after "minor" head injury and occurs even in the absence of morphopathologic change in any other vascular, neural, or glial elements. This confirms earlier, uncontrolled pathologic studies in humans and makes such axonal damage the most likely organic basis for the "postconcussion syndrome" and for the cumulative effects of repeated concussion, as seen in some boxers.[34,47]

Interestingly, one major feature of the pathology of dementia pugilistica is the presence of neurofibrillary tangles (NFT) but not Alzheimer plaques. NFT in Alzheimer's disease and in other conditions such as Guamanian amyotrophic lateral sclerosis have been postulated to result from abnormalities in axonal flow, in the latter case probably related to aberrant calcium metabolism.[22] Some of the challenges posed in these seemingly disparate areas of neurology may eventually find common ground and similar solutions.

Hypoxia-ischemia. The classical pathology of hypoxia-ischemia, involving mainly the hippocampus and the vascular border zones of the brain, is all too often superimposed on the other pathologic features that are more specific for TBI. The traumatized brain is particularly sensitive to hypoxia-ischemia, and the relationship is probably more than just additive.[32] When present, such pathology, including the concomitant brain swelling, can obviously become a major determinant of ultimate clinical outcome; the most significant recent improvements in the management of the TBI patient have resulted from recognition of the importance of this component and its prevention. Thus, as is further alluded to below, challenges that are relevant to the problem of cerebral ischemia and infarction will also have an impact on the problem of TBI.

Diffuse microvascular damage also has been recently implicated as a major component of both closed and penetrating TBI.[2,43] Diffuse perivascular damage with astrocytic footplate swelling is a prominent feature at both the light and electron microscopic levels within minutes of high-velocity gunshot wounds in nonhuman primates. In CHI the vascular response appears to be biphasic. Depending on the severity of the trauma, early changes include an initial transient systemic hypertension (probably related to brainstem effects), an early loss of cerebrovascular autoregulation with a decreased response to changes in PCO_2, and a transient dysfunction of the blood-brain barrier (BBB), probably due to endothelial changes (although endothelial tight junctions may remain intact early). The loss of autoregulation makes the brain particularly susceptible to fluctuations in systemic blood pressure; for example, systemic hypertension can increase the risk of hyperemia and brain swelling, more commonly seen in younger

patients. The early dysfunction of the BBB results in rapid swelling of perivascular astrocytes, which peaks at about 1 hour postinjury but begins to recover by 6 hours. Later endothelial changes include formation of intraluminal microvilli or blebs and craters, which peak at about 6 hours postinjury but can persist as long as 6 days. Although the clinical significance of these changes is still not known, they are probably related to the loss of autoregulation, to the altered vascular sensitivity to circulating neurotransmitters, and to cerebral edema. Importantly, very similar endothelial changes can be induced in nontraumatized animals by applying various superoxide radical generators to the intact pial surface. Both cyclooxygenase inhibitors such as indomethacin and oxygen free radical scavengers such as superoxide dismutase will prevent or reverse these arteriolar changes experimentally in trauma models, suggesting that such drugs may eventually play a role in the management of TBI.[38]

Mechanisms of Secondary Tissue Injury

Over the past decade, delayed secondary injury at the cellular level has come to be recognized as a major contributor to the ultimate tissue loss after TBI. As alluded to above, a cascade of physiologic, vascular, and biochemical events is set in motion in injured tissue. This includes changes in arachidonic acid metabolites such as the prostaglandins and the leukotrienes;[16] the formation of oxygen free radicals;[38] and changes in neuropeptides,[17] electrolytes such as calcium and magnesium,[45] excitatory neurotransmitters such as glutamate or acetylcholine,[18] and lymphokines such as interleukin-1,[44] or lactic acid[57] (Table 4–1). These products can result in progressive secondary injury to otherwise viable brain tissue through a number of mechanisms: for example, by producing further ischemia or altering vascular reactivity, by producing brain swelling (edema or hyperemia), by injuring neurons and glia directly or activating macrophages that result in such injury, or by establishing conditions favorable to secondary infection. In other words, much of the

TABLE 4–1. **POSSIBLE MECHANISMS OF SECONDARY INJURY IN TBI**

A. Hypoxia-ischemia
B. Mass effect
   1. Delayed hematoma
   2. Brain swelling
      Cerebral edema
      Hyperemia
   3. Hydrocephalus
C. Infection
D. Potential cellular mechanisms
   1. Phospholipid metabolism
      Lipid peroxidation (arachidonic acid chain)
         Prostaglandins, leukotrienes
         Platelet activating factor (PAF)
   2. Oxygen free radicals
      Free iron catalysis
   3. Excitotoxic mechanisms
      Glutamate (NMDA) receptors
      Acetylcholine
   4. Neuropeptides
      Endorphins (dynorphin)
      Thyrotropin-releasing hormone (TRH)
   5. Calcium and magnesium metabolism
      abnormalities
   6. CNS lactic acidosis
   7. Axonal flow abnormalities

ultimate brain loss after TBI may be due not to the injury itself, but to an uncontrolled vicious cycle of biochemical events set in motion by the trauma. The control of this complex cascade of cellular events remains one of the most important challenges in the acute management of head injury. At the same time it offers a potential window of opportunity during which brain swelling and nerve cell death could be prevented by pharmacologic or other intervention in the first few hours after an injury.

Phospholipid – Arachidonic Acid Metabolites

Arachidonic acid (AA) is released by the action of phospholipases and is particularly plentiful in traumatized brain. Its metabolites are likely to play a role in secondary brain injury. AA is metabolized through two major pathways: the cyclooxygenase path, leading to formation of prostaglandins, and the lipoxygenase path, leading to the formation of leukotrienes. While both may play a role, the cyclooxygenase pathway appears to be the most important in TBI; among the

metabolites that may be most active are prostaglandin E2 and thromboxane. Animal studies have demonstrated marked elevations in cerebrospinal fluid and brain prostaglandins within minutes of injury.[6,16,55] Theoretically, these metabolites could produce secondary injury by inducing vasospasm, thrombosis, and/or edema. However, therapeutic trials using cyclooxygenase inhibitors in animals have been disappointing, particularly when these are administered more than a few minutes after the injury.[54,61]

Finally, preliminary studies suggest that another highly active phospholipid metabolite, platelet activity factor (PAF), may also play an important role in secondary injury through a variety of mechanisms.[37]

Oxygen Free Radicals

Oxygen free radicals are also a very active species biologically and have been shown to be produced early in ischemic and traumatic tissue injury, both in the central nervous system and elsewhere.[38] The superoxide radical ($O^{\cdot}$) is formed through a variety of mechanisms, including both the xanthine oxidase and the cyclooxygenase pathways, and results in tissue injury in its own right by combining directly with cellular elements (Fig. 4–1). However, when combined with its own breakdown product, hydrogen peroxide, in the presence of free iron it forms the hydroxyl radical, $OH^{\cdot}$, which is even more destructive. The hydroxyl radical's affinity for the abundant lipids in brain results in lipid peroxidation, with further release of arachidonic acid and a vicious cycle in which more free radicals are produced through the cyclooxygenase pathway (along with prostaglandins), overwhelming natural superoxide scavenging mechanisms. The continued presence of free iron is essential for this cycle, thus providing one likely explanation for the toxicity of free blood in TBI patients, including its possible relationship to posttraumatic epilepsy.

Pharmacologic intervention to reduce the formation of such radicals and/or to scavenge those already formed would be expected to reduce ultimate tissue injury, and the complexity of the biochemical events involved provides several potential therapeutic avenues. Animal models have con-

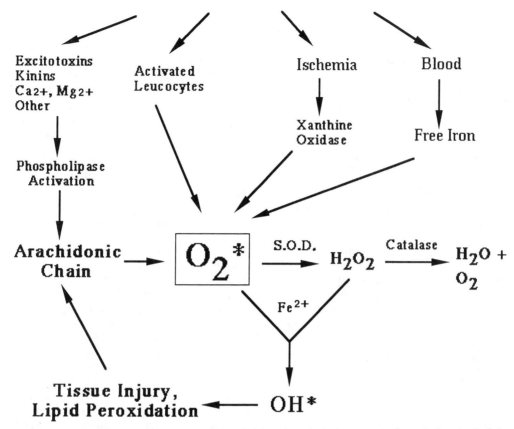

FIGURE 4-1. Oxygen free radicals in traumatic brain injury: hypothetical sequence of events (see text). $O_2^* =$ Oxygen radical; $OH^* =$ hydroxyl radical; S.O.D. = superoxide dismutase.

firmed this potential benefit in several systems. These include the use of steroids (especially the nonglucocorticoid 21-aminosteroids or "lazaroids") to inhibit lipid peroxidation and the release of arachidonate,[29] cyclooxygenase inhibitors to block prostaglandin formation, xanthine oxidase inhibitors such as allopurinol,[59] iron chelators such as deferoxamine, enzymes such as superoxide dismutase and catalase,[7] and various other free radical scavengers such as mannitol and tocopherol.

Excitotoxins

Another potential mechanism of secondary injury that has received increasing attention, particularly in the stroke and ischemia literature, is the role of excitotoxins, and especially of agonists of the NMDA subclass of glutamate receptors.[18] Theoretically, the sustained release of excess amounts of such naturally occurring neurotransmitters after an injury can lead to eventual neuronal death. The mechanisms for this effect are not yet clear, but they may involve alterations in calcium and magnesium metabolism and activation of various enzyme systems. Among these might be phospholipase-A, with consequent release of arachidonic acid and activation of the superoxide cycle discussed above. Experimental therapeutic interventions aimed at the excitotoxin mechanism include NMDA receptor antagonists such as dextromethorphan and acetylcholine antagonists such as scopolamine.[30]

Other endogenous agents that have received attention in recent years are various neuropeptides such as the endorphins (particularly dynorphin) and thyrotropin-releasing hormone (TRH). However, both

animal and clinical studies of opiate antagonists such as naloxone and its analogues
have been disappointing, although TRH and
its analogues still hold some promise.[17,19]

MANAGEMENT

Acute

Initial Evaluation and Resuscitation in Severe Traumatic Brain Injury

Present-day acute management of TBI is
primarily directed at the prevention of
secondary injury, especially that related
to hypoxia-ischemia or to expanding mass
lesions. Experience has shown that an organized team approach is essential to accom-
plish this goal, from prehospital through intensive care unit (ICU) and postacute care.
The cornerstone of early neurologic evaluation is the use of the Glasgow Coma Score
(GCS), along with checks of lateralization,
brainstem function, and pupillary response;
a system for easily recording sequential
changes in these and other vital parameters
is an integral part of care.[33] Although the
GCS has been criticized for its simplicity, it
has proved to be very reproducible across
individual examiners and institutions and
thus serves as a solid basis for evaluation of
potential deterioration over time. More detailed neurologic examination is probably
not warranted until the patient is well stabilized in the ICU; neurologists in particular
should resist the temptation. A history from
witnesses, particularly with regard to the
onset of coma, is important not only for decisions on acute care but also for long-term
prognosis. For example, the presence of an
initial "lucid" or "semilucid" interval in a
now-comatose patient suggests a possible
hematoma requiring prompt surgery, but it
also makes severe diffuse axonal injury unlikely and points to a relatively favorable
prognosis, provided there is no further secondary damage.

The importance of cardiopulmonary resuscitation and management in TBI care
cannot be overstated; airway and shock management should be the top priority in any
trauma patient. Superimposed hypoxia-ischemia can be the single most important determinant of ultimate outcome in severely
head-injured patients. We know from animal experiments that the traumatized brain
is particularly sensitive to hypoxia-ischemia, and levels of hypercarbia tolerated by
the normal brain can lead to critical mar-
ginal increases in intracranial pressure
(ICP) after TBI. As noted earlier, among the
most important improvements in TBI patient care over the past decade has been the
introduction of emergency care and transport systems that include paramedic training in early, on-site fluid resuscitation and
intubation.

The comatose TBI patient is often hypoxic
or hypercarbic, even though he or she may
appear to be ventilating normally. Patients
in coma (GCS <8) should thus be intubated
and hyperventilated, if possible, to a PCO_2 of
25 to 30 (but preferably not below that level
for more than brief periods). Sedation with
morphine 4 to 12 mg IV every 2 to 4 hours to
prevent systemic hypertension, or paralysis
with pancuronium bromide 4 mg every 2 to
4 hours, should be used as needed. The
stomach should be emptied to prevent aspi-
ration. Immobilization of the head in the
plane of the body is advisable, not only because of the possibility of associated cervical fracture (about 5%), but also for airway
maintenance and prevention of venous occlusion that might raise ICP. Elevation of the
head may further facilitate cranial venous
return, although its value is controversial.

Shock should suggest the possibility of
hemorrhage elsewhere in the body. Fluid resuscitation should rely on normal saline or
lactated Ringer's solution, but TBI patients
should not be overly hydrated; central
venous pressure monitoring can be helpful
in this regard. Dextrose and water should be
avoided, not only because it is hypotonic,
but because of the potential for increased
lactic acidosis and infarction in the hy-
poxic-ischemic patient with elevated blood
sugars.[49] Although formal studies have not
been done on the latter issue in head-injured
patients, we prefer to avoid maintenance
with any dextrose solutions in the early
acute phase.

Radiologic Examination

Computed tomography (CT) has become
standard in the management of mass lesions

in the head-injured patient, and it should be used when available in all patients with GCS <12 ("does not obey commands") or when focal signs are present. This should be done as soon as possible after the patient has been resuscitated and stabilized. As noted previously, delays of greater than 4 hours postinjury in evacuation of hematomas have been associated with significant deterioration in outcome. Comatose patients, however, must remain accompanied by a physician or critical care nurse; it is all too common to hear of a "stabilized" patient who suffers cardiac arrest or irreversible brain damage because of a simple airway problem in the elevator on the way to the CT suite. The usefulness of magnetic resonance imaging in the acute situation is limited in part by the difficulty of managing the comatose patient in most scanners.

In conscious patients with mild confusion and no lateralizing signs, a skull x-ray and observation may be sufficient. However, a fracture on x-ray markedly increases the risk of a surgical lesion and is indication for CT, even in the alert TBI patient. In any case, a high index of suspicion for delayed hematomas is imperative. One recent study found that the large differences in mortality of TBI patients found across a variety of hospitals with different resources was accounted for not by the high-risk ICU patient, but by deterioration of patients initially obeying commands and considered to be at "low" risk.[36]

Intensive Care Unit

Once a surgical mass lesion has been treated or excluded, the comatose patient should be managed in the ICU. The avoidance of secondary insults to the brain remains the principal goal of therapy. Principles of care and treatments discussed above for earlier stages are generally continued, and, as before, organization, training, and adherence to relatively simple principles are the mainstay of care. In addition to standard laboratory tests, evaluation for coagulopathies with platelet count, prothrombin time/partial thromboplastin time (PT/ PTT), thrombin time, fibrinogen, and fibrinogen split products may also be indicated.[35]

Intracranial Pressure Monitoring. Although many physicians, in particular, neurologists, may be reluctant to give up the neurologic examination as the principal measure of patient progress, recent studies suggest that the ICP, which is one determinant of cerebral perfusion pressure, is a more sensitive parameter.[40] For example, the classical Cushing triad has been shown to occur less than 25% of the time in patients with ICP > 30 mm Hg, a level that almost invariably proves fatal if not controlled. Yet it is much easier to prevent a rise to that level by treating when the patient is at 15 mm Hg than it is to bring ICP down from a level of 25 to 30 mm Hg. ICP has repeatedly been shown to correlate significantly with outcome, and its monitoring is increasingly used in the care of the comatose TBI patient. In one recent study, survival was 92% for patients with their ICP controlled, as opposed to 17% for those without.[14] The particular monitoring technique used is determined by the neurosurgeon and the facilities available. Choices include an intraventricular catheter, a subarachnoid screw, or the more recent fiber-optic epidural transducers.

One relatively simple algorithm in use for treating rises in intracranial pressure, the therapeutic intensity level (TIL), has the advantage of also providing a standard measure of severity of ICP elevations in TBI patients[46] (Table 4–2). It outlines an orderly increase

TABLE 4–2. INTRACRANIAL PRESSURE MANAGEMENT IN HEAD INJURY
Therapeutic Intensity Level (TIL)*

		Score
Sedation	(Morphine)	1
Paralysis (as needed)	(Pancuronium bromide)	1
Hyperventilation	$PCO_2 > 30$	1
	$PCO_2 < 30$	2
Ventricular drainage	<4 mL/h	1
	>4 mL/h	2
Mannitol	<1 g/kg per 8 h	3
	>1 g/kg per 8 h	6
Barbiturate coma	(Pentobarbital)	3

* Each new level is generally instituted when the previous level fails to control ICP below 15–20 mm Hg (see text).
The sum points for each of the modalities in use at a particular time is the TIL score at that time. Maximum = 15, Minimum = 0.

in therapeutic vigor from simple sedation through barbiturate coma (see below). Although treatment is always individualized for each patient, a new level of therapy is generally instituted when the previous level has failed to control ICP below 20 mm Hg. Each specific therapy is assigned a point value; the TIL score at a given time is the sum of points for the interventions in use at that time. Thus, a patient with an ICP of 20 at a TIL of 12 is quite different from a patient with the same ICP at a TIL of 3. It should be emphasized, however, that use of the TIL algorithm must not lull the physician into ignoring the possibility that progressive ICP elevations may also be due to surgical lesions such as delayed hematoma or hydrocephalus. Similarly, seizures, hyponatremia, and airway problems will raise the ICP.

Medical Therapy for Prevention of Secondary Injury. In addition to measures discussed above, specific medical therapy aimed at minimizing secondary injury is still in its infancy and is an area in which active clinical research begs to be integrated with clinical care. Such treatments should generally be started as soon as possible after the injury, ideally even before the patient goes to surgery or the ICU. Mannitol is the most valuable of the agents presently available, perhaps because, in addition to its osmotic effects, it is also an oxygen free radical scavenger. The usual initial dose is 1 g/kg in the adult. Patients are then maintained on 0.25-g boluses every 4 hours as necessary to control ICP (see above) as long as serum osmolarity is less than 310. Some surgeons advocate the continued use of low-dose mannitol. Other diuretics, such as furosemide, are still used by some practitioners in specific situations.

Barbiturate coma is the last step in the recommended nonsurgical control of ICP and has recently been confirmed to improve outcome in patients with otherwise uncontrolled ICP. In a recent large controlled study, patients under age 45 who were randomized to barbiturate were almost twice as likely to have ICP controlled; in the absence of cardiovascular risks, barbiturate therapy was over five times as likely to control ICP as was nonbarbiturate therapy.[14] Barbiturate coma is induced with pentobarbital at an initial loading dose of 10 mg/kg IV over 30 minutes. An additional 5 mg/kg is then given every hour for three doses, always with close monitoring of blood pressure. Serum levels should then be maintained at 3 to 4 mg/dL with doses of about 1 mg/kg per hour.

The use of corticosteroids for acute TBI remains all too common; 42% of over 1000 neurosurgeons responding to a recent US Army survey report using steroids routinely in head-injured patients. Nevertheless, several recent, well-conducted, controlled studies have failed to show any benefit of steroids at various doses, and other studies have shown a deleterious effect on the metabolism in these patients. However, nonglucocorticoid steroids (the "lazaroids") currently under investigation may soon offer a useful approach. Other experimental agents discussed above may also enter the therapeutic armamentarium shortly.

Posttraumatic Epilepsy

The overall risk of epilepsy in patients with closed head injury is relatively small: 2% to 5% overall and about 11% for patients with severe CHI.[3] Some studies, however, have shown a higher incidence in patients with depressed skull fracture (15%), hematoma (31%), or penetrating brain wounds (50%).[33,53] In all cases, the risk decreases markedly as time passes. Although the relative risk of developing epilepsy after penetrating head injury (PHI) is still about 25 times higher than the normal age-matched population at 10 to 15 years postinjury, patients with PHI can be 95% certain of remaining seizure free if they have no seizures for the first 3 years postinjury.[62]

The ongoing debate over the use of prophylactic anticonvulsants in head-injured patients must be separated into two questions: (1) Are anticonvulsants indicated in a patient with posttraumatic epilepsy (PTE)? and (2) Do prophylactic anticonvulsants prevent the onset of PTE? In light of data suggesting that most patients with one posttraumatic seizure will have recurrent seizures for some time, the answer of most clinicians to the first question is probably yes. The use of prophylactic anticonvulsants to prevent the onset of PTE is the more controversial issue; it has been predicated on several uncontrolled studies over the past four decades. However, one recent large uncontrolled study and three recent controlled, randomized studies have shown that phenytoin, even when given under carefully monitored conditions with maintenance of adequate blood levels, does not prevent the development of PTE beyond the first week after injury.[48,53,60,65] Prophylactic phenobarbital is theoretically preferable because of its suppressant effect on the kindling phenomenon and its reported superoxide radical scavenging effect; although the clinical data on its potential value remain equivocal, it is the agent of choice in much of Europe.[46] Further controlled studies of this and other agents are clearly needed. In any case, in light of the sensitivity of the acutely traumatized brain to the secondary insult of a grand mal seizure, at present we recommend routine acute use of phenytoin or phenobarbital in high-risk CHI and in PHI patients for a period of 2 to 4 weeks only. Because of the sometimes subtle cognitive effects of phenytoin and phenobarbital, however, carbamazepine may be the agent of choice for longer-term therapy in patients who have manifested PTE with one or more seizure.

Postacute and Long-Term Rehabilitation

Neurologic rehabilitation is reviewed elsewhere in this volume, but certain basic principles relevant to TBI should be discussed here. Rehabilitation is an area that has traditionally been ignored by neurosurgeons and neurologists, specialists whose knowledge of the central nervous system and whose diagnostic skills could be particularly valuable in this very important phase of management. Over the past few years, coincident with the increasing involvement of patient advocate groups and insurers, the field of TBI rehabilitation has grown exponentially. Multiple therapies, including coma stimulation, reality orientation, cognitive rehabilitation, speech therapy, occupational therapy, art therapy, and recreation therapy have been applied to the TBI patient. Yet their use has been largely empirical, and there has been a paucity of scientific validation for these sometimes expensive

interventions (including comparison with minimal-care, supportive models). If progress is to be made in this area, rehabilitation modalities must be subject to the same scrutiny for indications, dosage, duration of treatment, and efficacy as are other medical treatments such as drugs. The most important present-day challenge in the field is the development of reproducible, universally accepted measures of function and ultimate outcome with which to compare the value of various interventions.[4,52]

One of the most encouraging aspects of TBI rehabilitation is the amazing ability of the young adult brain to *compensate* for many aspects of injury naturally. This is particularly apparent in head injury, as opposed to progressive conditions such as multiple sclerosis or even stroke in older individuals. Disabilities such as hemiparesis, seizures, and certain language disorders may appear more dramatic initially, but they are more readily compensated for than the cognitive, and especially the attentional and behavioral, deficits, which often are more devastating in the long run. The goal of therapy should be the independence and community reintegration of the patient within his or her new limits, rather than the specialized treatment of specific deficits simply because "they are there." All too often, scarce resources available to the patient are used up in the early acute and postacute phases on evaluation and therapy of deficits that will improve anyway or that are relatively unimportant to the ultimate goal of independence. Some therapies may be actually counterproductive insofar as they foster continued dependence. Interventions that may be more cost effective, such as training in specific community reintegration skills, decision making, and certain forms of behavioral modification, may end up being omitted for lack of funds.

Rehabilitation facilities and the medical insurance industry are increasingly turning to the use of "case managers" or "care managers" in this field. The care manager should be a physician or health care professional who is responsible for the integration of various modalities of care and the allocation of resources for the head-injured patient. One of the principal roles of the neurologist or neurosurgeon should be to help place the entire rehabilitation process on a firm footing by providing care managers with an accurate pathologic diagnosis (e.g., focal contusions, DAI, hypoxia-ischemia), and an ongoing assessment of status and prognosis in terms that are useful to the entire rehabilitation team.[1] No less important are the identification of neurologic complications such as delayed hematoma or hydrocephalus and the monitoring of other medical conditions and medications that may be affecting recovery. Magnetic resonance imaging (MRI) may be especially useful at this stage in identifying clinically significant focal contusions, but electro-physiologic studies such as EEG and evoked responses have not proved to be as helpful. Evaluation at this stage should include particular attention to input from family and attendants who spend much time with the patient. Psychometric testing is an important part of the evaluation but is of very limited value in the confused patient and should focus on measurement of expected deficits for guiding therapy and evaluating progress (attentional deficits, mood and behavioral changes), rather than on standard batteries that seek to confirm anatomic deficits already identified on MRI or CT or that investigate in detail cognitive domains of limited practical interest to the case.

The use of pharmacologic agents (and particularly psychotropic medications) in TBI rehabilitation continues to hold much promise, but treatment remains largely empirical at present.[27] Properly controlled therapeutic trials are lacking, again largely because of the difficulty of defining patient groups and measuring outcomes. The sensitivity of the traumatized brain or the confused patient to medication must always be considered, and treatment must be tailored to each individual. Overmedication with anticonvulsants, sedatives, or stimulants is more often a problem than not; paradoxical responses to sedation in confused patients are especially common. Nevertheless, judicious use of adequate sedation can help reestablish sleep-wake cycles, and ritalin, dextroamphetamine, or bromocriptine may be useful as adjuncts in the management of the lethargic or apathetic patient.[28] Carbamazepine is also beginning to emerge as a possible useful adjunct in the management of certain behavioral problems.

Recent clinical and animal studies have suggested that the combination of dextroamphetamine with physical therapy in the early phases of rehabilitation can permanently improve ultimate motor scores.[10,20] The most interesting feature of these studies is that it is the combination of the two modalities that is crucial for the effect; it is not just an additive phenomenon. These findings have given new life to the study of the role of neurotransmitters in structural neural recovery. Other challenging aspects of neural recovery research include the interaction of various trophic factors, such as nerve growth factor, glial growth factors, and interleukin-1, in the process of axonal sprouting and reinnervation.[9]

"Minor" Head Injury

One group of patients that has been frequently mismanaged in the past is that group with so-called mild or minor head injury. As noted previously, however, not only has axonal damage been demonstrated in animal models of mild concussion, but MRI as well as positron emission tomography (PET) have repeatedly shown structural and metabolic changes in humans with minor head injury as well. The most important element in the management of these cases is the recognition that there is usually an organic, pathologic basis for their complaints, at least in the early postinjury period, and that it usually resolves over a few months. If mishandled, however, these patients often develop an overlying neurosis that makes evaluation and management infinitely more difficult. There is nothing more frustrating to the intelligent minor-head-injury victim than to be told there is "nothing wrong" by his physician, his family, and his employer. Proper counseling should thus include not only the patient but also the family, school, or employer. MRI, auditory evoked potentials, and specific neuropsychologic tests such as choice reaction time early in the course can help delineate the deficits.[15,25] One important research challenge in this area is better defining the anatomic, physiologic, and behavioral criteria for recognizing and measuring the severity of mild head injury.[12]

The basic elements of the postconcussion

syndrome are cognitive, somatic, and affective. Clinically significant neuropsychologic impairments have been documented repeatedly, even after minor "dings" without loss of consciousness.[5] The most frequent somatic complaints in one large recent study were headache (71%); decreased energy or "fatigue" (60%); and dizziness (53%). These had all markedly improved at 3 months.[39] The proper management of the fatigue element (which may relate to orbitofrontal injury) is a major factor in recovery, and it requires the cooperation of the school or employer.[64] We suggest a graded return to full workload over a period of 4 to 8 weeks.

REFERENCES

1. Alexander, M: Diagnosis and long-term management of severe head injury. American Academy of Neurology, Annual Course 420: Head Injury. Chicago, IL, 1989.
2. Allen, I, Kirk, J, Maynard, R, Cooper, G, Scott, R, and Crockard, A: An ultrastructural study of experimental high velocity penetrating head injury. Acta Neuropathol (Berl) 59:277–282, 1983.
3. Annegers, J, Grabow, J, Groover, R, Laws, EJ, Elveback, L, and Kurland, L: Seizures after head trauma: A population study. Neurology 30:683–689, 1980.
4. Bach-y-Rita, P: A conceptual approach to neural recovery. In Bach-y-Rita, P (ed): Traumatic Brain Injury. Demos, New York, 1989.
5. Barth, JT, Alves, WM, Ryan, TV, Macciocchi, SN, Rimel, RW, Jane, JA, and Nelson, WE: Mild head injury in sports: Neuropsychological sequelae and recovery of function. In Levin, HS, Eisenberg, HM, and Benton, AL (eds): Mild Head Injury. Oxford, New York, 1989, p 257.
6. Carey, ME, Sarna, GG, and Farrell, JB: The effect of an experimental missile wound to the brain on brain electrolytes, regional cerebral blood flow and blood brain barrier permeability. Louisiana State University Annual Final Report submitted to US Army Medical Research and Development Command, Fort Detrick, MD, 1985, pp 66–78.
7. Cerchiari, EL, Hoel, TM, Safar, P, and Sclabassi, RJ: Protective effects of combined superoxide dismutase and deferoxamine on recovery of cerebral blood flow and function after cardiac arrest in dogs. Stroke 18:869–878, 1987.
8. Clifton, GL, Robertson, CS, and Grossman, RG: Management of the cardiovascular and metabolic responses to severe head injury. In Becker, DP, and Povlishock, JT (eds): Central Nervous System Trauma Status Report. NINCDS, NIH, Bethesda, MD, 1985, p 139.
9. Davis, JN: Neuronal rearrangements after brain injury: A proposed classification. In Becker, DP and Povlishock, JT (eds): Central Nervous System Trauma Status Report. NINCDS, NIH, Bethesda, MD, 1985, p 491.
10. Davis, JN, Crisostomo, EA, Duncan, PW, Propst, M, and Feeney, DM: Amphetamine and physical therapy facilitate recovery from stroke: Correlative animal and human studies. In The 15th Princeton Conference on Cerebrovascular Disease. Raven Press, New York, in press.
11. Deardeu, M, Gibson, J, and McDowall, DG: Effect of high dose dexamethasone on outcome from severe head injury. J Neurosurg 64:81–88, 1986.
12. Department of Health and Human Services: Interagency Head Injury Task Force Report. NINCDS, NIH, Public Health Service, Bethesda, MD, 1989.
13. Deutschman, CS, Konstantinides, FN, Raup, S, and Cerra, FB: Physiological and metabolic response to isolated closed-head injury: Part 2. Effects of steroids on metabolism. Potentiation of protein wasting and abnormalities of substrate utilization. J Neurosurg 66:388–395, 1987.
14. Eisenberg, H, Frankowski, R, Contant, C, Marshall, L, Walker, M, and The Comprehensive CNS Trauma Centers: High-dose barbiturate control of elevated intracranial pressure in patients with severe head injury. J Neurosurg 69:15–23, 1988.
15. Eisenberg, HM and Levin, HS: Computed tomography and magnetic resonance imaging in mild to moderate head injury. In Levin, HS, Eisenberg, HM, and Benton, AL (eds): Mild Head Injury. Oxford, New York, 1989, p 133.
16. Ellis, E, Wright, K, and Wei, E: Cyclooxygenase products of arachidonic acid metabolism in cat cerebral cortex after experimental concussive brain injury. J Neurochem 37:892–896, 1981.
17. Faden, A: Neuropeptides and CNS injury. Arch Neurol 43(5):501–504, 1986.
18. Faden, A, Demediuk, P, Panter, S, and Vink, R: The role of excitatory amino acids and NMDA receptors in traumatic brain injury. Science 244:798–800, 1989.
19. Faden, A, Vink, R, and McIntosh, TK: Thyrotropin-releasing hormone and central nervous system trauma. Ann NY Acad Sci 553:380–384, 1989.
20. Feeney, DM and Sutton, RL: Pharmacotherapy for recovery of function after brain injury. CRC Critical Review in Neurobiology 13:135–197, 1987.
21. Gadisseaux, P: Nutrition and CNS trauma. In Becker, DP and Povlishock, JT (eds): Central Nervous System Trauma Status Report. NINCDS, NIH, Bethesda, MD, 1985, p 207.
22. Gajdusek, D: Hypothesis: Interference with axonal transport of neurofilament as a common pathogenetic mechanism in certain diseases of the central nervous system. N Engl J Med 312:714–718, 1985.
23. Gennarelli, TA and Thibault, LE: Biological models of head injury. In Becker, DP and Povlishock,

JT (eds): Central Nervous System Trauma Status Report. NINCDS, NIH, Bethesda, MD, 1985, p 391.

24. Gennarelli, T, Thibault, L, Adams, J, Graham, D, Thompson, C, and Marcincin, R: Diffuse axonal injury and traumatic coma in the primate. Ann Neurol 12:564–574, 1982.

25. Gentilini, M, Nichelli, P, and Schoenhuber, R: Assessment of attention in mild head injury. In Levin, HS, Eisenberg, HM, and Benton, AL (eds): Mild Head Injury. Oxford, New York, 1989, p 163.

26. Gildenberg, PL and Frost, EAM: Respiratory care in head injury. In Becker, DP and Povlishock, JT (eds): Central Nervous System Trauma Status Report. NINCDS, NIH, Bethesda, MD, 1985, p 161.

27. Gualtieri, CT: Pharmacotherapy and the neurobehavioral sequelae of traumatic brain injury. Brain Inj 2:101–129, 1988.

28. Gualtieri, CT and Evans, RW: Stimulant treatment for the neurobehavioural sequelae of traumatic brain injury. Brain Inj 2(4):273–290, 1988.

29. Hall, ED, Yonkers, PA, McCall, JM, and Braughler, JM: Effects of the 21-aminosteroid U74006F on experimental head injury in mice. J Neurosurg 68:456–461, 1988.

30. Hayes, RL, Lyeth, BG, and Jenkins, LW: Neurochemical mechanisms of mild and moderate head injury: Implications for treatment. In Levin, HS, Eisenberg, HM, and Benton, AL (eds): Mild Head Injury. Oxford University Press, New York, 1989, p 54.

31. Hume Adams, J, Graham, DI, and Gennarelli, TA: Contemporary neuropathological considerations regarding brain damage in head injury. In Becker, DP and Povlishock, JT (eds): Central Nervous System Trauma Status Report. NINCDS, NIH, Bethesda, MD, 1985.

32. Ishige, N, Pitts, LH, Hashimoto, T, Nishimura, MC, and Bartkowski, HM: Effect of hypoxia on traumatic brain injury in rats: Part 1. Changes in neurological function, electroencephalograms, and histopathology. Neurosurgery 20:848–853, 1987.

33. Jennett, B and Teasdale, G: Management of Head Injuries. FA Davis, Philadelphia, 1981.

34. Jordan, B: Neurologic aspects of boxing. Arch Neurol 44:453–459, 1987.

35. Kaufman, HH and Mattson, JC: Coagulopathy in head injury. In Becker, DP and Povlishock, JT (eds): Central Nervous System Trauma Status Report. NINCDS, NIH, Bethesda, MD, 1985, p 187.

36. Klauber, MR, Marshall, LF, Luerssen, TG, Frankowski, R, Tabaddor, K, and Eisenberg, HM: Determinants of head injury mortality: Importance of the low risk patient. Neurosurgery 24:31–36, 1989.

37. Kochanek, PM, Nemoto, EM, Melick, JA, Evans, RW, and Burke, DF: Cerebrovascular and cerebrometabolic effects of intracarotid infusion of platelet-activating factor in rats. J Cereb Blood Flow Metab 8(4):546–551, 1988.

38. Kontos, HA and Wei, EP: Superoxide production in experimental brain injury. J Neurosurg 64(5):803–807, 1986.

39. Levin, H, Mattis, S, Ruff, R, Eisenberg, H, Marshall, L, Tabaddor, K, High, WJ, and Frankowski, R: Neurobehavioral outcome following minor head injury: A three-center study. J Neurosurg 66:234–243, 1987.

40. Marshall, LF, Smith, RW, and Shapiro, HM: The outcome with aggressive treatment in severe head injuries. J Neurosurg 50:20–30, 1979.

41. Marshall, L, Toole, B, and Bowers, S: The National Traumatic Coma Data Bank, Part II: Patients who talk and deteriorate: Implications for treatment. J Neurosurg 59:285–288, 1983.

42. Maset, AL, Marmarou, A, Ward, JD, Choi, S, Lutz, HA, Brooks, D, Moulton, RJ, DeSalles, A, Muizelaar, JP, Turner, H, et al.: Pressure-volume index in head injury. J Neurosurg 67:832–840, 1987.

43. Maxwell, W, Irvine, A, Adams, J, Graham, D, and Gennarelli, T: Response of cerebral microvasculature to brain injury. J Pathol 155:327–335, 1988.

44. McClain, CJ, Cohen, D, Ott, L, Dinarello, CA, and Young, B: Ventricular fluid interleukin-1 activity in patients with head injury. J Lab Clin Med 110:48–54, 1987.

45. McIntosh, T, Faden, A, Yamakami, I, and Vink, R: Magnesium deficiency exacerbates and pretreatment improves outcome following traumatic brain injury in rats. J CNS Trauma 5(1):17–31, 1988.

46. Murri, L: Prophylaxis with phenobarbital. Presented at the National Congress of the Italian League against Epilepsy, Satellite Meeting: Pharmacological Prophylaxis of Posttraumatic Epilepsy, Pisa, Italy, 1989.

47. Oppenheimer, DR: Microscopic lesions in the brain following head injury. J Neurol, Neurosurg Psychiatry 31:299–306, 1968.

48. Penry, JK, White, BG, and Brackett, CE: A controlled prospective study of the pharmacologic prophylaxis of posttraumatic epilepsy. Neurology 29:600, 1979.

49. Plum, F: What causes infarction in ischemic brain?: The Robert Wartenberg lecture. Neurology 33:222–233, 1983.

50. Povlishock, JT: The morphopathologic responses to head injuries of varying severity. In Becker, DP and Povlishock, JT (eds): Central Nervous System Trauma Status Report. NINCDS, NIH, Bethesda, MD, 1985, p 443.

51. Povlishock, JT and Coburn, TH: Morphopathological change associated with mild head injury. In Levin, HS, Eisenberg, HM, and Benton, AL (eds): Mild Head Injury. Oxford University Press, New York, 1989, p 37.

52. Prigitano, G: Rehabilitation interventions after traumatic brain injury. In Bach-y-Rita, P (ed): Traumatic Brain Injury. Demos, New York, 1989.

53. Salazar, A, Jabbari, B, Vance, S, Grafman, J, Amin, D, and Dillon, J: Epilepsy after penetrating head injury, I: Clinical correlates. Neurology 35:1406–1414, 1985.

54. Shapira, Y, Davidson, E, and Weidenfeld, Y: Dexa-

methasone and indomethacin do not affect brain edema following head injury in rats. J Cereb Blood Flow Metab 8:395–402, 1988.

55. Shohami, E, Shapira, Y, Sidi, A, and Cotev, S: Head injury induces increased prostaglandin synthesis in rat brain. J Cereb Blood Flow Metab 7:58–63, 1987.

56. Strich, S: The pathology of brain damage due to blunt head injuries. In Walker, AE, Caveness, WF, and Critchley, M, (eds): The Late Effects of Head Injury. Charles C Thomas, Springfield, IL, 1969.

57. Suguru, I, Marmarou, A, Clarke, GD, Andersen, BJ, Fatouros, PP, and Young, HF: Production and clearance of lactate from brain tissue, cerebrospinal fluid, and serum following experimental brain injury. J Neurosurg 69:736–744, 1988.

58. Swann, KW: Management of severe head injury. In Ropper, AH and Kennedy, SF (eds): Neurological and Neurosurgical Intensive Care. Aspen Publishers, Rockville, MD, 1988, pp 165–185.

59. Taylor, MD, Palmer, GC, and Callahan, AS: Protective action by methylprednisolone, allopurinol and indomethacin against stroke-induced damage to adenylate cyclase in gerbil cerebral cortex. Stroke 15(2):329–335, 1984.

60. Tempkin, N, Dikmen, S, Keihm, J, Chabal, S, and Winn, H: Does phenytoin prevent posttraumatic seizures? One-year follow-up results of a randomized double-blind study. American Association of Neurological Surgeons, Annual Meeting 106, 1989.

61. Wei, EP, Kontos, HA, Dietrich, WD, Povlishock, JT, and Ellis, EF: Inhibition by free radical scavengers and by cyclooxygenase inhibitors of pial arteriolar abnormalities from concussive brain injury in cats. Circ Res 48(1):95–103, 1981.

62. Weiss, G, Salazar, A, Vance, S, Grafman, J, and Jabbari, B: Predicting posttraumatic epilepsy in penetrating head injury. Arch Neurol 43: 771–773, 1986.

63. Woolf, PD, Hamill, RW, Lee, LA, Cox, C, and McDonald, JV: The predictive value of catecholamines in assessing outcome in traumatic brain injury. J Neurosurg 66:875–882, 1987.

64. Wrightson, P: Management of disability and rehabilitation services after mild head injury. In Levin, HS, Eisenberg, HM, and Benton, AL (eds): Mild Head Injury. Oxford University Press, New York, 1989, p 245.

65. Young, B, Rapp, R, Norton, A, Haack, D, Tibbs, PA, and Bean, JR: Failure of prophylactically administered phenytoin to prevent late posttraumatic seizures. J Neurosurg 58:236–241, 1983.

CHAPTER 5

• •

UNEXPECTED DEMISE: SUDDEN DEATH IN NEUROLOGY

Martin A. Samuels, M.D.

Stressed middle-aged men, cocaine addicts, and epileptics have something in common: they are all at risk of sudden death.

Samuels, with remarkable command of the historical literature, weaves a compelling synthesis of neurogenic influences on the cardiovascular system, including lethal malfunctions.

While there is some evidence for all the points that Samuels makes, there is no proof that all the phenomena he describes are in fact linked. Reperfusion injury of the heart, for example, may occur through free radical production and mechanisms that have little to do with the author's postulates.

The risk of sudden death varies from low in epileptics to high in patients with subarachnoid hemorrhage. A minority of patients with stroke recover from stroke only to succumb to a cardiac complication or sudden death. Clearly, this is an important but understudied area.

VCH

Sudden unexpected death (SUD) is a problem of major importance, but very little is known about its cause. Of the many sudden death syndromes, in only one (sudden unexpected death in middle-aged men) has a likely pathogenesis been clarified: functional cardiac arrest due to ventricular arrhythmia. Electrocardiographic abnormalities have been known for a long time to occur in the context of neurologic disease. These changes fall into two categories: arrhythmias and repolarization changes. It is now believed that these changes represent one end of a spectrum of pathologic physiology that can alter cardiac repolarization, predispose to sudden death, and/or produce a characteristic form of cardiac damage known as myofibrillar degeneration or contraction band necrosis. This lesion can be caused by four classes of etiologies: cate-cholamine infusion, stress plus or minus steroids, nervous system stimulation, and reperfusion. These four apparently disparate etiologies are tied together by a common thread, the essential feature of which is sympathetic overactivity with secondary catecholamine toxicity. A unifying hypothesis is proposed to explain all forms of sudden death based on the anatomic connection between the nervous system and the heart and lungs.

DEFINITION OF THE PROBLEM

Although SUD is now recognized as a medical problem of major epidemiologic importance,[13] it has generally been assumed that neurologic disease rarely results in SUD. In fact, it has been traditionally taught that neurologic illnesses almost never cause sudden demise, with the only exceptions being the occasional patient who dies during an epileptic convulsion or rapidly following a subarachnoid hemorrhage. Further, it has been assumed that the various SUD syndromes — for example, sudden death in middle-aged men[13]; sudden infant death syndrome (SIDS); sudden unexpected nocturnal death syndrome (SUNDS)[45,46]; scared to death (also known as "voodoo" death)[8]; sudden death during a seizure[27]; sudden death during natural catastrophe[58]; sudden death associated with drug abuse; sudden death in wild and domestic animals[19,30,48]; sudden death during asthma attacks[2,15]; sudden death associated with the alcohol withdrawal syndrome[60]; sudden death during grief after a major loss; and sudden death during panic attacks[10] — are entirely separate and have no unifying mechanism. For example, it is generally accepted that sudden death in middle-aged men is usually caused by a cardiac arrhythmia (i.e., ventricular fibrillation,[32] which results in functional cardiac arrest), whereas most work on SIDS focuses on respiratory failure.

An alternative line of reasoning argues that the connection between the nervous system and the cardiopulmonary system provides the unifying link that allows a coherent explanation for most, if not all, of the forms of SUD.[43,56] Powerful evidence from multiple disparate disciplines allows for a neurologic explanation for SUD and is the subject of this chapter.[51]

NEUROANATOMY OF THE HEART AND LUNGS

Many visceral structures are highly autoregulated. The gut and heart are examples of organs that have evolved their own partially autonomous nervous system. In the case of the heart, the "nervous system" is actually adapted cardiac muscle that allows the organ a fair degree of independent function. The heart has its own intrinsic rhythms, and its contractile force can be varied depending on the amount of stretch. Starling's law of the heart articulates the rule by which this highly adapted muscle matches cardiac output to venous return. It is well known that

isolated cardiac muscle can be demonstrated to show an extensive array of behavior independent of any innervation by the nervous system. However, in real-life situations the heart is in fact richly innervated by both the sympathetic and parasympathetic limbs of the autonomic nervous system. This nervous system connection has been preserved over eons of evolution, a fact that argues strongly that this innervation, at least at some time, conferred an evolutionary advantage. It is logical to assume that this advantage can be summarized in the concept of *anticipation*. Above and beyond the autoregulatory capacity of the organ, the nervous system connection allowed our primitive ancestors to prepare for *perceived* threats. Whether in the present environment this innervation remains an advantage or instead has become an evolutionary disadvantage (i.e., a disease) can only be settled over many more generations.

There are a few unusual circumstances in which the heart can be presumed to be functioning in a denervated autonomous fashion. Examples would be patients with cardiac transplants or with severe autonomic neuropathies as might occasionally be seen in diabetes mellitus, Guillian-Barré syndrome, or amyloidosis. There are also a number of patients who have had their hearts deliberately partially denervated, either surgically, as in the treatment of the long QT syndrome with stellate ganglion blockade, or pharmacologically, with the array of antiarrhythmic drugs that work either exclusively or partially via neural mechanisms. Aside from these few exceptions, however, most people's hearts are, for good or ill, connected to the nervous system, and this innervation can have profound effects on the electrocardiogram, the contractile function of the cardiac muscle, and the tone in the coronary vessels. The neuroanatomies of cardiac and pulmonary structures are closely related and thus can be discussed concomitantly.

Central Nervous System

It is likely that the nervous supply to the heart and lungs arises in the limbic cortex and descends to the hypothalamus, possibly via the basal ganglia, most likely the amygdala (Fig. 5–1). From the hypothalamus, the two limbs of the autonomic nervous system descend with intermediate synapses in cardiopulmonary control centers in the brainstem's reticular formation, where a number of cardiovascular and respiratory reflexes are likely mediated. From there the parasympathetic limb descends to the dorsal motor nucleus of the vagus and the sympathetic limb to the intermediolateral cell column of the thoracic spinal cord.[59]

There is evidence of centers in the medullary reticular formation in the region of the nuclei reticularis gigantocellularis and reticularis parvicellularis that mediate the hypertension and neurogenic pulmonary edema (NPE) seen with the Cushing or cerebral ischemic response.[12] Under normal circumstances these centers are inhibited by neurons in the nucleus solitarius, a medullary nucleus to which afferents from arterial baroreceptors and chemoreceptors project via the vagus and glossopharyngeal nerves. Thus bilateral lesions in the nucleus solitarius will produce systemic hypertension and NPE identical to that caused by the Cushing or ischemic response[16] (see below). Both of these forms of NPE and hypertension are prevented by cervical spinal

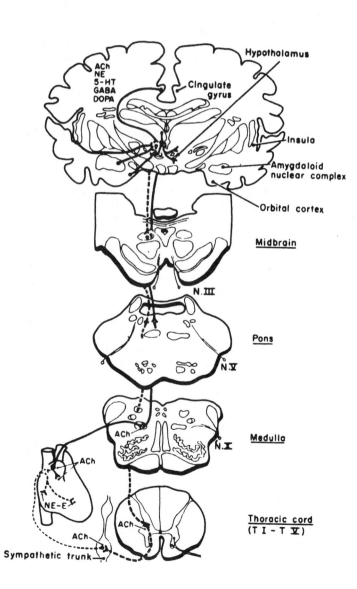

FIGURE 5–1. Neuroanatomy of the heart. Diagram of descending CNS autonomic pathways and the peripheral two-neuron chains that comprise the visceral motor innervation to the heart. Sympathetic neurons are indicated by the dotted pathway; parasympathetic and vagus neurons appear as solid lines. Release sites of norepinephrine (NE), epinephrine (E), and acetylcholine (ACh) are indicated. (From Truex,[59] p. 160, with permission.)

cord transection or sympathetic blockade with either ganglion blockade, alpha-adrenergic receptor blockade, or surgical sympathectomy.

Could systemic hypertension caused by sympathetic activity produce cardiogenic rather than neurogenic pulmonary edema? In theory, massive hypertension would cause a sudden rise in cardiac afterload. This would in turn lead to elevations of left atrial pressure, pulmonary venous pressure, and ultimately pulmonary capillary hydrostatic pressure (Pc). However, in this circumstance, left atrial pressure would have to exceed 50 mm Hg to elevate Pc to levels high enough to cause pulmonary edema. Bilateral lesions in the nucleus solitarius result in only a twofold increase in systemic blood pressure, levels that are not high enough to elevate left atrial pressures above 50 mm Hg. Furthermore, in at least some of the animal experiments, the protein content of the pulmonary edema fluid is high, thereby implicating a change in capillary permeability and not just a hemodynamic effect caused by systemic hypertension.[55]

A region in the caudal hypothalamus produces a similar form of systemic hypertension and pulmonary edema, which is prevented by sympathetic blockade. This center is under tonic inhibition from a nucleus in the lateral preoptic region, since lesions there will produce hypertension and NPE, a phenomenon prevented by prior lesions in the caudal hypothalamus.[35]

It seems clear that some balance exists between the sympathetic and parasympathetic limbs of the autonomic nervous system, since bilateral vagotomy, bilateral lesions in the dorsal motor nuclei of the vagus, and parasympatholytic drugs such as atropine enhance the pulmonary edema associated with volume overloading.[4,33]

Lastly, lesions in the A1 noradrenergic region of the caudal ventrolateral medulla also produce systemic hypertension and pulmonary edema, probably via loss of the tonic inhibition that these cells normally exert over vasopressin-secreting cells in the supraoptic and paraventricular nuclei of the hypothalamus.[3] The increased sympathetic activity characteristic of the development of systemic hypertension and NPE caused by lesions in other regions of the brainstem and hypothalamus is not associated with lesions in this area, however.[57]

Peripheral Nervous System

From the dorsal motor nucleus of the vagus, the parasympathetic fibers exit the central nervous system (CNS) with the vagus nerve and descend to the heart and lungs. These preganglionic fibers form the superior, middle, and inferior cardiac rami of the vagus nerve and as such contribute to the cardiac plexus. They synapse in the cardiac ganglia (where nicotinic receptors predominate) and thence via short postganglionic fibers to their muscarinic terminals in the sinoatrial (SA) and atrioventricular (AV) nodes, on the cardiac vessels, and on cardiac cells in all four chambers.

From the intermediolateral cell column of the thoracic spinal cord exit the axons of the sympathetic fibers. After leaving the cord in the anterior root, they immediately exit via the white rami communicantes and join the sympathetic chain that extends extraspinally along the length of the spinal cord bilaterally. Three major ganglia exist in the cervical region: the upper, middle, and lower cervical ganglia. There are ganglia for each thoracic segment designated T-1, T-2, and so on, in both the right and left sympathetic chains. In dogs and primates, the lower cervical and first thoracic ganglia are usually fused to form the large stellate ganglion. With respect to the heart, the left stellate ganglion contains neurons that reenter the peripheral nerves via the gray rami communicantes and terminate in the SA and AV nodes and on most of the left ventricle, while the right stellate contains cells that terminate in the septum, right ventricle, and atria. In general, the two stellate ganglia function inversely. For example, stimulation of the left stellate ganglion lengthens the QT interval of the ECG, while stimulation of the right stellate shortens the QT interval. Conversely, ablation of the left stellate shortens the QT interval, while ablation of the right stellate lengthens it. As in the parasympathetic limb, the ganglia have predominantly nicotinic neurotransmission. The postganglionic sympathetic fibers terminate on adrenergic receptors of both alpha and beta types. Evidence based on pharmacologic data indicates that each of these receptor types has at least two subtypes. It is likely that sympathetic activity has a major effect on coronary tone, with the alpha receptors being responsible for vasoconstriction and the beta receptors for vasodilation. On the other hand, heart rate is primarily controlled by parasympathetic tone. The appearance of the ECG is undoubtedly related to a complex interaction between parasympathetic and sympathetic tone, as well as right versus left stellate asymmetries (see Fig. 5 – 1).

The pulmonary vessels have both a sympathetic and parasympathetic nerve supply. The parasympathetic fibers rise from the trunk of the vagus nerve. Their stimulation results in some pulmonary vasodilation and a drop in Pc. It is not clear how important this innervation is in the normal physiologic functioning of the pulmonary vessels.[42]

The sympathetic supply probably arises from multiple thoracic levels and, via the segmental sympathetic ganglia, richly innervates the pulmonary vascular bed. There is pharmacologic evidence that alpha receptor – mediated innervation causes vasoconstriction, while beta receptor – mediated innervation causes vasodilation. Furthermore, there is evidence that the alpha receptor – mediated sympathetic activity has a greater effect on the venous side of the pulmonary circulation. Thus sympathetic nerve stimulation can cause a rise in Pc and pulmonary artery pressure without an associated rise in systemic blood pressure and left atrial pressures.[37]

Because alpha receptor – mediated sympathetic fibers are widely distributed throughout the vessels of the body, a nonspecific "sympathetic storm" could result in systemic hypertension as well as pulmonary venoconstriction with a rise in Pc and consequent pulmonary edema.

Thus NPE theoretically could result either from a potent generalized pulse of activity in the alpha receptor – mediated sympathetic fibers or from a segmental, more localized burst of similar activity affecting only the lungs. In the former case, systemic hypertension and left atrial hypertension would be present; in the latter, they would be absent. In other words, systemic hypertension is consistent with, but not necessary for, the development of NPE.

NEUROGENIC LUNG DISEASE

The Pulmonary Capillary-Tissue-Lymphatic System

NPE is a rapidly developing, protein-rich alveolar pulmonary edema that develops after a neurologic insult such as head injury, epileptic seizure, intracranial hypertension, subarachnoid hemorrhage, or autonomic dysreflexia. To understand the mechanisms by which NPE occurs, one must review the basic principles underlying the function of the pulmonary capillary – tissue – lymphatic system, schematically represented in Figure 5 – 2.[36] Transcapillary fluid migration is governed by the four Starling forces: capillary hydrostatic pressure (Pc) and interstitial tissue colloid osmotic pressure (πi) tend to favor movement of water *out* of the capillary; plasma colloid osmotic pressure (πp) and interstitial tissue hydrostatic pressure (P_i), tend to favor movement of water *into* the capillary.

Under normal circumstances, πp is maintained by virtue of the fact that there are interendothelial tight junctions that inhibit the movement of solute from the pulmonary capillary into the interstitial space. The major determinant of pulmonary Pc is the precapillary to postcapillary resistance ratio, which is largely regulated by the smooth muscle tone in the precapillary arterioles and the postcapillary venules.

Fluid may move into the interstitial tissue space, thereby producing interstitial pulmonary edema, when Pc rises or πp falls. For small amounts of fluid, the lymph outflow system acts as an overflow drain, preventing fluid from appearing in the air spaces. Thus the nature of the lymph outflow reflects the content of the interstitial fluid space. When the amount of edema exceeds the capacity of the lymph outflow to compensate, this fluid appears in the air spaces, producing alveolar pulmonary edema.

In cardiogenic pulmonary edema, the left heart has failed, leading to increased left atrial pressure and, in turn, increased pulmonary venous pressure. This results in a

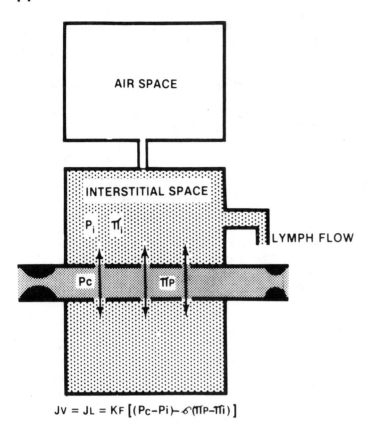

AIR SPACE

INTERSTITIAL SPACE

P_i π_i

LYMPH FLOW

Pc π_P

$$J_V = J_L = K_F \left[(P_C - P_i) - \sigma(\pi_P - \pi_i) \right]$$

FIGURE 5-2. Schematic representation of the pulmonary capillary-tissue-lymphatic system. Starling's forces represented in the Starling equation are capillary hydrostatic pressure (Pc), plasma colloid osmotic pressure (π_P), tissue hydrostatic pressure (Pi), and colloid osmotic pressure of tissue fluid (π_i). J_v = net transvascular fluid filtration rate, J_L = lymph flow, K_F = capillary filtration coefficient or hydraulic conductivity, and σ = protein reflection coefficient. The alveolar epithelial junctions are tight compared to the interendothelial junctions in lung and thereby restrict solute transport into the airspaces. The dots represent plasma proteins in plasma, tissue fluid, and lymph. The lymph flow represents the overflow in the system, i.e., the difference between the amount of fluid filtered and the amount reabsorbed. A major determinant of Pc is the precapillary to postcapillary resistance ratio as regulated by the smooth muscle tone of the arteries and veins. (From Malik,[36] p. 2, with permission.)

rise in Pc and a shift of water across the pulmonary capillary into the interstitial space and ultimately into the air spaces. The movement of pure water into the interstitial space will dilute the protein there, leading to a fall in the protein content of the lymph fluid.

By contrast, in many forms of noncardiac pulmonary edema (including NPE), the protein content in the lymph outflow and in the air spaces approaches that found in plasma, meaning that part or all of the mechanism of NPE must involve changes in pulmonary capillary permeability allowing for solute to leak out into the interstitial tissue. The presence of this change in pulmonary capillary permeability does not exclude the possibility that a rise in Pc may also be present in circumstances that lead to NPE. In fact, pulmonary artery pressures have sometimes been found to be elevated during NPE, a fact that reflects a high Pc.

The Mechanism of NPE

With this anatomic, physiologic, and pharmacologic background, it is possible to consider several mechanisms of NPE. These are not necessarily mutually exclusive and, in fact, probably frequently act together in a particular patient to produce NPE. Furthermore, it is likely that milder subclinical forms of this syndrome commonly occur, whereas full-blown NPE is quite rare. The following represents a summary of possible mechanisms of NPE, proposed by Malik.[36]

Several hemodynamic phenomena can lead to NPE. Left atrial hypertension may cause a sudden rise in Pc leading to pulmonary edema. If the rise is sudden and massive, it is possible that the pressure itself may be adequate to injure the pulmonary capillary endothelium, leading to high-protein pulmonary edema. However, left atrial pressures greater than 50 mm Hg are needed experimentally to produce pulmonary edema, and pressures in this range have rarely been measured in patients with NPE.[53] Furthermore, the protein leak appears to be reversible within hours, something that should not occur if the leak is caused by a mechanical disruption of the capillary endothelium. In other words, although left atrial hypertension is a common accompaniment of NPE, it appears that it alone is rarely, if ever, sufficient to cause it.

Systemic hypertension can clearly cause pulmonary edema if it is massive and sudden enough. When this occurs, it is always associated with greatly increased left atrial pressures. Because NPE can be seen when systemic blood pressure is normal, it is clear that systemic hypertension cannot be the sole cause of NPE.

Pulmonary venoconstriction may certainly result in a sudden rise in Pc without systemic hypertension or increased left atrial pressures. Pulmonary arterial vasoconstriction, if it occurs, could only result in a rise in Pc if it were nonuniform such that blood were shunted from areas of vasoconstriction to other areas, thereby resulting in a rise in Pc in the latter areas.

There is evidence that sympathetic overactivity results in a reduction in pulmonary vascular compliance. If this occurs, then even a small shift of volume from systemic to pulmonary circulation could result in an inordinate rise in Pc.[50]

Of great importance in the mechanisms leading to NPE is the fact that sympathetic nerve stimulation actually leads to an increase in pulmonary capillary permeability to protein, possibly because sympathetic nerve fibers innervate contractile elements in the endothelial cells. Thus sympathetic activity may actually lead to physical opening of the right junctions in the capillary, allowing protein flux.[50,53]

Lastly, there is some evidence that sympathetic stimulation may cause lymphatic constriction. This could lead to alveolar pulmonary edema with only a small shift of fluid from the capillaries to the interstitial tissue space.[38]

In summary, NPE is probably caused by a combination of factors, the common denominator of most of which is increased sympathetic activity.

NEUROGENIC HEART DISEASE

A wide variety of changes in the electrocardiogram (ECG) is seen in the context of neurologic disease. Two major categories of change are regularly noted: (1) arrhythmias and (2) repolarization changes. It is likely that the increased tendency for life-threatening arrhythmias found in patients with acute neurologic disease is due to the repolarization change, which increases the vulnerable period during which an extrasystole would be likely to result in ventricular tachycardia and/or ventricular fibrillation. Thus the essential and potentially most lethal features of the ECG that are known to change in the context of neurologic disease are the ST segment and T wave, reflecting abnormalities in repolarization.

Brief History of the Understanding of Neurogenic Electrocardiographic Changes

Although the effect of the nervous system on the cardiovascular system has been known for a long while, the clinical association in the Western literature between ECG abnormalities and CNS disease goes back only 40 years, when Byer and colleagues[7] reported on five patients (four with strokes and one with hypertensive encephalopathy) with large upright T waves and long QT intervals. In 1953, Levine[31] reported on a patient with subarachnoid hemorrhage whose ECG showed an apparent myocardial infarction. The heart was said to be normal at autopsy. Levine felt that the abnormalities were due to vagal stimulation and referred to Fulton's work, which suggested that area 13 in the orbital-frontal cortex was the major cortical representation of the vagus nerve. This hypothesis was based on stimulation studies in which bradycardia could be elicited with stimulation of Brodmann area 13.[18] Burch and co-workers[6] drew attention to peaked T waves, long QT intervals, and U waves as manifestations of CNS disease, primarily but not exclusively in subarachnoid hemorrhage patients. It is from this article that the popular term "cerebral T waves" probably arose. Since that time, a large number of cases of so-called neurogenic ECG changes have been reported in the world's literature. Despite the many case reports, little is known about the mechanism of these changes. The major landmarks in our present understanding of this phenomenon are as follows:

Cropp and Manning[11] reported on a series of 15 patients with subarachnoid hemorrhage with ECG changes. Four of these patients died, and each was said to have a normal heart at autopsy. The authors postulated that the ECG changes resulted from autonomic nervous system abnormalities arising from area 13 in the orbital-frontal cortex. Hugenholtz[25] reported on six patients with various neurologic lesions (including metastatic cancer, cerebral emboli, subdural hematoma, multiple strokes, and subarachnoid hemorrhage) who had striking prolongation of the QT interval, deeply inverted and widened T waves, and prominent U waves. Electrolyte determinations were normal, and it was the author's belief that the changes resulted from an abnormality in cerebral control or cardiac repolarization. The question was raised as to whether this hypothalamic effect is mediated by a neural or a humoral mechanism. However, no data were available at the time to make any postulate in this regard.

Some studies have shown postmortem evidence of myocardial damage, whereas others have failed to show such histologic lesions. It is likely that failure to recognize myocardial lesions in many of the older studies was a result of insensitivity of observation techniques. Clearly, gross examination of the heart will fail to reveal the vast majority of lesions now known to be present in such hearts. Even light microscopy may sometimes be too insensitive, in that electron microscopy shows widespread lesions when light microscopic examination is unimpressive or equivocal. The myofibrillar necrosis noted in the more recent studies is identical histologically to the cardiac lesion of catecholamine infusion, stress plus or minus steroids, nervous system stimulation in animals, and reperfusion of transiently ischemic cardiac muscle. Furthermore, it is identical to the so-called catecholamine cardiomyopathy described in human beings with pheochromocytoma.[29]

However, the rapid appearance and disappearance of these ECG changes with perturbations of the nervous system strongly suggest that these effects, even in humans, are due to neural rather than humoral factors. Hammer and colleagues[21] reported on a patient who had sudden appearance and disappearance of ECG abnormalities during resection of a basilar artery aneurysm. The effects appeared and disappeared too rapidly to be attributed to any humoral abnormality. A similar phenomenon was reported by Cropp and Manning[11] in 1960. Intraoperative recordings showed evidence of rapidly reversible arrhythmias during surgical treatment of a cerebral aneurysm. Although they may be imitated and perhaps even exacerbated by excessively high circulating catecholamines, these ECG abnormalities can occur without elevations of systemic catecholamines, presumably by release of norepinephrine directly into cardiac muscle by sympathetic nerve terminals. Of course, in the human being, one cannot separate the effect of systemic elevations of catecholamine due to "stress" and that of local cardiac catecholamines due to specific release from cardiac nerves. The two are presumably additive with regard to the production of cardiac lesions. Systemic catecholamines have been elevated when measured in patients with neurologically induced ECG changes.

Cardiac enzymes also are elevated in many but not all patients with presumed neurogenic ECG changes. The isoenzyme creatine kinase myocardial band (CK MB) is felt by many researchers to be cardiospecific, although low levels (less than 2% of total CK) may be found in normal subjects, depending on the specific assay used. Despite this methodologic problem, it is clear that CK MB is often elevated in patients with neurogenic ECG abnormalities.[44] This provides further support to the notion that there is a myocardial cell injury resulting in release of CK MB enzyme. Patients with CNS insults but a normal ECG usually have undetectable CK MB in the serum.

A typical case illustrating some of the classic findings is summarized as follows:

A 44-year-old previously healthy right-handed women came to the emergency department complaining of abdominal pain. An ECG was interpreted as normal. Seven days later she returned with a mild left hemiparesis, and the ECG showed marked anterolateral T wave inversions "consistent with ischemia or subendocardial myocardial infarction." A CT scan was performed and showed a hemorrhagic mass in the right cerebral hemisphere. Despite therapy for increased intracranial pressure, the patient became progressively more comatose. While she was deeply comatose (and just prior to death), the ECG showed marked improvement. At autopsy there was a large hemorrhagic tumor (anaplastic carcinoma, unknown primary) that produced a significant shift of midline structures.

The case illustrates many of the features of neurogenic ECG changes. Nearly every type of ECG abnormality has been reported, but all of them may be divided into two major categories: cardiac arrhythmias and repolarization abnormalities. Most often, the changes are seen best in the anterolateral or inferolateral leads. If such an ECG is read by pattern recognition by an individual who is not aware of the clinical history, it will often be said to represent subendocardial infarction or anterolateral ischemia. The ECG abnormalities usually improve, often dramatically, with brain death.

The phenomenon is not rare. In a series of 100 consecutive stroke patients, 90% showed abnormalities on the ECG, compared with 50% of a control population of 100 patients admitted for carcinoma of the colon.[14] This, of course, does not mean that 90% of stroke patients have neurogenic ECG changes. Obviously, stroke and coronary artery disease have common risk factors, so that many ECG abnormalities in stroke patients represent concomitant atherosclerotic coronary disease. Nonetheless, a significant number of stroke patients have authentic neurogenic ECG changes.

Although neurogenic ECG changes have been most commonly reported in subarachnoid hemorrhage cases, they do occur frequently in other stroke syndromes and in many other neurologic diseases, including neoplasms, infections, epilepsy, and psychiatric disorders.

To understand the possible mechanism underlying these various ECG abnormalities, it would be worthwhile to review the historical background of our present understanding of the neurologic influence over the cardiovascular system. The concept of the trophic influence of the nervous system (i.e., the neurologic control of the metabolism of visceral organs) begins with the works of Magendie[34] more than 150 years ago. In the latter half of the 19th century, there were several descriptions of damage to visceral organs caused by stimulation of the nervous system either centrally or peripherally. These pathologic processes were thought to be results of an abnormality in the trophic influence of the nervous system and thus were dubbed *neurogenic dystrophies*, a subject that Pavlov and his students found extremely interesting.

The Mechanism of Neurogenic Heart Disease

Catecholamine Infusion

Clues to the mechanism of the so-called trophic influence of the nervous system over the heart may be obtained by analyzing the various methods of producing myofibrillar degeneration (also known as contraction band necrosis and coagulative myocytolysis). These methods can be divided into four categories: catecholamine infusion, stress (plus or minus steroids), nervous system stimulation, and reperfusion.

As long ago as 1907, Josué[28] showed that epinephrine infusions could cause cardiac hypertrophy. This observation has been reproduced on many occasions, documenting the fact that systematically administered catecholamines are associated not only with ECG changes reminiscent of widespread ischemia but also with a characteristic pathologic picture in the cardiac muscle that is distinct from myocardial infarction. An identical picture may be found in human beings with chronically elevated plasma catecholamines, such as occurs with pheochromocytoma. Patients with stroke often have elevated systemic catecholamine levels, a fact which may, in part, account for the high incidence of cardiac arrhythmias and ECG changes seen in these patients.[41] On light microscopy, these changes range from increased eosinophilic staining with preservation of cross-striations to total transformation of the myocardial cell cytoplasm into dense eosinophilic transverse bands with intervening granularity, called by some *myofibrillar degeneration*. In severely injured areas, infiltration of the necrotic debris by mononuclear cells is often noted, sometimes with hemorrhage. Ultrastructurally, the changes in cardiac muscle are even more widespread than they appear to be with light microscopy. Nearly every muscle cell shows some pathologic alteration ranging from a granular appearance of the myofibrils to profound disruption of the cell architecture with relative preservation of ribosomes and mitochondria. Intracardiac nerves can be seen, identified by their external lamina, microtubules, neurofibrils, and the presence of intracytoplasmic vesicles. These nerves can sometimes be seen immediately adjacent to an area of myocardial cell damage. The pathologic changes in the cardiac muscle are usually closer to the nerve, often returning completely to normal by a distance of 2 to 4 μm away from the nerve ending.[26]

Myofibrillar degeneration is an easily recognizable form of cardiac injury distinct in several major respects from coagulation necrosis, the major lesion of myocardial infarction.[1] In coagulation necrosis, the cells die in a relaxed state without prominent contraction bands. This is not visible by any method for many hours or even days. Calcification occurs only late, and the lesion elicits a polymorphonuclear cell response. In stark contrast, in myofibrillar degeneration the cells die in a hypercontracted state, with prominent contraction bands. The lesion is visible early, perhaps within minutes of its onset. It elicits a mononuclear cell response and may calcify almost immediately.[49]

Stress (Plus or Minus Steroids)

A similar, if not identical, cardiac lesion can be produced using various models of "stress." This concept was first articulated by Selye,[52] but it was not directly applied to the heart until Selye published his monograph *The Chemical Prevention of Cardiac Necrosis* in 1958. He found that cardiac lesions probably identical to those described above could be regularly produced in animals that were pretreated with certain steroids, particularly 2-alpha-methyl-9-alpha-fluorohydrocortisone (fluorocortisol), and then subjected to various types of stress. Other hormones, such as dihydrotachysterol (calciferol) and thyroxine, also could sensitize animals for stress-induced myocardial lesions, but less potently than fluorocortisol. This so-called stress could be of multiple types, including restraint, surgery, bacteremia, vagotomy, toxins, and others. He believed that the "first mediator" in translating these widely disparate stimuli into a stereotyped cardiac lesion was the hypothalamus and that it, by its control over the autonomic and principally sympathetic nervous system, caused the release of certain agents that were toxic to the myocardial cell. Since Selye's original work, similar experiments have been repeated in many different types of laboratory animals with comparable results. Although the administration of exogenous steroids facilitates the production of cardiac lesions, stress alone can result in the production of morphologically identical lesions.

Whether a similar pathophysiology could ever be operable in human beings is, of course, of great interest. Many investigators have speculated on the role of stress in the pathogenesis of human cardiovascular disease, particularly on its relationship to the phenomenon of sudden unexpected death.

A few autopsies on patients who experienced sudden death have shown myofibrillar degeneration. In 1980, Cebelin and Hirsch[9] reported on a careful retrospective analysis of the hearts of 15 victims of physical assault who died as a direct result of the assault, but without sustaining internal injuries. Eleven of the 15 individuals showed myofibrillar degeneration. Age- and cardiac disease–matched controls showed little or no evidence of this change. This appears to represent a human stress cardiomyopathy.[9] Whether such assaults can be considered murder has become an interesting legal correlate of the problem.

Since the myofibrillar degeneration is predominantly subendocardial, it may involve the cardiac conducting system, thus predisposing to cardiac arrhythmias. This lesion, combined with the propensity of catecholamines to produce arrhythmias even in a normal heart, may well raise the risk of a serious arrhythmia considerably. This may be the major immediate mechanism of sudden death in many neurologic circumstances, such as subarachnoid hemorrhage, stroke, epilepsy, head trauma, psychologic stress, and increased intracranial pressure. Even the arrhythmogenic nature of digitalis may be largely mediated by the nervous system. Further evidence for this mechanism is the antiarrhythmic effect of sympathetic denervation of the heart for cardiac arrhythmias of many types.

Furthermore, it is known that the stress-induced myocardial lesions can be prevented by sympathetic blockade using many different classes of antiadrenergic agents, most notably ganglionic blockers such as mecamylamine and catecholamine-depleting agents such as reserpine.[47] This suggests that catecholamines, either released directly into the heart by sympathetic nerve terminals or reaching the heart through the bloodstream after release from the adrenal medulla, are toxic to myocardial cells.

Nervous System Stimulation

Nervous system stimulation produces cardiac lesions histologically indistinguishable from those just described for cardiac damage induced by stress (plus or minus steroids) and catecholamines. It has been known for a long time that stimulation of the hypothalamus can lead to autonomic cardiovascular disturbances, and many years ago, lesions in the heart and gastrointestinal tract had been produced using hypothalamic stimulation. It has been clearly demonstrated that stimulation of the lateral hypothalamus produces hypertension or ECG changes reminiscent of those seen in patients with CNS damage of various types. Furthermore, this effect on the blood pressure and ECG can be completely prevented by C-2 spinal section and stellate ganglionectomy, but not by vagotomy, suggesting that the mechanism of the ECG changes is

sympathetic rather than parasympathetic or humoral. Stimulation of the anterior hypothalamus produces bradycardia, an effect that can be blocked by vagotomy. Unilateral hypothalamic stimulation does not result in histologic evidence of myocardial damage by light microscopy, but bilateral prolonged stimulation regularly produces myofibrillar degeneration indistinguishable from that produced by catecholamine injections and stress, as previously described.[40]

Other methods of producing cardiac lesions of this type include stimulation of the limbic cortex, mesencephalic reticular formation, stellate ganglion, and regions known to elicit cardiac reflexes, such as the aortic arch. Experimental intracerebral and subarachnoid hemorrhages can also result in cardiac contraction band lesions. These neurogenic cardiac lesions will occur even in an adrenalectomized animal, although they will be somewhat less pronounced.[22] This evidence argues strongly against an exclusively humoral mechanism in the intact organism. High levels of circulating catecholamines exaggerate the ECG findings and myocardial lesions, but high circulating catecholamine levels are not required for the production of pathologic changes. These ECG abnormalities and cardiac lesions are stereotyped and identical to those found in the stress and catecholamine models already outlined. They are not affected by vagotomy, and they are blocked by maneuvers that interfere with the action of the sympathetic limb of the autonomic nervous system, such as C-2 spinal section, stellate ganglion blockade, and administration of antiadrenergic drugs such as propranolol.

On light microscopy, the histologic changes in the myocardium range from normal muscle to severely necrotic (but not ischemic lesions with secondary mononuclear cell infiltration. The findings on ultrastructural examination are invariably more widespread, often involving nearly every muscle cell, even when the light microscopic appearance is unimpressive. The ECG findings undoubtedly reflect the total amount of muscle membrane affected by the pathophysiology process. Thus the ECG may be normal when the lesion is early and demonstrable only by electron microscopy. Conversely, the ECG may be grossly abnormal when only minimal findings are present on light microscopy, since the cardiac membrane abnormality responsible for the ECG changes may be reversible. Cardiac arrhythmias of many types may also be elicited by nervous system stimulation along the outflow of the sympathetic nervous system.

Reperfusion

The fourth, and last, model for the production of myofibrillar degeneration is reperfusion, as is commonly seen in patients dying after time on a left ventricular assist pump for cardiac surgery. Similar lesions are seen in hearts that were reperfused using angioplasty or fibrinolytic therapy. The mechanism by which reperfusion of ischemic cardiac muscle produces myofibrillar degeneration is related to the cellular entry of calcium after a period of relative deprivation.[5]

Zimmerman and Hulsmann[61] found that perfusion of rat hearts in a calcium-free medium for a short time followed by readmission of calcium causes a massive entry of calcium into the cell, resulting in irreversible contracture. This has become known as the calcium paradox.[61] Some years later it was reported that reoxygenation of hypoxic myocardium induces a similar series of events, as does reperfusion after a period of ischemia.[23,24]

Sudden calcium influx by one of several possible mechanisms (e.g., a period of calcium deficiency with loss of intracellular calcium, a period of anoxia followed by reoxygenation of the electron transport system, a period of ischemia followed by reperfusion, or opening of the receptor-operated calcium channels by excessive amounts of locally released norepinephrine) may be the final common pathway by which the irreversible contractures occur, leading to myofibrillar degeneration.

The precise cellular mechanism for the ECG change and the histologic lesion may well reflect the effects of large volumes of norepinephrine released into the myocardium from sympathetic nerve terminals.[17] The fact that cardiac necrosis is greatest near the nerve terminals in the endocardium and is progressively less severe as one samples muscle approaching the epicardium provides further evidence that catecholamine

toxicity produces the lesion.[20] This locally released norepinephrine is known to stimulate synthesis of adenosine $3',5'$-cyclic phosphate, which in turn results in the opening of the calcium channel with influx of calcium and efflux of potassium. This efflux of potassium could explain the peaked T waves (a hyperkalemic pattern) often seen early in the evolution of neurogenic ECG changes.[26] The actin and myosin filaments interact under the influence of calcium but do not relax unless the calcium channel closes. Continuously high levels of norepinephrine in the region may result in failure of the calcium channel to close, leading to cell death, and finally to leakage of catecholamines and enzymes out of the myocardial cell. Free radicals released as a result of reperfusion after ischemia or by the metabolism of catecholamines to the known toxic metabolite adrenochrome may contribute to cell membrane destruction, leading to leakage of cardiac enzymes into the blood.[39,54] Thus the cardiac toxicity of locally released norepinephrine would represent a continuum ranging from a brief reversible burst of ECG abnormalities to a pattern resembling hyperkalemia and then to an irreversible failure of the muscle cell with permanent repolarization abnormalities or even to the occurrence of transmural cardiac necrosis with Q waves on the ECG.

Histologic changes would also represent a continuum ranging from complete reversibility in a normal heart, through mild changes seen best on electron microscopy, to severe myocardial cell necrosis with mononuclear cell infiltration and even hemorrhages. The level of cardiac enzymes released and the ECG changes would roughly correlate with the severity and extent of the pathologic process. This explanation, summarized in Figure 5–3, would tie together all the observations in the catecholamine infusion, stress, nervous system stimulation, and reperfusion models.

THE UNIFYING (NEUROCARDIOPULMONARY) HYPOTHESIS OF SUDDEN UNEXPECTED DEATH

In conclusion, there is powerful evidence suggesting that overactivity of the sympa-

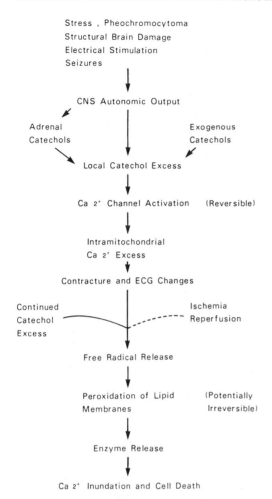

FIGURE 5-3. Proposed pathogenesis of neurogenic cardiopulmonary disease. (Adapted from Drislane et al,[15] p. 500.)

Investigations aimed at altering the natural history of these events using catecholamine receptor blockade, calcium channel blockers, free radical scavengers, and antioxidants are ongoing in many centers around the world.

REFERENCES

1. Baroldi, F: Different morphological types of myocardial cell death in man. In Fleckenstein, A and Rona, G (eds): Recent Advances in Studies in Cardiac Structure and Metabolism. Pathophysiology and Morphology of Myocardial Cell Alteration. University Park Press, Baltimore, Vol. 6, 1975, pp 385–397.
2. Bateman, JRM and Clarke, SW: Sudden death in asthma. Thorax 34:40–44, 1979.
3. Blessing, WW, Sved, AF, and Reis, DJ: Destruction of noradrenergic neurons in rabbit brainstem elevates plasma vasopressin causing hypertension. Science 217:661–662, 1982.
4. Borison, HL and Kovacs, BA: Central mechanisms in pulmonary edema of nervous origin in guinea pigs. J Phys (Lond) 145:374–383, 1959.
5. Braunwald, E and Kloner, RA. Myocardial reperfusion: A double-edged sword? J Clin Invest 76:1713–1719, 1985.
6. Burch, GE, Myers, R, and Adildskov, JA: A new electrocardiographic pattern observed in cerebrovascular accidents. Circulation 9: 719–726, 1954.
7. Byer, E, Ashman, R, and Toth, LA: Electrocardiogram with large upright T wave and long Q-T intervals. Am Heart J 33:796–801, 1947.
8. Cannon, WB: "Voodoo" death. Psychosom Med 19:182–190, 1957.
9. Cebelin, M and Hirsch, CS: Human stress cardiomyopathy. Hum Pathol 11:123–132, 1980.
10. Coryell, W, Noyes, R, and House, JD: Mortality among outpatients with anxiety disorders. Am J Psychiatry 143:508–510, 1986.
11. Cropp, CF and Manning, GW: Electrocardiographic change simulating myocardial ischemia and infarction associated with spontaneous intracranial hemorrhage. Circulation 22:25–38, 1960.
12. Dampey, RAL, Kumada, M, and Reis, DJ: Central neural mechanisms of the cerebral ischemic response. Circ Res 44:48–62, 1979.
13. DeSilva, RA: Central nervous system risk factors for sudden cardiac death. Ann NY Acad Sci 382: 143–161, 1982.
14. Dimant, J and Grob, D: Electrocardiographic changes and myocardial damage in patients with acute cerebrovascular accidents. Stroke 8:448–455, 1977.
15. Drislane, FW, Samuels, MA, Kozakewich, H, Schoen, FJ, and Strunk, RC: Myocardial contraction band lesions in patients with fatal asthma: Possible neurocardiologic mechanisms. Am Rev Resp Dis 135:498–501, 1987.

thetic limb of the autonomic nervous system is the common phenomenon that links the major cardiac and pulmonary pathologies seen in neurologic catastrophes. These profound effects on the heart and lungs may contribute greatly to the mortality rates of many primarily neurologic conditions such as subarachnoid hemorrhage, status epilepticus, and head trauma. These phenomena may also be important in the pathogenesis of SUD in adults, sudden infant death, sudden death during asthma attacks, cocaine- and amphetamine-related deaths, and sudden death associated with the alcohol withdrawal syndrome, all of which may be linked by stress and catecholamine toxicity.

16. Doba, N and Reis, DJ: Role of central and peripheral adrenergic mechanisms in neurogenic hypertension produced by brainstem lesions in the rat. Circ Res 34:293–301, 1974.

17. Eliot, RS, Todd, GL, Pieper, GM, and Clayton, FC: Pathophysiology of catecholamine-mediated myocardial damage. J S Med Assoc 75:513–518, 1979.

18. Fulton, JF: Functional Localization in the Frontal Lobes. Oxford, London, 1949.

19. Gelberg, HB, Zachary, JF, Everitt, JI, Jensen, RC, and Smetzer, DL: Sudden death in training and racing thoroughbred horses. J Am Vet Med Assoc 12:1354–1356, 1985.

20. Greenhoot, JH and Reichenbach, DD: Cardiac injury and subarachnoid hemorrhage. J Neurosurg 30:521–531, 1969.

21. Hammer, WJ, Leussenhop, AJ, and Weintraub AM: Observations on the electrocardiographic changes associated with subarachnoid hemorrhage with special reference to their genesis. Am J Med 59:427–433, 1975.

22. Hawkins, WE and Clower, BR: Myocardial damage after head trauma and simulated intracranial haemorrhage in mice: The role of the autonomic nervous system. Cardiovasc Res 5:524–529, 1971.

23. Hearse, DJ, Humphrey, SM, and Chain, EG: Abrupt reoxygenation of the anoxic potassium arrested perfused rat heart: A study of myocardial enzyme release. J Mol Cell Cardiol 5:39–407, 1973.

24. Hearse, DJ, Humphrey, SM, and Bullock, GR: The oxygen paradox and the calcium paradox: Two facets of the same problem? J Mol Cell Cardiol 10:641–668, 1978.

25. Hugenholtz, PG: Electrocardiographic abnormalities in cerebral disorders: Report of six cases and review of the literature. Am Heart J 63:451–461, 1962.

26. Jacob, WA, Van Bogaert, A, and DeGroot-Lasseel, MHA: Myocardial ultrastructural and haemodynamic reactions during experimental subarachnoid hemorrhage. J Mol Cell Cardiol 4:287–298, 1972.

27. Jay, GW, and Leestma, JE: Sudden death in epilepsy. Acta Neurologica Scand (Suppl 82)63:1–66, 1981.

28. Josué, O: Hypertrophie cardiaque causée par l'adrénaline et la toxine typhique. C R Soc Biol (Paris) 63:285–287, 1907.

29. Karch, SB and Billingham, ME: Myocardial contraction bands revisited. Hum Pathol 17:9–13, 1986.

30. King, JM, Roth, L, and Haschek, WM: Myocardial necrosis secondary to neural lesions in domestic animals. J Am Vet Med Assoc 180:144–148, 1982.

31. Levine, HD: Non-specificity of the electrocardiogram associated with coronary heart disease. Am J Med 15:344–350, 1946.

32. Lown, B, DeSilva, RA, and Lenson, R: Roles of psychologic stress and autonomic nervous system changes in provocation of ventricular premature complexes. Am J Cardiol 41:979–985, 1978.

33. Luisada, AA and Sarnoff, SJ: Paroxysmal pulmonary edema consequent to stimulation of cardiovascular receptors: Pharmacologic experiments. Am Heart J 13:293–307, 1946.

34. Magendie, F: L'influence de la cinquième paire des nerfs sur la nutrition et les fonctions de l'oeil. J Physiol (Paris) 4:176–179, 1924.

35. Maire, FW and Patton, HD: Neural structures involved in the genesis of preoptic pulmonary edema, gastric erosions and behavior changes. Am J Physiol 184:345–350, 1956.

36. Malik, AB: Mechanisms of neurogenic pulmonary edema. Circ Res 57:1–18, 1985.

37. Maron, MB and Dawson, CA: Pulmonary venoconstriction caused by elevated cerebrospinal fluid pressure in the dog. J Appl Physiol 49:73–78, 1956.

38. McHale, NG and Roddie, IC: Peripheral lymph flow during intravenous noradrenaline infusion in sheep. J Physiol (Lond) 334:350, 1983.

39. Meerson, FZ: Pathogenesis and prophylaxis of cardiac lesions in stress. In Chazov E, Saks, V, and Rona, G (eds): Advances in myocardiology, Vol. 4. Plenum, New York, pp 3–21, 1983.

40. Melville, KI, Blum, B, Shister HE, and Silver, MD: Cardiac ischemic changes and arrhythmias induced by hypothalamic stimulation. Am J Cardiol 12:781–791, 1963.

41. Myers, MG, Norris, JW, Hachinski, VC, and Sole, MJ: Plasma norepinephrine in stroke. Stroke 12:200–204, 1981.

42. Nandiwada, P, Hyman, AL, and Kadowitz, PJ: Pulmonary vasodilatory response to vagal stimulation and acetylcholine in the cat. Circ Res 53:86–95, 1983.

43. Natelson, BH: Neurocardiology: An interdisciplinary area for the 80's. Arch Neurol 42:178–184, 1985.

44. Norris, JW, Hachinski, VC, Myers MG, et al.: Serum cardiac enzymes in stroke. Stroke 10:548–553, 1979.

45. Parrish, RG, Tucker, M, Ing, R, and Encaracion, C: Sudden unexplained death syndrome in Southeast Asian refugees: A review of CDC surveillance. MMWR 36:43ss–55ss, 1987.

46. Paulozzi, LJ and Munger, R: Sudden unexpected nocturnal deaths in Washington, JAMA 253:2645–2647, 1985.

47. Raab, W, Stark, E, MacMillan, WH, et al.: Sympathogenic origin and anti-adrenergic prevention of stress-induced myocardial lesions. Am J Cardiol 8:203–211, 1961.

48. Richter, CP: On the phenomenon of sudden death in animals and man. Psychosom Med 19:191–198, 1957.

49. Rona, G: Catecholamine cardiotoxicity. J Mol Cell Cardiol 17:291–306, 1985.

50. Rosell, S: Neuronal control of microvessels. Ann Rev Physiol 42:359–371, 1980.

51. Samuels, MA: Electrocardiographic manifestations of neurologic disease. Seminars in Neurology 4:91–99, 1984.

52. Selye, H: The Chemical Prevention of Cardiac Necrosis. Ronald Press, New York, 1958.

53. Simon, RP and Bayne, LL: Pulmonary lymphatic

flow alterations during intracranial hypertension in sheep. Ann Neurol 15:188–194, 1984.

54. Singal, PK, Kapur, N, Dhillon, KS, Beamish, RE, and Dhalla, NA: Role of free radicals in catecholamine-induced cardiomyocaphy. Can J Physiol Pharmacol 60:1390–1397, 1982.

55. Stein, PM, MacAnenspie, CI, and Rothe, CF: Total body vascular capacitance changes during high intracranial pressure. Am J Physiol 245:947–956, 1983.

56. Talman, WT: Cardiovascular regulation and lesions of the central nervous system. Ann Neurol 18:1–12, 1985.

57. Theodore, J and Robin, ED: Speculations on neurogenic pulmonary edema (NPE). Am Rev Respir Dis 113:405–411, 1976.

58. Trichopoulos, D, Katsouyanni, K, Zavitsanox, X, Tzonou, A, and Dalla-Vorgia, P: Psychological stress and fatal heart attack: The Athens (1981) earthquake natural experiment. Lancet 1:441–443, 1983.

59. Truex, RC: Neurogenic and humoral influences on the heart. In Dreifuss, LS and Likoff, W (eds): Cardiac Arrhythmias. Grune & Stratton, New York, 1972.

60. Vetter, WR, Cohn, LH, and Reichgott, M: Hypokalemia and electrocardiographic abnormalities during acute alcohol withdrawal. Arch Intern Med 120:536–541, 1967.

61. Zimmerman, ANA and Hulsmann, WC: Paradoxical influence of calcium ions on the permeability of the cell membranes of the isolated rat heart. Nature 211:616–647, 1966.

SECTION THREE

· · · · · · · · · · · · ·

PROFESSIONAL CHALLENGES

EDITOR'S COMMENTARY

Scherokman quotes evidence that the biomedical literature grows at a compound rate of 6% to 7% per year, doubling every 10 to 15 years. Medical wisdom does not. The challenge is to incorporate knowledge that makes a difference to the framework that every well-trained physician has. Luckily the framework does not have to be discarded but updated. Progress has made it both more difficult and easier to keep up to date—more difficult because of the sheer volume of new information; easier because of the many modern ways of accessing this information. Physicians need not fret about missing something important. If it is important enough, it is bound to appear in one of the media and it will be repeated in publications, conferences, or pronouncements. It has become difficult to do anything important in medicine anonymously. If the doctors miss it, the patients will point it out.

VCH

CHAPTER 6

• •

KEEPING UP WITHOUT STAYING UP: UNDERSTANDING THE LITERATURE, TECHNOLOGY, AND CLINICAL TRIALS

Barbara Scherokman, M.D.

The scientific method consists essentially of observation, hypothesis generation, and verification. The approaches that Scherokman outlines so clearly serve to verify questions arising from the bedside, and they may also generate a differential diagnosis and a broader knowledge base on which to consider the patient's problem. However, in clinical medicine most of the errors are made at the observation stage. If the key elements of the history are not elicited and the crucial findings are missed, no amount of literature can redress proceeding along the wrong track.

The author emphasizes the desirability of "blind" comparisons with "gold standards" for diagnostic tests. Sound advice, except that for some tests the "gold standard" is only 10 karats.

VCH

Growing evidence indicates that our effectiveness as clinicians begins to decline as soon as we complete our clinical training.[1,2] Serious consequences of not keeping up with advances have been documented;[3] however, neurologists attempting to keep informed of medical advances face an arduous task. With the biomedical literature expanding at a compound rate of 6% to 7% per year,[4] the literature doubles every 10 to 15 years. The practicing neurologist must therefore keep up to date with advances in medicine by using scanning and reading strategies that stress efficiency as well as assess validity and applicability. A related and valuable technique involves using a personal computer to scan a large fraction of current journal literature rapidly.

This chapter summarizes methods described in detail by Sackett, Haynes, and Tugwell[5] and in articles by Sackett[6] and by Haynes and associates.[7-12] Neurologists, indeed all physicians, can profit from the clinical reading paradigm developed by these researchers and epidemiologists at McMaster University.

Although physicians use various methods in trying to stay informed, journal reading consistently ranks higher than other means of continuing education in several large surveys.[13-16] Many clinicians turn to reading review articles and editorials to handle the large volume of literature. Reviews and editorials do have a place in clinical reading inasmuch as they are the best sources to consult when attempting to gather all the relevant original references on a particular subject. The reader must be cautious, however, about the opinions stated in reviews and editorials; the reviewer's opinion frequently differs from the conclusion drawn following one's own critical analysis of the original article. This chapter emphasizes keeping up with the literature by focusing only on *original* journal articles.

APPROACHES TO CLINICAL LITERATURE

Two basic approaches can be used to deal with the immense number of original articles. The choice of method depends on the intent of the reader.

If the purpose is to survey large volumes of literature to keep up to date with important advances in clinical medicine, then highly selective criteria should be used to find articles that are both useful and scientifically valid. With this approach, the *surveillance method*, many articles are discarded. As stated by Sackett, "It is only through the early rejection of *most* articles that busy clinicians can focus on the *few* that are both valid and applicable in their own practices."[6]

When trying to solve a particular clinical problem, the reader uses the *problem-solving approach* of applying specific critical reading techniques. With this approach, one does not initially discard any of the articles found on a subject. The goal is to read every article on a subject critically so as to decide which one is the most scientifically valid (see The Problem-Solving Method, p. 89).

The Surveillance Method

The surveillance method helps the busy clinician sort through a large volume of literature and find articles that are both applicable to his or her own practice and of sufficient rigor to be scientifically valid. Fortunately, the volume of medical litera-

ture can be reduced to a manageable size because most of what is published has little clinical relevance or not enough scientific merit to justify a change in clinical action.

Figure 6–1 is a flow diagram of the first four steps used in surveying large volumes of literature.[6] If the answer to any of the questions is no, the reader should throw out the article and go on to the next one.

Step 1: Is the title interesting? If the article is of interest, readers go on to the next step.

Step 2: Would the results be useful? If the conclusions, if valid, would be important in the readers' practice, they go on to the next step.

Step 3: Would the results apply to your patients? This question can be answered by looking at the site where the study was done. Readers determine whether the conclusions, if valid, would apply to the types of patients they see in practice. Also, by comparing the site with their own, they can decide if the diagnostic and therapeutic procedures described in the study could be carried out at their own institution.

Step 4: Is the study scientifically valid? The answer to this question depends on the type of article, as standards to determine if the study fulfills the main methodologic criterion for scientific validity differ.

If the article is on diagnosis, the major question is whether there was a "blind" comparison with a "gold standard." The gold standard is an accepted test that establishes a definitive diagnosis. The reader must first accept the gold standard as being the best test to establish the diagnosis. In a diagnostic test study, patients who either have the disease or do not have the disease by the gold standard are subjected to the diagnostic test in question. Interpretation of the diagnostic test is done by clinicians who do not know whether a given patient really has the disease (blind). Afterward, the diagnostic test results are compared with the gold standard.

For a therapy article, the major consideration is whether the patients were

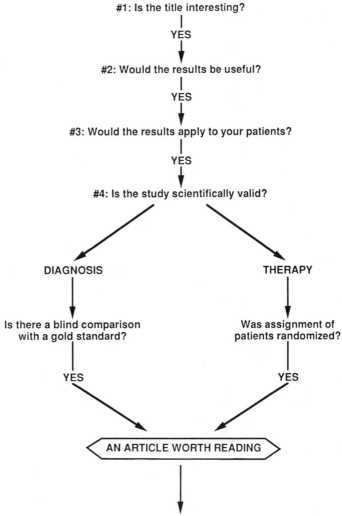

#1: Is the title interesting?

YES

#2: Would the results be useful?

YES

#3: Would the results apply to your patients?

YES

#4: Is the study scientifically valid?

DIAGNOSIS   THERAPY

Is there a blind comparison   Was assignment of
with a gold standard?   patients randomized?

YES   YES

AN ARTICLE WORTH READING

Read the "Methods" section

FIGURE 6–1. Surveillance method. (Adapted from Sackett,[6] p. 557.)

assigned to treatment groups in a randomized fashion.

If all the answers to the above questions are yes, then the article is worth keeping. The reader would next look at the "Methods" section and use the tactics described under The Problem-Solving Method to read the article critically.

By using these guidelines, busy readers can separate the articles worth keeping and reading from the studies that are neither useful nor scientifically valid. These techniques can greatly expand the volume of clinical literature reviewed.

The Problem-Solving Method

Routes Used to Gather Information

Reading to solve clinical problems differs from surveying a large volume of literature. In this instance, the reader must find the best and most recent information published on the problem. Although there are several routes for gathering information on a particular clinical problem (Table 6–1), some sources serve the reader's needs better than others. The first three routes listed in Table 6–1 — clinical monographs, textbooks, and experts' opinions — reflect someone

1. Textbooks of medicine
2. Clinical monographs
3. Consultation with an expert
4. Recent issues of journals
5. Personal reprint collection
6. "Bibliography of Reviews" in *Index Medicus*
7. *Index Medicus* subject section
8. Computer searches of the literature

Source: Adapted from Haynes, et al.,[10] p. 637.

else's ideas on a subject. If the author or expert is not a critical reader of the medical literature, one may get biased opinions rather than a scientifically valid view of the subject. Furthermore, books are commonly published a year or more following manuscript preparation.

Numbers 4 and 5 in Table 6–1 are directed at finding original journal articles. Browsing through recent issues of journals, however, may be unrewarding unless the reader is lucky enough to run across an article on his or her specific clinical question. Likewise, perusing a personal reprint collection may yield few relevant articles because the surveillance method used to compile the collection selected a limited number of valid and applicable articles.

Review articles can save time in answering clinical questions, but they must be read selectively and critically, since an unscientific literature review can come to incorrect conclusions. Table 6–2 lists guidelines for

TABLE 6–2. **GUIDELINES FOR ASSESSING RESEARCH REVIEWS**

1. Questions and methods stated clearly?
2. Comprehensive search methods used to locate relevant studies?
3. Explicit methods used to determine which articles to include?
4. Validity of primary studies assessed?
5. Assessment of primary studies reproducible and nonbiased?
6. Variation in findings of relevant studies analyzed?
7. Findings of primary studies combined appropriately?
8. Reviewer's conclusions supported by data cited?

Source: Adapted from Oxman and Guyatt,[17] p. 698.

assessing review articles.[17] Reviews are not as timely as original articles, however, because they are written long after a series of studies have been published.

The best information on a subject comes from original journal articles, which can be located by surveying the subject section of the *Index Medicus*. Monthly issues of the *Index Medicus* generally are received by libraries within 3 to 6 months after the date of publication of an article.[10] Searching can be done by hand or electronically by using a computer, which is the fastest method of searching.

Using a Computer to Search the Literature

All the routes discussed above can be time-consuming, time-delayed, and nonexhaustive. Electronic searching is much faster, and citations are available much closer to the time of their publication. Citations from "priority" journals appear in computerized data bases within 2 to 6 weeks after publication. Also, because of their vast storage capacity, computerized medical data bases have detailed indexing that is impossible in printed indexes.

Index Medicus is one of a class of general printed indexes of the biomedical literature. The on-line version of this index is called MEDLINE. The two major competitors of *Index Medicus* are *Excerpta Medica* (on-line version is EMBASE) and *Science Citation Index* (on-line version is SCISEARCH). These indexes cover a slightly different but overlapping body of literature. *Excerpta Medica* contains more of the European literature, and *Science Citation Index* has more basic-science references. The MEDLINE service of the US National Library of Medicine (NLM) is the optimal route for best yield at the lowest time and price.[18]

Computerized searching can be done in many libraries or from one's office or home. When using the MEDLINE search capabilities in a library, it is important to be present during the actual search so as to guide it along specific areas of interest.

It is now possible to retrieve pertinent information from large literature data bases, resulting in faster solutions to clinical problems. The basic equipment needed for online searching consists of either a "dumb" terminal or a personal computer with at least 256K memory (preferably more), at least one double-sided, double-density disk drive, a Hayes Smartmodem or completely compatible modem, communication software, and a standard plug-in jack for a household telephone. A printer is needed if a hard copy of literature searches is desired.

Software Options. Many software options (see Appendix) enable access to large literature data bases. Although all of these access programs lead to the same data base, they differ in several characteristics. Haynes[18] compared the performance characteristics of MEDLINE search systems in terms of cost, on-line time, and difficulty to learn. PaperChase was the easiest system to use but the most expensive per search. Dialog provides the widest range of services.

The most popular software appears to be GRATEFUL MED, recently developed by the NLM. This program automatically calls the NLM computer, logs into the NLM computer with personal user code and password, enters the search request and stores any references found, and disconnects from the NLM computer. The average cost of a GRATEFUL MED search is $2 to $4.

Additional information on on-line searching systems and services can be obtained from several sources.[19-25] The NLM and some commercial vendors offer short courses of instruction in many locations. Also, in many medical school libraries, experienced searchers offer on-site training.

Critical Reading Guidelines for Specific Types of Articles

Searching a literature data base often yields a number of articles pertaining to a specific clinical problem. The next step is to determine which study is the most scientifically valid. Many clinicians assume that if a study is published in an important journal, it must be true and accurate. Unfortunately, the review and editorial policies of even the most highly respected journals provide incomplete protection from error. The busy clinician who quickly reads only the abstract and conclusions does so at considerable risk to his or her patients. Guidelines have been published for assessing the appli-

cability and scientific validity of original articles on diagnostic tests,[5,26-28] prognosis,[5,29] causation,[5,30] and treatment.[5,31] These guidelines focus on examination of the "Materials and Methods" section of papers. Discussed here are the guidelines developed at McMaster University Health Sciences Center that apply to articles on diagnosis and therapy.

Articles on Diagnostic Tests. There are eight questions to ask when critically reading articles on diagnostic tests (Table 6-3).[5,26]

1. *"Blind" comparison with a "gold standard"?* (See p. 88.) Diagnostic test results compared with the gold standard are usually displayed as a "two-by-two" table (Fig. 6-2). By using this table, one can determine the sensitivity, specificity, and likelihood ratios.[5,26-28]

2. *Appropriate spectrum of mild and severe disease, treated and untreated disease, and individuals with different but commonly confused disorders?* The value of a diagnostic test lies in its ability to detect equivocal cases and to distinguish between commonly confused disorders. Therefore, when a new diagnostic test is being tested, a wide spectrum of diseases as well as different but similar disorders must be used.

3. *Setting of the study?* To be a useful test for readers, the study population should match the prevalence in their own practices. The clinical value of a diagnostic test changes with the prevalence of the target disease, and tertiary care centers

TABLE 6-3. **CRITICAL READING GUIDELINES FOR ARTICLES ON DIAGNOSTIC TESTS**

1. "Blind" comparison with a "gold standard"?
2. Appropriate spectrum of mild and severe, treated and untreated disease and individuals with different but commonly confused disorders?
3. Setting for the study?
4. Reproducibility of the test result and interpretation determined?
5. *Normal* defined sensibly?
6. Contribution to a cluster determined?
7. Test described in enough detail?
8. "Utility" of the test determined?

Source: Adapted from Haynes,[26] p. 704.

By Gold Standard, Patient

	Has the Disease	Does Not Have Disease	
Positive	a	b	
Negative	c	d	

TEST (label to the left of Positive/Negative rows)

$$\text{Sensitivity} = \frac{a}{a + c}$$

$$\text{Specificity} = \frac{d}{b + d}$$

$$\text{Prevalence} = \frac{a + c}{a + b + c + d}$$

$$\text{Likelihood Ratio for Positive Test} = \frac{\text{Sensitivity}}{1 - \text{Specificity}}$$

$$\text{Likelihood Ratio for Negative Test} = \frac{1 - \text{Sensitivity}}{\text{Specificity}}$$

FIGURE 6-2. Two-by-two table for comparison of a diagnostic test with the gold standard. (Adapted from Haynes,[26] p. 704.)

tend to have a higher prevalence of disease. Thus one needs to know about the study site.

4. *Reproducibility of the test result and interpretation determined?* Validity of a diagnostic test depends both on the absence of deviation from the truth (accuracy) and the presence of reproducibility (precision). This is especially important when expertise is needed in performing or interpreting the test.

5. *"Normal" defined sensibly?* The authors should state what they mean by normal, and readers should be satisfied

that such a definition makes clinical sense.

6. *Contribution to a cluster determined?* Any single component of a sequence of diagnostic tests should be evaluated in the framework of its clinical utility.

7. *Test described in enough detail?* The authors should give details of performing the test and interpreting its results so readers can reproduce the test in their own practices.

8. *"Utility" of the test determined?* The outcome of the cases of patients who had false-positive and false-negative results

should be stated and an indication given of whether the time taken to perform the test caused any delay in treatment.

These guidelines for critical analysis of articles on diagnostic tests can help readers decide which articles are the most valid and applicable. Although all criteria may not be fulfilled by a given article, those that satisfy the most criteria are the most scientifically sound.

Articles on Therapy. In addition to analyzing articles critically to find useful diagnostic tests, it is equally important to distinguish useful from useless, or even harmful, therapy. In the history of medicine there are numerous examples of randomized trials proving that an accepted therapy is actually harmful. Clinicians should use a therapy not because it *should* work but because it actually *does* work. There are six guidelines to follow when trying to determine if a therapy article is both valid and applicable (Table 6–4).[5,31]

1. *Assignment of patients randomized?* The basic design of a therapy study is to start with two groups that are very similar in clinical characteristics, so that when the treatment received by each group is varied, the outcome will be due only to the treatment difference. The best way to ensure clinically similar groups is to randomize the entry of patients into either the treatment or the control group. Randomization gives every patient an equal chance of receiving the treatment or placebo. Unfortunately, randomization does not guarantee that the two groups will be clinically similar. It is important,

therefore, for the authors to give the clinical characteristics of both groups and to state if there are any significant differences between groups.

2. *All relevant outcomes reported?* Because a reader's decision about therapy depends on both beneficial and harmful effects of the treatment, authors must state all of the clinically relevant outcomes. Objective criteria for outcomes should be stated, and these endpoints should be determined by observers who are unaware of the patients' treatment ("blind" outcome assessment).

3. *Study patients similar to yours?* The characteristics of the study patients must be stated in enough detail so that readers can tell if the study would apply to their own patients.

4. *Statistically and clinically significant?* Statistical significance indicates how likely it is that a difference could be due to chance alone. The *P* value is the probability of a difference being due to chance alone and not to the treatment. Therefore, a *P* value should be as low as possible, usually <0.05. But *statistical* significance does not indicate how *clinically* significance the difference is, and clinical significance is really what clinicians are interested in. If a study turns out not to be statistically significant, then the next question is: Are there enough patients to show a clinically significant difference if it should occur? A "no" answer indicates what is referred to as a type II error or a study with a low power.[32]

5. *Therapeutic maneuver feasible?* The authors must describe the therapeutic maneuver in enough detail to allow clinicians to reproduce it in their own practices.

6. *All patients accounted for?* Similarities between treatment and placebo groups can be changed if patients drop out of either group. For this reason, authors should state exactly what happened to the dropouts in each group. One should be skeptical if 10% of patients are unaccounted for at the end of the study. The paper should be discarded if 20% of patients are lost at the end of the study.

TABLE 6–4. CRITICAL READING GUIDELINES FOR ARTICLES ON THERAPY

1. Assignment of patients randomized?
2. All relevant outcomes reported?
3. Study-patients similar to yours?
4. Statistically and clinically significant?
5. Therapeutic maneuver feasible?
6. All patients accounted for?

Source: Adapted from Sackett,[31] p. 1157.

Using these guidelines enables the reader to determine whether a particular therapy causes more good than harm, and thus which articles on therapy are best.

DECIDING WHICH JOURNALS TO READ REGULARLY

Another time-saving procedure is to prioritize the journals chosen for reading. Top priority should be given to journals that consistently provide valid and applicable articles.

According to two studies, physicians claim to read journals from 1 to 3 hours per week.[13,14] Unfortunately, there may be no way to increase the time busy clinicians have to read journals. Therefore the strategies for keeping up must be designed to increase the readers' efficiency during this fixed amount of reading time.

One way to increase efficiency is to survey journals that are likely to have a large number of useful and valid studies, rather than waste time on low-yield journals. The time saved can be used to survey more of the world's biomedical literature and thereby do a better job of keeping up to date.

How does one determine the yield from journals? It seems reasonable that specialty journals in neurology would be most likely to have the highest yield of useful and valid articles. This is not always the case, however, since many articles are reports of experiments or preliminary investigations in humans. These reports are mainly communications between researchers and are not directly applicable to clinicians.

Another method is to survey journals that have a large circulation. The larger the circulation, the more likely that clinically important studies will be included. Readers can determine the circulation of most journals from *Ulrich's International Periodicals Directory*[33] or from *Business Publication Rates and Data*.[34]

The best method to determine the yield of neurology journals is to assess the actual yield of valid articles that have direct relevance to one's own clinical practice. The four strategies described for the surveillance method can be used to determine the yield of a given journal. By looking at the table of contents, one can decide which articles may be interesting and useful. After this initial screening, the site of the study and the scientific validity can be obtained from a quick perusal of the original article. Reject studies on diagnostic tests that do not have a blind comparison with a gold standard, as well as therapy articles that are not randomized.

By keeping track of how many articles are rejected compared with the number of original studies (that is, preplanned investigations) in each journal, one can decide which journals have the highest yield. Several issues of a journal should be used for a personal survey to determine yield, because the number of relevant articles varies from issue to issue. After the yield is determined, one can rank the different journals in order of highest to lowest yield and decide how many can be read regularly.

When the screening criteria of applicability and validity were applied to the issues for 6 months of three major neurology journals, 24 (9%) of 284 original articles were found to be on diagnosis and therapy. Of these 24 articles, only 8 made it through the screening procedure. This low percentage does not reflect on the quality of the journals; rather, it is an indication of how well the journal articles fit the clinician's needs.

In developing a personal journal reading list, it is important to include nonneurologic journals. Most articles of clinical importance in any medical field are published not in specialty journals, but in general medical journals with wide circulation. This is because researchers want their studies to reach the widest possible audience. Again the four Surveillance criteria can be used to generate a monthly reading list.

SUMMARY

Reading strategies that stress efficiency as well as validity and applicability of studies can help the busy neurologist keep up to date with the expanding literature. Computerized literature searching is the quickest and most reliable method for solving clinical problems. Only through the critical assessment of original articles generated by an in-depth literature review can a neurologist be sure that more good than harm is being done for the patient. The most important criterion for a valid study on a new diagnostic test is a blind comparison with a gold standard. Similarly, randomized patient assignment is essential for a credible article on therapy.

APPENDIX: SELECTED ADDRESSES FOR ACCESS ROUTES TO MEDLINE

MEDLINE: National Library of Medicine, Medlars Management System, 8600 Rockville Pike, Bethesda, MD 20209 (301-496-6913). In Canada: Health Sciences Research Center, Canada Institute for Scientific and Technical Information (CISTI), National Research Council, Montreal Road, Ottawa, Ontario K1A 0S2 (613-993-1604). Accessible via dumb terminal or personal computer.

GRATEFUL MED: US Department of Commerce, National Technical Information Service, 5285 Port Royal Road, Springfield, VA 22161 (703-487-4650). In Canada consult CISTI (see above). Available for IBM PC or compatibles and for Macintosh.

PAPERCHASE: Longwood Galleria, 350 Longwood Avenue, Boston, MA 02215 (617-278-3900). Available for IBM PC or compatible.

DIALOG and Knowledge Index: 3460 Hillview Avenue, Palo Alto, CA 94304 (415-858-3785). In Canada: Micromedia Ltd., 144 Front Street, Toronto, Ontario (416-593-5211). Data base accessible via any computer; access software runs on IBM PC or compatible but is expected to be available for the Macintosh as well.

REFERENCES

1. Evans, CE, Haynes, RB, Birkett, NJ, Gilbert, JR, Taylor, DW, Sackett, DL, Johnston, ME, and Hewson, SA: Does a mailed continuing education program improve physician performance? Results of a randomized trial in antihypertensive care. JAMA 255:501–4, 1986.
2. Evans, CE, Haynes, RB, Gilbert, JR, Taylor, DW, Sackett, DL, and Johnston, M: Educational package on hypertension for primary care physicians. Can Med Assoc J 130:719–722, 1984.
3. Stross, JK and Harlan, WR: The dissemination of new medical information. JAMA 241:2622–2624, 1979.
4. de Solla Price, D: The development and structure of the biomedical literature. In Warren, KS (ed): Coping with the Biomedical Literature. Praeger, New York, 1981.
5. Sackett, DL, Haynes, RB, and Tugwell, P: Clinical Epidemiology: A Basic Science for Clinical Medicine. Little, Brown and Co, Boston, 1985. *(A classic general reference on critical reading and keeping up to date.)*
6. Sackett, DL: How to read clinical journals: I. Why to read them and how to start reading them critically. Can Med Assoc J 124:555–558, 1981. *(Introduction to critical reading and the surveillance method.)*
7. Haynes, RB, McKibbon, KA, Fitzgerald, D, Guyatt, GH, Walker, CJ, and Sackett, DL: How to keep up with the medical literature: I. Why try to keep up and how to get started. Ann Intern Med 105:149–153, 1986. *(Strategies to enhance the efficiency and effectiveness of journal reading.)*
8. Haynes, RB, McKibbon, KA, Fitzgerald, D, Guyatt, GH, Walker, CJ, and Sackett, DL: How to keep up with the medical literature: II. Deciding which journals to read regularly. Ann Intern Med 105:309–312, 1986. *(How to determine the yield of journals.)*
9. Haynes, RB, McKibbon, KA, Fitzgerald, D, Guyatt, GH, Walker, CJ, and Sackett, DL: How to keep up with the medical literature: III. Expanding the number of journals you read regularly. Ann Intern Med 105:474–478, 1986. *(Tactics for formulating a personalized journal-reading list.)*
10. Haynes, RB, McKibbon, KA, Fitzgerlad, D, Guyatt, GH, Walker, CJ, and Sackett, DL: How to keep up with the medical literature: IV. Using the literature to solve clinical problems. Ann Intern Med 105:636–640, 1986. *(Comparison of various means, from textbook to computers, that provide access to information of potential value in addressing clinical problems.)*
11. Haynes, RB, McKibbon, KA, Fitzgerald, D, Guyatt, GH, Walker, CJ, and Sackett, DL: How to keep up with the medical literature: V. Access by personal computer to the medical literature. Ann Intern Med 105:810–824, 1986. *(Describes many of the options available to clinicians who wish to do their own computer searching of MEDLINE.)*
12. Haynes, RB, McKibbon, KA, Fitzgerald, D, Guyatt, GH, Walker, CJ, and Sackett, DL: How to keep up with the medical literature: VI. How to store and retrieve articles worth keeping. Ann Intern Med 105:978–984, 1986. *(Assists the reader in the development of a tailor-made system for filing.)*
13. Stinson, ER and Mueller, DA: Survey of health professionals' information habits and needs: Con-

ducted through personal interviews. JAMA 243:140–3, 1980.

14. Curry, L and Putnam, RW: Continuing medical education in Maritime Canada: The methods physicians use, would prefer, and find most effective. Can Med Assoc J 124:563–566, 1981.

15. Council on Medical Education: Survey of the current status of continuing medical education. Association of American Medical Colleges Continuing Medical Education Newsletter 10:2–20, 1981.

16. Currie, BF: Continuing education from medical periodicals. Journal of Medical Education 51: 420, 1976.

17. Oxman, AD and Guyatt, GH: Guidelines for reading literature reviews. Can Med Assoc J 138:697–703, 1988. (*Review articles must be read selectively and critically.*)

18. Haynes, RB, McKibbon, KA, Walker, CJ, Mousseau, J, Baker, LM, Fitzgerald, D, Guyatt, G, and Norman, GR: Computer searching of the medical literature: An evaluation of MEDLINE searching systems. Ann Intern Med 103:812–816, 1985.

19. Marchall, JG: Computers: How to choose the online medical database that's right for you. Can Med Assoc J 134:634–638, 1986.

20. Baker, CA: Colleague: A comprehensive online medical library for the end user. Medical Reference Services Quarterly 3:13–26, 1984.

21. Batson, E: AMA/NET: Telecommunications network for physicians. Postgrad Med J 77:109–110, 1985.

22. Hawkins, DT and Levy, LR: Front end software for online database searching: Part I: Definitions, system features, and evaluation. Online 9:30–37, 1985.

23. Fenichel, CH: The Microcomputer User's Guide to Information Online. Hayden Book Co, Hasbrouck Heights, NJ, 1984.

24. The Basics of Searching MEDLINE: A Guide for the Health Professional. National Library of Medicine, Bethesda, MD, 1985. (Available from the National Technical Information Service, 5285 Port Royal Road, Springfield, VA 22161.)

25. Feinglos, SJ: MEDLINE: A Basic Guide to Searching. Medical Library Association, Chicago, 1985.

26. Haynes, RB: How to read clinical journals: II. To learn about a diagnostic test. Can Med Assoc J 124:703–710, 1981. (*Eight critical reading guidelines for reading articles on diagnostic tests.*)

27. Sackett, DL: Interpretation of diagnostic data: 5. How to do it with simple maths. Can Med Assoc J 129:947–954, 1983. (*The use of likelihood ratios in clinical decision making with diagnostic tests.*)

28. Longstreth, WT, Doepsell, TD, and van Belle, G: Clinical neuroepidemiology. I. Diagnosis. Arch Neurol 44:1091–1099, 1987. (*Discusses sources of information on which a diagnosis is based, reliability and validity of information collected, and likelihood ratios.*)

29. Tugwell, P: How to read clinical journals: III. To learn the clinical course and prognosis of disease. Can Med Assoc J 124:869–872, 1981. (*Six critical reading guidelines for reading articles on prognosis.*)

30. Kilgore, ST: How to read clinical journals: IV. To determine etiology or causation. Can Med Assoc J 124:985–990, 1981. (*Nine critical reading guidelines for reading articles on causation.*)

31. Sackett, DL: How to read clinical journals: V. To distinguish useful from useless or even harmful therapy. Can Med Assoc J 124:1156–1162, 1981. (*Six critical reading guidelines for reading articles on therapy.*)

32. Detsky, AS, Sackett, DL: When was a "negative" clinical trial big enough? How many patients you needed depends on what you found. Arch Intern Med 145:709–712, 1985. (*Guidelines for determining whether a study had enough patients to prove a difference between groups, if a difference does exist.*)

33. Ulrich's International Periodicals Directory, ed. 23. RR Bowker, New York, 1984.

34. Business Publication Rates and Data. 67(12), 1985. (Provides information about most journals, including circulation figures.)

SECTION FOUR

. . . .

EPILEPSY

EDITOR'S COMMENTARY

Epilepsy is not only one of the commonest neurologic problems in the world but one of the most resented. Loss of awareness and control, coupled with the uncertainty of its next occurrence, impose a psychologic burden difficult to redress. Whereas disbelief and denial are common reactions to the diagnosis of epilepsy, the converse phenomenon, that is, individuals seeking the diagnosis of epilepsy through their behavior, also occurs. Burnstine and Lesser address the difficult problem of pseudoseizures in a systematic and common-sense manner. Their table setting out the differences between epileptic and psychogenic seizures is particularly helpful. One must bear in mind, however, that a patient may manifest both types of seizures, and the physician must be prepared to diagnose and manage both.

Even when patients comply, seizures cannot always be controlled. McLachlan evaluates the available antiepileptic drugs, discusses factors determining their choice, and outlines principles of drug administration and monitoring. The fact that so many drugs are used highlights their limitations. The best antiepileptic drugs are yet to come.

A correct diagnosis does not guarantee appropriate treatment. Willmore reviews the prophylactic use of anticonvulsant drugs after head trauma, absence epilepsy, cerebral infarction, febrile seizure, and a single seizure. He finds strong views and weak data. He advocates preventive anticonvulsants only for the most serious head injury patients and only at the time immediately following trauma, for patients with epilepsy and risk factors for the development of convulsive seizures, and for patients with a complicated convulsive seizure. In the last case it may take a second seizure before the patient is ready to comply with a therapeutic regimen.

Patients may cease to need medication after surgery, or may require discontinuation to attain monotherapy after surgery, or a drug-free state. Porter discusses the scientific bases for discontinuing anticonvulsants and gives much practical advise on how best to achieve this. A special circumstance of discontinuation is when a patient attempts to cut down or discontinue medication without the benefit of medical advice and gets into difficulties with seizures without acknowledging the experiment. Probably there are as many patient- as doctor-initiated attempts at discontinuation. Physicians may prevent some of this insidious noncompliance by reviewing periodically the need for medications with the patient.

Blume identifies the circumstances under which seizures prove refractory to treatment and provides a detailed, comprehensive, and systematized approach to the management of therapeutically unresponsive seizure disorders. Sometimes the distress and drama associated with recurrent seizures compel action and *leave less time for thought. When all else fails, retake the history and rethink the problem.*

Patients refractory to the medical management of their seizures were the classic candidates for epilepsy surgery. Girvin argues convincingly that surgery should be considered earlier, and he highlights some of the changes in understanding and thinking that underlie the trend toward more frequently surgery. A problem with evaluating surgical results is that surgery is carried out at only a few highly specialized centers, after perceived failure of more conventional management and after inordinately long waiting periods, so that not only the patients but the physicians acquire tremendous expectations. All these factors create selection biases and difficulties with objective evaluation. Girvin calls for some standardization to allow for comparison of results among centers. Perhaps the suggestion should go a step further: for defined categories of patients, surgery should be undertaken only in the context of a randomized, clinical trial. This could provide proof for the benefits of an approach that at the moment thrives on a strong rationale and encouraging results.

VCH

CHAPTER 7

• •

PSYCHOGENIC SEIZURES

Thomas H. Burnstine, M.D. and Ronald P. Lesser, M.D.

Absence of proof is no proof of absence. This is the quandary posed by some patients with obvious nonorganic seizures, in whom doubt remains as to whether in addition they may also have epileptic seizures.

Pseudoseizures are a well-recognized phenomenon among Siberian shamans and members of certain religious sects, who believe themselves possessed by spirits. The setting of clinical pseudoseizures is often different, but the results are similar: bringing attention to the individual.

The diagnosis and management of pseudoseizures demand of physicians the best that they can deliver in the art and science of medicine, the empathy to gain the patient's confidence, and the expertise to justify it.

VCH

Psychogenic seizures are episodic patterns of behavior that may be thought to be due to epilepsy by the patient, family or friends, or medical personnel. Actually, however, they are of emotional origin and are not accompanied by the paroxysmal cerebral depolarization known to accompany epileptic seizures. They must be differentiated from other episodic disorders, both psychiatric and nonpsychiatric, and proper treatment initiated. It is important to recognize that psychogenic seizures and epileptic seizures may or may not coexist within an individual.[21,22]

DIAGNOSIS

Clinical Manifestations

The differentiation of epileptic from psychogenic seizures begins with observing the behavioral manifestations of the episode or obtaining a detailed description from witnesses. The clinical presentations of psy-

chogenic seizures are quite varied, although often stereotyped in an individual patient.[11] Because psychogenic seizures may resemble epileptic seizures, differentiation can be difficult even for experienced observers.[18,21] Several features, however, can help to distinguish the two disorders (Table 7–1).

Psychogenic seizures can begin gradually, a feature that may help to distinguish them from epileptic attacks. As with epilepsy, patients with psychogenic seizures might have an increased number of episodes associated with stress[16,27] or precipitated by various sensory stimuli.[27]

Common subjective phenomena at onset include palpitations, malaise, choking, dizziness, pain,[11] and peripheral sensory disturbances.[27] Olfactory, gustatory, and visual phenomenology have also been described.[11,27]

The motor manifestations of psychogenic seizures are varied, and some only superficially resemble those seen in epilepsy. Findings include side-to-side movements of the

TABLE 7–1. **FEATURES USEFUL FOR DIFFERENTIATING BETWEEN EPILEPTIC AND PSYCHOGENIC SEIZURES**

	Epileptic Seizure	*Psychogenic Seizure*
Exciting cause	Rare	Often emotional disturbance, sometimes other environmental factors
In sleep or when alone	Common	Sometimes reported by patients
Onset	Usually relatively short	Can be short but often gradual, over several minutes
Aura	Any, but particularly special senses; unilateral sensory or motor or epigastric	Palpitations, malaise, choking, dizziness, acral paresthesias, altered mental status May be similar to epilepsy
Cry	At onset	During ictus, quasi-volitional
Talking	With complex partial seizures, often unintelligible	Occasional. Often unintelligible
Movement	Rarely, tonic alone. If bilateral tonic or clonic, synchronus	Rigidity may be opisthotonic. Quasi-clonic movements often asynchronous, flailing, thrashing, quivering. Side-to-side movements of head, body. Pelvic thrushing
Injury	Often, especially to tongue. Directed violence rare	Sometimes, may bite lips, hands, sustain bruises, lacerations. Directed violence not unusual
Restraint	To prevent accident	To control violence and prevent accident
Consciousness	Loss of consciousness with generalized tonic-clonic seizures, profound confusion or complete unresponsiveness/unconsciousness with complex partial seizures, maintained consciousness with simple partial seizures	Often poorly responsive
Avoidance testing	No response with generalized tonic-clonic seizures, may respond post-ictally or during complex partial seizures	Often react, including by terminating episode
Micturition	Frequent	Sometimes
Defecation	Occasional	Reported
Duration	Usually a few minutes	Some similar to epilepsy. Others much longer
Termination	Usually over a relatively short period. Differentiation of ictal from postictal phrase of complex partial seizures may be difficult at times without EEG	May be similar to epilepsy or very gradual
Ictal epileptiform EEG abnormality	Usual	Never

Source: Lesser,[21] p. 274, with permission.

head and body[8]; out-of-phase clonic activity[8,11]; forward pelvic motions[8,11]; trembling[27]; quivering and thrashing of the extremities[20]; atonic,[11,27] hypertonic,[8,11] and opisthotonic[8,11] postures; vocalizations such as screams, cries, grunts, and sobs,[11] as well as more complex speech[34]; and eye movement such as upward deviation, convergence,[11] and quivering of eyelids.[8]

Decreased responsiveness,[7,8,11] as well as purposeful or semipurposeful directed or nondirected motor activity are commonly seen.[8,11,18] There may be self-injury and aggression toward others.[11] By comparison, directed aggression is very rare in epileptic seizures.[38,39] However, such violence may occur in a variety of psychiatric illnesses,[12,41] and violent, although nonpurposeful and nondirected, behaviors may occur in other conditions, such as certain sleep disorders.[30] Each of these, if suspected, should be diagnosed separately.

Various autonomic[11,36] and alimentary[7,8,11] changes have been documented during psychogenic seizures, including cardiorespiratory changes, choking, hyperventilation, coughing, increased salivation, swallowing, chewing, licking, and lip-smacking. The pupils may dilate during a psychogenic seizure, probably due to increased sympathetic nervous system activity during the episode. Riley and Brannon[34] commented that both urinary and fecal incontinence may occur.

The duration of psychogenic seizures is often similar to that of epileptic seizures.[8,18] However, just as epileptic seizures may be prolonged, so may psychogenic seizures. Consequently, psychogenic seizures have been misdiagnosed and treated as status epilepticus.[19,24,35]

Psychogenic seizures end gradually more often than abruptly.[11] Postictal confusion or lethargy may be described, although this was found only in a minority of patients in one study.[27]

The social, interactive origin of many emotionally based symptom complexes, such as psychogenic seizures, would lead to the prediction that most would occur in the presence of other people. As with any conversion symptom, however, one cannot exclude the possibility of an occurrence while the patient is alone. Patients sometimes report episodes during sleep, but, in our experience, electroencephalographic (EEG) recording has revealed arousal followed by the episode.

Psychologic Aids to Diagnosis

Some psychologic techniques may be useful for diagnostic purposes. Suggestion often can be used to induce or abort a psychogenic seizure, but it rarely has this effect on epileptic seizures. A variety of techniques have been used, including verbal suggestion[27,32]; visual stimulation such as flickering and stroboscopic light[27]; and intravenous saline administration.[3,22,27]

Avoidance testing, such as resistance to eye opening and to dropping of the hand on the face, may be used.[16] The rationale is that a truly unconscious patient would not resist these actions, but a patient undergoing a psychogenic seizure would resist or terminate the episode. However, an epileptic patient could react to such maneuvers during a complex partial seizure or a postictal confusion state, whereas not all of those with psychogenic seizures will react in the manner described to such procedures, even if they are painful.[21,25] Such criteria are, at best, strongly suggestive.

The physician must be sure that any episode that occurs duplicates those that the patient has previously experienced. Also, the manifestations of epileptic seizures may be very unusual, easily mistaken for pseudoepilepsy, and may occur during attempts to induce psychogenic seizures. For example, one patient[23] had bilateral ictal sensory phenomena, including during a saline induction protocol. The episodes were clearly epileptic, as evidenced by left "temporal" ictal EEG patterns that never occurred interictally. These episodes were most likely due to seizures originating in the second sensory area.

Differential Diagnosis

The differential diagnosis of psychogenic seizures includes epilepsy and all other forms of pseudoepilepsy, such as syncope (including hyperventilation syndrome) intoxications, metabolic derangements/delirium, transient ischemic attacks, migraine, and sleep disorders. We and others[31] have found that episodes due to hyperventilation syndrome are often thought to be due to epilepsy. Many symptoms of hyperventilation are similar to the subjective phenomena previously described for psychogenic seizures,[4,28] and the two conditions probably overlap in some cases. The patients are usually unaware that they are overbreathing. However, because the symptoms and signs easily will be reproduced by having the patient overbreathe, all patients with suspected psychogenic seizures should undergo 4 to 5 minutes of vigorous hyperventilation unless this is contraindicated by other medical conditions.

Ancillary Testing Procedures

The difficulty of differentiating some psychogenic versus epileptic seizures on clinical grounds underscores the important supportive role of ancillary testing procedures, of which EEG is the most important. Almost all recent reports have used EEG recording to document the nature of questionable seizures.[21] Prolonged inpatient monitoring, using combined video/EEG analysis, may be necessary for proper diagnosis in some cases.[43]

When assessing either ictal or interictal records, it is important to realize that only unequivocal epileptiform activity, including spikes, polyspikes, sharp waves, and spike-and-slow-wave complexes, may be used to support the diagnosis of epilepsy. Several normal variants may be confused with epileptiform patterns, including wicket spikes, fourteen- and six-per-second spikes and sharp waves, six-per-second spike-and-wave pattern, benign epileptiform transients of sleep or small sharp spikes, hyperventilation effects, hypnagogic and hypnopompic hypersynchrony, and subclinical rhythmic electroencephalographic discharges of adults.[21,17]

Interictal epileptiform activity is very rare in patients who do not have epilepsy,[47] except for relatives of patients with primary generalized epilepsy[14] or benign focal epilepsy of childhood.[26] The presence of such activity, however, does not exclude the possibility of psychogenic seizures.

Conversely, the absence of abnormalities on an EEG does not always rule out the possibility that an episode was epileptic in origin. Many focal seizures, especially if they do not alter consciousness (e.g., simple partial seizures), will not alter the EEG as recorded by routine scalp electrodes.[6] However, added noninvasive electrodes may increase the diagnostic yield of the test in this setting.[1] Furthermore, the presence of abnormalities does not always rule out the possibility that an episode was psychogenic. Paroxysmal EEG activity, which may be mistakenly thought to be epileptic in nature, may be mimicked by artifacts such as rhythmic shaking of the EEG electrodes or the electrode board ("head box"). Video analysis may be necessary to confirm the nonepileptic nature of such findings.[2] Moreover, there are many causes of slowing on an EEG that are not epileptic. Such nonepileptic slowing has occasionally accompanied psychogenic seizures.[29]

Because an EEG may not be available at the time of a seizure, there has long been interest in the possibility of documenting the occurrence of an epileptic attack on the basis of biochemical tests. Serum prolactin levels have been found to increase immediately after epileptic, but not psychogenic, seizures.[40] However, postictal serum prolactin elevations do not occur after all seizures, especially simple partial seizures.[46] Therefore an increased serum prolactin concentration may be used to support, but its absence may not always be used to refute, the diagnosis of epilepsy.

ETIOLOGY

Previous descriptions of the underlying psychologic profiles of patients with psychogenic seizures are varied, and no common set of diagnostic criteria has been developed. Often a psychogenic seizure is thought to be a conversion disorder. However, in addition to representing a somatiform disorder, or Briquet's syndrome per se, psychogenic seizures can be manifestations of other diagnostic categories[21] including affective disorders[5,33,37]; personality disorders[13,33,37]; anxiety disorders[9]; schizophrenia[10,37]; and Munchausen's syndrome[35]; as well as other types of episodes with suspected volitional control.[16]

Efforts to detect a pattern of neuropsychologic and emotional deficits in patients with psychogenic seizures that would reliably distinguish them from those with epilepsy have yielded mixed results. Recent studies have tried to use the Minnesota Multiphasic Personality Inventory (MMPI) to reliably differentiate the two groups. Studies have[15,45] and have not[42] found a consistent pattern of MMPI scores. Wilkus and Dodrill[44] suggested that this discrepancy was due to differences among the types of psychogenic seizure patients studied: Those with either significant affectual expression or little motor activity had MMPI scores that differed from patients with partial seizures, whereas psychogenic seizure patients with either little affectual expression or prominent motor activity had MMPI scores that did not differ from those of epileptic patients with generalized seizures.

Therefore, a wide spectrum of patients

may develop psychogenic seizures. These episodes may be conversion symptoms, which are unconsciously generated and reactive, or they may be part of a conscious effort by patients to manipulate the environment around them.

TREATMENT

Because of the heterogeneity of factors associated with the occurrence of psychogenic seizures, it is likely that a variety of approaches would be helpful, even for patients with similar underlying etiologies.

We have found that a useful initial approach following diagnosis is a counseling session. First we outline the differential diagnosis of seizures. We state that there are many different types of seizures; some are due to epilepsy, but some are not. Then we explain that some or all (depending on the case) of the patient's seizures are psychogenic in origin. We begin to explore the reasons for these physical manifestations and discuss treatment options. It is important that the health professionals involved maintain a sympathetic and nonjudgmental atmosphere: the best interests of the patients will be served by allowing them to save face. We have been surprised at how often patients or their families are accepting of this diagnosis when presented in this manner. They also may begin to discuss previous psychologic trauma that they now realize is pertinent to their problem.[35a] Patients without epilepsy can discontinue their anticonvulsant medications. Subsequent treatment may vary and includes behavioral modification techniques, supportive psychotherapy, milieu-related techniques, and hypnosis.[9,21] However, even some patients who have had no, or very little, psychotherapy may cease having psychogenic seizures once the nature of their episodes is explained to them.[22] Therefore, even strategies of very limited scope may be successful in individual cases.

EPIDEMIOLOGY

In a patient with psychogenic seizures, a frequent issue is whether epilepsy coexists, requiring anticonvulsant therapy. A recent literature review found that the two disorders definitely coexisted in 12% of patients with psychogenic seizures and possibly coexisted in another 24%.[21] Furthermore, epilepsy was well controlled or had been present only in the past in some of these patients. Therefore epilepsy does not have to accompany psychogenic seizures, but it may be present in some patients. If two diagnoses are suspected, they both should be confirmed whenever possible. This has important treatment implications: up to 22% of patients with psychogenic seizures have been found to experience toxicity on anticonvulsant drugs[19]; and respiratory arrest has occurred due to treatment of psychogenic status epilepticus.[24]

The sex and age distribution of patients with psychogenic seizures reflects that of conversion symptoms in general. About three fourths of the cases occur in women.[21] It has been reported in all age groups, with a range of from 4 years[7] to 73 years of age.[21] Most commonly, patients are in their third or fourth decade of life.[21]

CONCLUSION

Psychogenic seizures are one form of pseudoepilepsy. Their characteristics allow presumptive clinical diagnosis in some cases, but in most, ancillary testing is required to define the etiology of the episode and demonstrate or disprove the existence of epilepsy. Once psychogenic seizures have been diagnosed, a variety of methods may help in treating the disorder, but a nonjudgmental and supportive approach to the patient is the important first therapeutic step.

REFERENCES

1. Bare, M, Burnstine, T, Lesser, R, Fisher, R, Vining, E, Cole, A, and Kaplan, P: Electroencephalographic changes during simple partial seizures. Epilepsia 30:643–644, 1989.
2. Burnstine, TH, Lesser, RP, and Cole, AJ: Synchronized video and EEG analysis is needed to differentiate psychogenic from epileptic seizures. J Epilepsy 1991, in press.
3. Cohen, RJ and Suter, C: Hysterical "seizures": Suggestion as a provocative EEG test. Ann Neurol 11:391–395, 1982.
4. Compernolle, T, Hoogduin, K, and Joele, J: Diagnosis and treatment of the hyperventilation

syndrome. Psychosomatics 20:612–625, 1979.

5. Desai, BT, Porter, RJ, and Penry, JK: Psychogenic seizures: A study of 42 attacks in six patients, with intensive monitoring. Arch Neurol 39:202–209, 1982.

6. Devinsky, O, Kelley, K, Porter, RJ, and Theodore, WH: Clinical and electroencephalograhic features of simple partial seizures. Neurology 38:1347–1352, 1988.

7. Finlayson, RE, and Lucas, AR: Pseudoepileptic seizures in children and adolescents. Mayo Clin Proc 54:83–87, 1979.

8. Gates, JR, Ramani, V, Whalen, S, and Loewenson, R: Ictal characteristics of pseudoseizures. Arch Neurol 42:1183–1187, 1985.

9. Goodyer, IM: Epileptic and pseudoepileptic seizures in childhood and adolescence. J Am Acad Child Adolesc Psychiatry 24:3–9, 1985.

10. Gross, M: Pseudoepilepsy: A study in adolescent hysteria. Am J Psychiatry 136:210–213, 1979.

11. Gulick, TA, Spinks, RP, and King, DW: Pseudoseizures: Ictal phenomena. Neurology 32:24–30, 1982.

12. Gumnit, RJ: Behavior disorders related to epilepsy. In Gotman, J, Ives, JR, and Gloor, P (eds): Long Term Monitoring in Epilepsy (EEG Suppl 37). Elsevier, New York, 1985, pp 313–323.

13. Gumnit, RJ and Gates, JR: Psychogenic seizures. Epilepsia (Suppl 2) 27:S124–S129, 1986.

14. Hauser, WA and Anderson, VE: Genetics of epilepsy. In Pedley, TA and Meldrum, BS (eds): Recent Advances in Epilepsy, Vol 3. Churchill Livingstone, New York, 1986, pp 273–296.

15. Henrichs, TF, Tucker, DM, Farha, J, and Novelly, RA: MMPI indices in the identification of patients evidencing pseudoseizures. Epilepsia 29:184–187, 1988.

16. Holmes, GL, Sackellares, JC, McKiernan, J, Ragland, M, and Dreifuss, FE: Evaluation of childhood pseudoseizures using EEG telemetry and video monitoring. J Pediatr 97:554–558, 1980.

17. Klass, DW and Westmoreland, BF: Nonepileptogenic epileptiform electroencephalographic activity. Ann Neurol 18:627–635, 1985.

18. King, DW, Gallagher, BB, Murvin, AJ, Smith, DB, Marcus, DJ, Hartlage, LC, Ward, C III: Pseudoseizures: Diagnostic evaluation. Neurology 32:18–23, 1982.

19. Krumholz, A and Niedermeyer, E: Psychogenic seizures: A clinical study with follow-up data. Neurology 33:498–502, 1983.

20. Lennox, WG: Epilepsy and Related Disorders, Vol 1. Little, Brown & Co, Boston, 1960.

21. Lesser, RP: Psychogenic seizures. In Pedley, TA and Meldrum, BS (eds): Recent Advances in Epilepsy, Vol 2. Churchill Livingstone, New York, 1985, pp 273–296.

22. Lesser, RP, Lueders, H, and Dinner, DS: Evidence for epilepsy is rare in patients with psycho-

genic seizures. Neurology 33:502–504, 1983.

23. Lesser, RP, Lueders, H, Conomy, JP, Furlan, AJ, and Dinner, DS: Sensory seizure mimicking a psychogenic seizure. Neurology 33:800–802, 1983.

24. Levitan, M and Bruni, J: Repetitive pseudoseizures incorrectly managed as status epilepticus. Can Med Assoc J 134:1029–1031, 1986.

25. Levy, RS and Jankovic, J: Placebo-induced conversion reaction: A neurobehavioral and EEG study of hysterical aphasia, seizure and coma. J Abnorm Psychol 92:243–249, 1983.

26. Lüders, H, Lesser, RP, Dinner, DS, and Morris, HH III: Benign focal epilepsy of childhood. In Lüders, H and Lesser, RP (eds): Epilepsy: Electroclinical Syndromes. Springer-Verlag, New York, 1987, pp 303–346.

27. Luther, JS, McNamara, JO, Carwile, S, Miller, P, and Hope, V: Pseudoepileptic seizures: Methods and video analysis to aid diagnosis. Ann Neurol 12:458–462, 1982.

28. Missri, JC and Alexander, S: Hyperventilation syndrome. JAMA 240:2093–2096, 1978.

29. Niedermeyer, E, Blumer, D, Holscher, E, and Walker, BA: Classical hysterical seizures facilitated by anticonvulsant toxicity. Psychiatrica Clinic (Basel) 3:71–84, 1970.

30. Parkes, JD: Sleep and Its Disorders. WB Saunders, Philadelphia, 1985, p 209.

31. Perkin, GD, and Joseph, R: Neurological manifestations of the hyperventilation syndrome. J R Soc Med 79:448–450, 1986.

32. Ramani, V and Gumnit, RJ: Management of hysterical seizures in epileptic patients. Arch Neurol 39:78–81, 1982.

33. Ramani, V, Quesney, LF, Olson, D, and Gumnit, RJ: Diagnosis of hysterical seizures in epileptic patients. Am J Psychiatry 137:705–709, 1980.

34. Riley, TL, Brannon, WL Jr: Recognition of pseudoseizures. J Fam Pract 10:213–220, 1980.

35. Savard, G, Andermann, F, Teitelbaum, J, and Lehmann, H: Epileptic Munchausen's syndrome: A form of pseudoseizures distinct from hysteria and malingering. Neurology 38:1628–1629, 1988.

35a. Shen, W, Bowman, ES, and Markand, ON: Presenting the diagnosis of pseudoseizure. Neurology 40:756–759, 1990.

36. Standage, KF: The etiology of hysterial seizures. Can Psychiatric Assoc J 20:67–73, 1975.

37. Stewart, RS, Lovitt, R, and Steward, M: Are hysterical seizures more then hysteria? A research diagnostic criteria, DSM-III, and psychometric analysis. Am J Psychiatry 139:926–929, 1982.

38. Treiman, DM: Epilepsy and violence: Medical and legal issues. Epilepsia (Suppl 2) 27:S77–S104, 1986.

39. Treiman, DM and Delgado-Escueta, AV: Violence and epilepsy: A critical review. In Pedley, TA and Meldrum, BS (eds): Recent Advances in

Epilepsy, Vol 1. Churchill Livingstone, New York, 1983, pp 179–209.

40. Trimble, MR: Serum prolactin in epilepsy and hysteria. Br Med J 2:1682, 1978.

41. Trimble, MR: Neuropsychiatry, Part 2: Differential diagnosis of non-epileptic attacks. In Laidlaw, J, Richens, A, and Oxley, J (eds): A Textbook of Epilepsy, ed 3. Churchill Livingstone, New York, 1988, pp 385–393.

42. Vanderzant, CW, Giordani, B, Berent, S, Dreifuss, FE, and Sackellares, JC: Personality of patients with pseudoseizures. Neurology 36:664–668, 1986.

43. Wada, JA: Differential diagnosis of epilepsy. In Gotman, J, Ives, JR, and Gloor, P (eds): Long-Term Monitoring in Epilepsy (EEG Suppl 37). Elsevier, New York, 1985, pp 285–311.

44. Wilkus, RJ and Dodrill, CB: Factors affecting the outcome of MMPI and neuropsychological assessments of psychogenic and epileptic seizure patients. Epilepsia 30:339–347, 1989.

45. Wilkus, RJ, Dodrill, CB, and Thompson, PM: Intensive EEG monitoring and psychological studies of patients with pseudoepileptic seizures. Epilepsia 25:100–107, 1984.

46. Wylie, E, Lüders, H, MacMillan, JP, and Gupta, M: Serum prolactin levels after epileptic seizures. Neurology 34:1601–1604, 1984.

47. Zivin, L and Ajmone-Marsan, CA: Incidence and prognostic significance of "epileptiform" activity in the EEG of non-epileptic subjects. Brain 91:751–778, 1968.

CHAPTER 8

• •

SELECTION OF ANTIEPILEPTIC DRUG THERAPY

Richard S. McLachlan, M.D., F.R.C.P(C)

Much has happened since Paracelsus prescribed opium for epilepsy, but not enough. Despite the widening repertoire, we still lack drugs that combine high antiepileptic effect with minimal side effects.

McLachlan emphasizes that much thought should be given to the initial choice of drug, that monotherapy should precede polytherapy, and that close monitoring is essential for both.

He points out that there is no proof that magnesium sulfate is any more effective than, or even equal in effect to, more standard antiepileptic therapy. The continuing widespread use of magnesium sulfate in eclampsia proclaims the triumph of custom over evidence.

VCH

The decision to begin treatment of seizures with antiepileptic drugs is based on first making a diagnosis of epilepsy. There are, of course, exceptions to this rule, as described elsewhere in this text, but in the majority of patients, drug therapy is prescribed when a history of recurrent seizures has been obtained. To begin antiepileptic medication in a patient thus implies a diagnosis of epilepsy, with all of the emotional, psychologic, social, and vocational implications associated with that disorder. Although the diagnosis of epilepsy is seemingly straightforward and indeed obvious in some cases, one must resist the temptation to reach this conclusion too quickly, particularly when sufficient documentation of the patient's spells is unavailable. Once embarked on, the course of treatment is not easy to reverse if the diagnosis proves to be incorrect. With this reservation in mind, the purpose of this chapter is to outline the drug treatment alternatives and to review the factors that should be considered in determining which antiepileptic drug to use once the diagnosis of epilepsy has been established.

AVAILABILITY OF ANTIEPILEPTIC DRUGS

Epilepsy is a relatively common neurologic disorder affecting between 0.5% and 1% of the population, or more than 2.5 million people in North America. Because at some point the majority of individuals so affected seek medical treatment, a number of anticonvulsant, or more appropriately, antiepileptic or antiseizure drugs have been developed and marketed over the years. The current selection provides the physician with more flexibility in treating seizure disorders than has ever before been available.

In 1857 potassium bromide was introduced as the first widely effective anticonvulsant, and it maintained that position until it was eclipsed by phenobarbital in 1912. Notable additions to the treatment of epilepsy since then have been phenytoin in 1938, carbamazepine in 1974, and valproic acid in 1978. Table 8–1 shows the drugs currently approved for the treatment of epilepsy in the United States and Canada,[20] and a number of other compounds have been used with variable efficacy for the treatment of seizures (Table 8–2). Details regarding the pharmacology, toxicity, and clinical use of these medications are available from any pharmacopoeia and from a number of other sources.[1,6,10,11,14,17,18] Additional drugs are available in other countries, where the treatment of epilepsy may be influenced by various unique medical, pharmacologic, social, and economic factors. During the 25 years from 1935 to 1960, 15 new antiepileptic drugs were approved in the United States, compared to only 5 in the next 25 years, reflecting in part the 10 years of development and $100 million in investment currently required before the average new pharmaceutical is licensed for use.

TABLE 8–1. ANTIEPILEPTIC DRUGS IN NORTH AMERICA

Generic Name	Trade Name
Carbamazepine	Tegretol
Clobazam*	Frisium
Clonazepam	Klonopin, Rivotril
Clorazepate†	Tranxene
Ethosuximide	Zarontin
Ethotoin†	Peganone
Mephenytoin	Mesantoin
Mephobarbital‡	Mebaral
Methsuximide*	Celontin
Nitrazepam*	Mogadon
Paramethadione	Paradione
Phenacemide†	Phenurone
Phenobarbital	Luminal
Phensuximide‡	Milontin
Phenytoin	Dilantin
Primidone	Mysoline
Trimethadione‡	Tridione
Valproic acid	Depakine§

* Not licensed in the United States.
† Not licensed in Canada.
‡ Emergency release in Canada.
§ Depakote or Epival as sodium valproate preparation.

TABLE 8–2. OTHER MEDICAL THERAPIES FOR EPILEPSY*

Corticotropin (ACTH)	Amantadine
Corticosteroids	Allopurinal
Medroxyprogesterone	Imipramine
Acetazolamide	Methysergide
Magnesium sulfate	Diazepam†
Vitamin B$_6$	Lorazepam†
Vitamin D	Paraldehyde†
Vitamin E	Lidocaine†
Gamma globulin	Pentobarbital†
Nimodipine	

* Some of these are of questionable use; see text for further description.
† For status epilepticus.

FACTORS DETERMINING CHOICE OF ANTIEPILEPTIC DRUG

Satisfactory control of seizures can be obtained with medication in the majority of patients with epilepsy, in most cases relatively easily but in some individuals only after a number of changes in anticonvulsant drug selection and adjustments in dosage have been made. A rational plan for drug management individualized for each patient should therefore be devised based on the factors outlined in Table 8–3. By tailoring the treatment to each patient based on these considerations, the goal of maximum drug efficacy with a minimum of side effects or toxicity can be obtained in even the most difficult-to-control seizure disorders.

TABLE 8–3. FACTORS THAT INFLUENCE CHOICE OF ANTISEIZURE MEDICATION

1. Type of seizure
2. Potential drug side effects
3. Age of patient
4. Sex of patient
5. Pharmacologic properties of drug
6. Cost of medication

Seizure Type

The primary consideration in determining the choice of anticonvulsant is the type of seizure to be treated. The International Classification of Seizures, first proposed in 1969 and later revised in 1981, is now the most widely used guide to distinguish seizures on the basis of their clinical and electroencephalographic (EEG) characteristics.[5] The choice of anticonvulsants based on seizure type has been determined more or less empirically, but the reason for the differences in drug effectiveness may relate chiefly to differences in the underlying pathophysiology of the seizures. In contrast to normal neurons, which discharge action potentials at about 20 Hz, many of the neurons recorded during seizures or interictal EEG spikes fire in bursts of high-frequency discharge in the range of 200 to 900 Hz. Both this burst activity and EEG spikes and seizures result from a large depolarization of neuronal membranes, called a depolarizing shift, which occurs synchronously in thousands of neurons. There is evidence that this depolarizing shift can result from a decrease in inhibitory synaptic activity involving mainly gamma-aminobutyric acid (GABA), an increase in synaptic drive involving excitatory amino acids such as glutamate, or an endogenous defect in neuronal membrane function involving calcium and other ion channels.[7] The specific pharmacological effects of anticonvulsant drugs at the cellular level are only partially understood, but there is considerable evidence that they suppress or counteract these various abnormal mechanisms, with the emphasis of effect determined by the choice of drug.[15]

A potential scheme for antiepileptic drug selection based on seizure type, including some epilepsy syndromes with characteristic seizures, is illustrated in Table 8–4. It should be recognized that such a protocol is far from rigid and must take into consideration the other factors discussed below. In addition, the empirical biases of physicians who treat many patients with epilepsy will influence their choice of medication. Only the drugs of first choice are indicated, as the possibilities for alternative treatment are even more variable and are therefore less amenable to wide generalization.

TABLE 8–4. ANTIEPILEPTIC DRUG OF CHOICE BASED ON SEIZURE TYPE AND IN SOME EPILEPSY SYNDROMES

Generalized Seizures

Tonic-clonic	CBZ = PHT = VPA
Absence	ESM = VPA
Myoclonic, tonic, atonic	VPA
Multiple types	VPA

Partial Seizures

Simple or complex	CBZ = PHT
Secondarily generalized	CBZ = PHT

Syndromes

Febrile convulsions	PB = VPA
Infantile spasms	COR = NZM
Lennox-Gastaut syndrome	VPA
Myoclonic epilepsy of Janz	VPA
Benign rolandic epilepsy	CBZ = PHT

Abbreviations: CBZ = carbamazepine; COR = corticosteroids/corticotropin; ESM = ethosuximide; NTM = nitrazepam; PHT = phenytoin; PB = phenobarbital; VPA = valproic acid.

Side Effects

Because several drugs may be effective in controlling a certain seizure type, a second important consideration in the choice of treatment is the potential for drug toxicity. For example, carbamazepine, phenytoin, phenobarbital, primidone, and valproic acid are all effective in the treatment of generalized seizures but differ in the frequency and intensity of side effects.[12,16] Bromide therapy can be very effective for the treatment of epilepsy, but it is seldom used because toxicity is more severe and more frequent than with other antiepileptic drugs. Such a narrow therapeutic index also accounts for the limited use of some other drugs, such as trimethadione. Side effects increase when more than one drug is used, occurring in 20% to 30% of patients on monotherapy, 30% to 40% on two antiepileptic drugs, and 40% to 50% on three or more.[4] Of the most commonly used anticonvulsants, carbamazepine and valproic acid have the lowest incidence of overall side effects.

Age

The choice of antiepileptic drug, and particularly adjustments in dosage, will be influenced by the age of the patient. Because many aspects of drug metabolism are age-related, especially in the first decade, considerable variation in the pharmacokinetics of antiepileptic drugs can occur, depending on the age of the patient. In contrast to the first weeks of life, when the half-lives of most anticonvulsants are prolonged, young children aged 1 to 10 years require comparatively higher doses because they have a high metabolic rate. During adolescence, the half-lives again increase. Furthermore, because greater individual variability in the toxicity of antiepileptic drugs occurs during childhood, flexibility in the approach to the treatment of seizures in young patients is essential. For example, phenobarbital, a widely used anticonvulsant in children, can be well tolerated but may also result in sedation or irritability in up to 50% of patients. Similarly, valproic acid monotherapy is usually very well tolerated in children, but it is associated with more than five times the risk of fatal hepatotoxicity in children less than 2 years of age, compared with those older than 2 years.[9] Similar problems with greater toxicity can emerge in patients over age 60 as well; these patients often have difficulty with cognitive and sedative side effects even at low doses of anticonvulsants, including such drugs as carbamazepine and valproic acid.

Sex

The findings of some published studies that cite a very high incidence of complications and developmental abnormalities with the use of antiepileptic drugs during pregnancy are contrary to the experience of most physicians who prescribe these medications. However, women of childbearing age who may use anticonvulsants during the first trimester of pregnancy should be apprised of the possible twofold to threefold increase in the risk of certain congenital malformations, with an overall incidence of 5% to 10%.[23] Low-dose monotherapy probably reduces the risk. Because valproic acid and possibly carbamazepine appear to increase the risk of spina bifida, it is recommended that women on these drugs who become pregnant should have amniocentesis and alpha-fetoprotein levels assessed. Although small amounts of anticonvulsants may be found in breast milk, breast-feeding is not contraindicated if the baby is well. Young women, particularly adolescents, do not appreciate the acne, hirsutism, and coarsening of facial features that can appear with phenytoin. It should therefore not be used as a drug of first choice in young women. There is suggestive evidence that anticonvulsant medication may interfere with the effectiveness of the birth control pill and vice versa, but any such interaction is small and should not be a reason to deny use of this form of contraception.

Pharmacologic Properties

The pharmacologic properties of antiepileptic drugs can at times influence the selection of treatment. For example, the nonlinear zero-order kinetics of phenytoin near or within its therapeutic range can result in much confusion in the use of this drug (Fig. 8-1). It is very easy to move from a subtherapeutic level to clinical intoxication by dose changes of only 50 to 100 mg/d if the patient is on the steep part of the dose-response curve. In addition, there is considerable variability among individuals in the pharmacokinetics of phenytoin. Occasionally patients who are slow metabolizers, despite being maintained at a constant dose, will have a gradual increase in phenytoin blood levels over several months until they become toxic. In contrast, some patients either metabolize phenytoin very rapidly or do not absorb it and therefore require a daily dose of 600 to 700 mg or higher to maintain adequate blood levels. These potential problems might be enough to suggest the selection of another antiepileptic drug in certain patients. On the other hand, because of its longer half-life in comparison to a drug such as carbamazepine, phenytoin can be given as a single daily dose, which is an advantage for some patients. Phenobarbital has the longest half-life of all the anticonvulsants, which makes it a good choice for non-

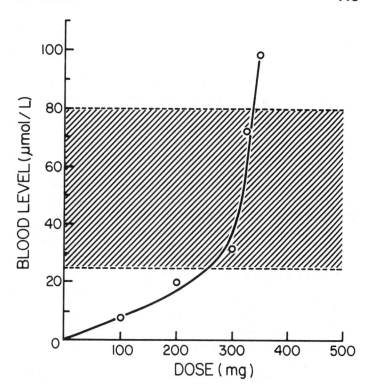

FIGURE 8-1. Relationship between phenytoin blood level and daily dosage. Serum concentrations of phenytoin for five different daily doses in a single patient are illustrated. Note the exponential increase in blood levels as the dose increases. Since the steep part of the curve occurs within the therapeutic range (*shaded area*), a small change in dosage of 25 mg/d determined the difference between seizure control with a high therapeutic level and drug toxicity.

compliant patients who either forget or refuse to take their medications for brief periods. These patients are less likely to experience withdrawal seizures when they do not take phenobarbital than with drugs that have shorter half-lives.

Slight differences in the pharmacologic properties of generic preparations, particularly involving bioavailability related to more rapid absorption, may be reflected in poorer seizure control or increased side effects. Patients who are sensitive to the side effects of medication or who have a difficult-to-control seizure disorder may experience fewer problems with a proprietary or trade name preparation. As already discussed, greater individual variability exists in the pharmokinetics of many drugs in children, which necessitates closer monitoring of blood levels.[8]

Cost

The expense of anticonvulsant medication can be a burden for patients who are not covered by a private or government-spon-

sored drug plan. There is a considerable range in the price of anticonvulsants, with the more recently introduced drugs costing many times more than cheaper preparations such as phenobarbital. The proprietary anticonvulsants are also more expensive, and this should be pointed out to individuals who pay for their own drugs. Although the cost of a medication is not a determining factor in the choice of anticonvulsants for the majority of patients, who are willing to pay more if the treatment is effective, there are some individuals for whom a less expensive drug such as phenobarbital is prescribed purely for financial reasons.

MONOTHERAPY VERSUS POLYPHARMACY

The initial management of a patient with epilepsy should always be based on the use of a single anticonvulsant: the majority of patients require only one drug to control seizures, the side effects are minimized, drug interactions are eliminated, compliance is better, and the cost is less than with polypharmacy.[19] Even if the patient has more than one type of seizure, the goal should be to achieve control using a single antiepileptic drug. If the drug of first choice fails, then monotherapy should be continued by switching to a second drug and discontinuing the first, rather than adding to the initial treatment. Only when monotherapy with several anticonvulsants has failed should polypharmacy be considered. Less than one fourth of the patients uncontrolled with monotherapy will achieve improved seizure control when a second drug is added, and this is often at the expense of greater side effects.[21] Conversely, a reduction in the number of anticonvulsants in patients already on polypharmacy may not only reduce toxicity but also effect improved seizure control by removing adverse drug interactions and by increasing compliance. However, excessive zeal in the quest for monotherapy should be avoided, because there are clearly some patients who do require two or more anticonvulsants to maintain acceptable seizure control.

MONITORING ANTIEPILEPTIC DRUG THERAPY

The widespread availability of therapeutic anticonvulsant blood level monitoring has contributed considerably to the successful pharmacologic management of epilepsy.[13,22] Although the majority of patients take a single drug and have no further seizures or major side effects, the 20% to 30% whose seizures are not controlled, who have side effects, or who are receiving multiple drugs can pose a difficult management problem. Serum levels of anticonvulsants that can be expressed in either total or free (non–protein bound) components allow more precise dosage adjustments in these cases. The blood level, however, is only a guide for treatment, and one should remember that the therapeutic range is an empirically derived mean for a group of patients. Therefore, the therapeutic levels of individual patients may lie outside this mean range. Furthermore, serum levels do not take into account the possible anticonvulsant effects of some of the metabolites of antiepileptic drugs. The clinical state of the

patient—whether he is having seizures or side effects—is thus the major determinant of any changes to be made in anticonvulsant therapy, with blood levels acting only as a guide to the type and magnitude of these changes.[3] If (1) seizures are controlled, (2) there are no side effects, and (3) compliance is not a problem, then routine monitoring of anticonvulsant blood levels is not required, apart from a single baseline level one month after the initiation of therapy in case subsequent problems develop. If that baseline level is above or below the average therapeutic range and the patient is doing well, an alteration in dose is not necessarily required. Other indications for monitoring, apart from uncontrolled seizures and drug toxicity, are unexplained illness, pregnancy, and changes in the dose or type of medication (including non-anticonvulsants). Phenytoin will be monitored more frequently than other antiepileptic drugs because of its nonlinear kinetics and the good correlation of serum levels with toxicity and seizure control. Serum levels of valproic acid, on the other hand, correlate relatively poorly with seizure control, as can those of drugs with short half-lives if early-morning trough levels are not obtained.

Another commonly used method of monitoring anticonvulsant therapy is that of routine screening for hematologic, hepatic, and renal toxic reactions. Repeated routine testing of this type is not necessary.[17a] The value of such monitoring in predicting these rare but serious complications is questionable, and reliance on normal results may provide false reassurance in some cases. The asymptomatic elevation in liver function tests, mild leukopenia, or thrombocytopenia that can occur with a number of antiepileptic drugs can also be misleading. In addition, the practical difficulties of drawing blood routinely, particularly in children, and the cumulative cost of such screening do not favor this approach. An alternative to routine screening is to inform patients of the possible adverse reactions; to carry out baseline complete blood count, platelet count, and liver and renal function tests prior to instituting therapy; and, most importantly, to advise the patient to seek medical attention immediately for any unusual or unexpected symptoms.[2] It is acknowledged that this approach, although in the best interest of patients in general, may not be in the best interest of the physician working under the constraints of a litigious society.

PRINCIPAL ANTIEPILEPTIC DRUGS

Most patients with seizures can be satisfactorily controlled using one of only three anticonvulsants: carbamazepine, phenytoin, or valproic acid. One of these drugs will therefore be the initial treatment of choice in the majority of patients. Phenobarbital and ethosuximide are often the drugs of choice in children under 10 years of age, although valproic acid is gradually emerging as the favored initial therapy in many of these cases as physicians become more familiar with it. Table 8–5 illustrates typical doses of those drugs generally used in adults and children, and it provides the therapeutic ranges for blood levels. Because the latter may vary somewhat, depending on the method used for determination of the levels, individual laboratories should provide their own values. If treatment with these medications proves ineffective, then one of the benzodiazepines, primidone, mephobarbital, mephenytoin, phensuximide, or methsuximide could be tried. The use of combination preparations such as phenytoin plus mephobarbital (Mebroin), or phenytoin plus phenobarbital plus methamphetamine (Phelantin) is not recommended.

Following are some comments about each of the commonly used antiepileptic drugs. Anyone not familiar with these medications should obtain more complete information from a pharmacopeia or other source before prescribing these drugs to patients. Parenteral therapy and the treatment of status epilepticus are not discussed in this chapter.

Carbamazepine

This is the drug of choice for both partial and generalized tonic-clonic seizures in female and in most male patients, because it avoids the cosmetic effects of phenytoin and generally is associated with low toxicity. Diplopia, ataxia, and headache are common features of overmedication with carbamazepine, and the drug can have an antidiuretic effect, resulting in fluid retention. Some patients will experience lethargy and other side effects with the initiation of therapy, but this usually can be overcome by starting with a low dose of 100 to 200 mg and working up to the full therapeutic dose over 1 or 2 weeks. Because carbamazepine produces autoinduction of its own metabolism, a paradoxic fall in blood levels often occurs as the dose is increased, with an associated reduction in the potential for side effects. There has been an overreaction to the risk of aplastic anemia and hepatitis, both of which are rare and probably no more common than with other anticonvulsants. For reasons stated above, the frequent blood sampling recommended by the pharmaceutical companies for patients taking carbamazepine is excessive. Elevated liver enzymes or lowered white blood cell count may occur but is not usually clinically significant. A recently introduced slow release formulation of carbamazepine provides less fluctuation in

TABLE 8–5. **DAILY DOSE OF COMMONLY PRESCRIBED ANTICONVULSANTS**

	ADULT		CHILD	THERAPEUTIC RANGE	
	Dose* (mg)	Range (mg)	(mg/kg)	μmol/L	μg/mL
Carbamazepine	600	400–1200	10–30	15–50	4–12
Phenytoin	300	200–400	5–10	25–80	10–20
Valproic acid	1500	750–3000	15–60	350–700	50–100
Phenobarbital	120	30–240	3–7	65–170	10–40
Primidone	750	500–1500	10–20	15–55	5–12
Ethosuximide	750	500–1500	15–30	300–750	40–100

* This is a very general target dose using monotherapy.

blood levels and allows less frequent administration, particularly in patients who do not like to take their medication during school or at work. A drawback to carbamazepine therapy is the lack of a parenteral preparation for use in patients with a tendency for sequential seizures or status epilepticus.

Phenytoin

Phenytoin is very effective in the control of partial seizures and all types of generalized seizures except absence. It is a reliable drug for severe, intractable, generalized tonic-clonic (grand mal) seizures that occur in association with mental retardation. The cosmetic side effects, including gum hypertrophy, hirsutism, and acne, can be troublesome, particularly in young women, and chronic therapy can occasionally result in osteomalacia, mild peripheral neuropathy, or cerebellar degeneration with irreversible gait ataxia. The latter tends to occur in patients who are difficult to control and may in part be related to frequent seizures. Vestibulocerebellar and cognitive dysfunction occur with high serum levels. In the elderly, when used at low doses of 100 to 200 mg (which is often all that is required to control a mild seizure tendency), phenytoin can produce less cognitive dysfunction than does carbamazepine. The availability of phenytoin in capsules, tablets, suspension, and an injectable solution provides flexibility in drug utilization. Intramuscular administration is not recommended because it results in crystallization of the drug at the injection site, with subsequent slow and erratic absorption. Serum level monitoring is particularly important with phenytoin to avoid the problems related to its nonlinear kinetics, discussed above.

Valproic Acid

The serendipitous discovery in 1963 that this carboxylic acid and organic solvent had anticonvulsant properties has led to its current wide acceptance as one of the major antiepileptic drugs. Initially proposed as a facilitator of inhibitory GABA activity, it more likely acts directly on neuronal membranes to reduce excitability. Although it is ap-

proved in North America only for the treatment of absence seizures, it has a broad spectrum of antiepileptic activity against most seizure types and therefore is extensively used for tonic-clonic, myoclonic, and atonic seizures as well. It is useful in patients with more than one seizure type, such as the combination of absence and generalized tonic-clonic convulsions, for which two anticonvulsants are otherwise usually required. Valproic acid is also effective for the treatment of partial seizures, particularly if these progress to secondary generalization, but superior efficacy to other anticonvulsants such as carbamazepine or phenytoin has not been demonstrated.

Toxicity is low, reversible, and generally mild in nature. Gastrointestinal complaints, which are the most common, can largely be abolished by using the enteric coated preparation to prevent gastric irritation. Weight gain, particularly in females, can be a problem, and some patients develop postural tremor, hair loss, and less frequently, lethargy. Hyperammonemia, which occurs in at least 50% of patients, is almost always asymptomatic but rarely can be associated with stupor or coma. This is a separate condition from the well-publicized but rare fatal hepatotoxicity, which has occurred primarily with polytherapy in children less than 2 years of age who have evidence of other neurologic dysfunction in addition to seizures.[9] Pancreatitis is another rare toxic reaction.

A disadvantage of valproic acid therapy is the relatively poor correlation of serum levels with clinical effectiveness compared with other drugs. Its pharmacologic activity can also persist for days to weeks after the drug is cleared from serum. Thus therapeutic monitoring does not predict clinical efficacy as accurately as with other antiepileptic drugs. Drug interactions, with resulting toxicity or increase in seizures, are not uncommon with valproic acid, particularly when combined with a barbiturate or phenytoin.

Barbiturates

Although seldom prescribed as a drug of first choice in adults, phenobarbital is still widely used (more than 75 years after its introduction) as the initial treatment for many seizure disorders in children, particularly in infants. It has broad effectiveness but is primarily used for generalized tonic-clonic seizures in children, as an alternative choice for partial epilepsy that is uncontrolled with other drugs in adults, and in status epilepticus. Studies indicate that cognitive and behavioral alterations in the form of sedation, hyperactivity, and impaired school performance will occur in up to 50% of children, but general experience suggests that most children tolerate the drug well. For this reason and because serious life-threatening toxic reactions are extremely rare, it remains in common use despite the availability of newer anticonvulsants. However, valproic acid is being used with increasing frequency in young patients who previously would have been treated with phenobarbital. A large-scale trial comparing the two drugs in childhood epilepsy would be of value.

Primidone is chemically almost identical to phenobarbital and metabolizes rapidly to phenobarbital and phenylethylmalonamide. Good evidence exists that all three of these components have independent antiepileptic activity,[14] indicating that a failure of phenobarbital to control seizures should not exclude a trial of primidine, which is best used as an alternative choice for uncontrolled generalized tonic-clonic or partial seizures in adults. Although occasional patients appear to achieve better seizure control with mephobarbital (methylphenobarbital), overall it is equal in clinical effect to phenobarbital. Sedation is the most common side effect of the barbiturates in adults, but another distressing and often unreported concern is impotence in men, particularly with the use of primidone. Development of tolerance is not usually a problem, but stopping these drugs after long-term use can be difficult; patients may develop withdrawal symptoms of transient irritability and sleeplessness.

Ethosuximide

Ethosuximide is used almost exclusively as the drug of choice for the treatment of absence seizures in childhood. However,

European physicians in particular favor valproic acid for these patients because, unlike ethosuximide, it provides protection against potential generalized tonic-clonic seizures as well. It has been suggested but never convincingly demonstrated that ethosuximide may precipitate grand mal seizures. Gastrointestinal symptoms, lethargy, and headache are the main dose-related side effects, and rarely an acute psychosis may appear, usually within a few days of starting therapy.

Benzodiazepines

The drugs in this class of antiepileptic compounds are used largely as alternative therapy (clobazam, clonazepam, chlorazepate, nitrazepam) for seizures uncontrolled by other drugs or as initial treatment (diazepam, lorazepam) for status epilepticus. In patients with epilepsy compounded by anxiety, the mood-altering properties of these medications can be used to provide a dual approach to the control of seizures. All seizure types will potentially respond to benzodiazepines, but their use is limited by the common sedative and cognitive side effects and the frequent development of tolerance with breakthrough of seizures, usually after several months of therapy. Drug holidays or alternating treatment with different benzodiazepines may delay the onset of the latter problem. Drooling is a frequent minor but annoying complication in children, particularly with nitrazepam. Although diazepam and lorazepam have shorter half-lives, they may occasionally be used as maintenance therapy or to prevent clusters of repetitive seizures, which occur in some patients. These drugs are, of course, most commonly used for the rapid treatment of status epilepticus.

OTHER MEDICAL TREATMENT

In addition to the commonly used drugs for status epilepticus, Table 8-2 lists a number of other medications that have been used for specific situations or as adjunctive treatment when more standard therapy fails to control seizures. Controversy continues as to whether corticotropin, prednisone, or nitrazepam should be used initially for infantile spasms, with recent comparative studies suggesting that they are all equally effective. Although pyridoxine dependency is a rare cause of seizures, pyridoxine hydrochloride (vitamin B_6) is commonly used as adjunctive therapy for infantile spasms, as well as other seizures of infancy and childhood, with occasional benefit. Both vitamin D and vitamin E have been described as treatment for epilepsy, but their effectiveness has yet to be confirmed. Attempts at hormonal manipulation with drugs such as medroxyprogesterone acetate in patients with catamenial epilepsy seldom result in a significant reduction in seizures. Only slightly more effective in these as well as some other patients with uncontrolled seizures is acetazolamide, which, in rare cases, produces definite improvement when added to existing therapy. Magnesium sulfate remains the mainstay of treatment of seizures in eclampsia by obstetricians, although there is no evidence that it is any more effective than, or even equal in effect to, more standard antiepileptic therapy. The calcium channel blockers nimodipine and flunarizine both have demonstrated antiepileptic properties, but only the former is commercially available. The other medications listed in Table 8–2 have all been described primarily in case reports as potential antiepileptic agents, but their usefulness, if any, has yet to be satisfactorily demonstrated in controlled studies.

FUTURE ANTIEPILEPTIC DRUGS

A large number of promising compounds are currently undergoing rigorous investigation as antiepileptic drugs at various levels, from testing on animal models in the laboratory to controlled trials in epilepsy patients. Increasing cooperation between the pharmaceutical industry, government agencies, and university-based clinical researchers has considerably reinforced the search for new, effective medications. Of the many drugs currently being assessed, some of the most promising are gabapentin, an amino acid related to GABA; lamotrigine, a weak antifolate compound that inhibits the release of excitatory amino acids; vigabatrin, an inhibitor of the GABA catabolic enzyme GABA transaminase; and felbamate, a dicarbamate related to meprobamate. Many of these drugs were developed on the basis of knowledge obtained in the research laboratory about the basic cellular mechanisms involved in the pathophysiology of seizures. Promising new potential antiepileptic drugs are now being developed, based on recent evidence of the involvement of excitatory amino acid neurotransmitters such as glutamate in the initiation and propagation of seizures. In particular, compounds acting to impede the function of the N-methyl-D-aspartate (NMDA) receptor, which mediates postsynaptic excitatory neurotransmission in many areas of the brain, have generated much interest as possible novel antiepileptic agents. The study of neuropeptides as modulators of seizure activity is also being pursued and may yield additional useful anticonvulsants. If the pace of development of new compounds in the laboratory continues, and the interest in carrying out clinical drug trials is maintained, it is quite conceivable that one of these as-yet unproven agents may well become the antiepileptic drug of choice in the near future.

ANNOTATED REFERENCES

1. Aicardi, J: Epilepsy in children. International Review of Child Neurology. Raven Press, New York, 1986, pp 319–340. (*A classic textbook by a single experienced author; anyone who treats seizures in children should have this book.*)
2. Camfield, C, Camfield, P, Smith, E, and Tibbles, JAR: Asymptomatic children with epilepsy: Little benefit from screening for anticonvulsant-induced liver, blood, or renal damage. Neurology 36:838–841, 1986.
3. Chadwick, DW: Overuse of monitoring of blood concentrations of antiepileptic drugs. Br Med J 294:723–724, 1987.
4. Collaborative Group for Epidemiology of Epilepsy: Adverse reactions to antiepileptic drugs: A follow-up study of 355 patients with chronic antiepileptic drug treatment. Epilepsia 29:787–793, 1988.
5. Commission on Classification and Terminology of the International League Against Epilepsy: Proposal for revised clinical and electroencephalographic classification of epileptic seizures. Epilepsia 22:489–501, 1981.

6. Delgado-Escueta, AV, Trieman, DM, and Walsh, GO: The treatable epilepsies (Part II). N Engl J Med 308:1576–1584, 1983.

7. Dichter, MA, and Ayala, GF: Cellular mechanisms of epilepsy: A status report. Science 237:157–164, 1987. (*A brief but comprehensive review of the basic neurophysiology of seizures.*)

8. Dodson, WE: Aspects of antiepileptic treatment in children. Epilepsia (Suppl 3)29:S10–S14, 1988.

9. Dreifuss, FE, Santilli, N, Sweeney, KP, Moline, BA, and Menander, KB: Valproic acid hepatic fatalities: A retrospective review. Neurology 37:379–385, 1987.

10. Eadie, MJ and Tyrer, JH: Anticonvulsant Therapy: Pharmacological Basis and Practice, ed 3. Churchill Livingstone, Edinburgh, 1989. (*The Australian approach to anticonvulsant therapy.*)

11. Engel, J: Seizures and Epilepsy. Contemporary Neurology Series, Vol 31. FA Davis, Philadelphia, 1989, pp 410–442. (*This text covers, in varying depth, virtually every aspect of epileptology; if your library is limited to one book on epilepsy, it should be this one.*)

12. Herranz, L, Armijo, JA, Arteaga, R: Clinical side effects of phenobarbital, primidone, phenytoin, carbamazepine, and valproate during monotherapy in children. Epilepsia 29:794–804, 1988.

13. Kutt, H and Penry, JK: Usefulness of blood levels of antiepileptic drugs. Arch Neurol 31:283–288, 1974.

14. Levy, RH, Dreifuss, FE, Mattson, RH, Meldrum, BS and Penry, JK: Antiepileptic Drugs, ed 3. Raven Press, New York, 1989. (*The most comprehensive book on antiepileptic drugs; an excellent reference text.*)

15. Macdonald, RL and McLean, MJ: Anticonvulsant drugs: Mechanisms of action. In Delgado-Escueta AV, Porter RJ, Ward AA, and Woodbury, DM (eds): Basic mechanisms of the epilepsies, molecular and cellular approaches. Advances in Neurology, Vol 44. Raven Press, New York, 1986, pp 713–736. (*This is only one of the chapters from this reference text, which describes in detail the "current" understanding of the cellular physiology, neuroanatomy, neurochemistry, and molecular biology of epilepsy.*)

16. Mattson, RH, Cramer, JA, Collins, JF, Smith, DB, Delgado-Escueta, AV, Browne, TR, Williamson, PD, Treiman, DM, McNamara, JO, McCutcheon, CB, Homan, RW, Crill, WE, Lubozynski, MF, Rosenthal, NP, and Mayersdorf, A: Comparison of carbamazepine, phenobarbital, phenytoin, and primidone in partial and secondarily generalized tonic-clonic seizures. N Engl J Med 313:145–151, 1985. (*More comparative drug trials of this type are required.*)

17. Morselli, PL, Pippenger, CE, and Penry, JK: Antiepileptic drug therapy in pediatrics. Raven Press, New York, 1983.

17a. Pellock, JM and Willmore, LJ: A rational guide to routine blood monitoring in patients receiving antiepileptic drugs. Neurology 41:961–964, 1991.

18. Reynolds, EH: Drug treatment of epilepsy. Lancet 2:721–725, 1978.

19. Reynolds, EH and Shorvon, SD: Monotherapy or polytherapy for epilepsy. Epilepsia 22:1–10, 1981.

20. Reynolds, JEF (ed): The Extra Pharmacopeia. Pharmaceutical Press, London, 1989, pp 400–415.

21. Schmidt, D: Two antiepileptic drugs for intractable epilepsy with complex-partial seizures. J Neurol Neurosurg Psychiatry 45:1119–1124, 1982.

22. Taylor, WJ and Caviness, MHD: A textbook for the clinical application of therapeutic drug monitoring. Abbott Laboratories, Irving, 1986, pp 207–281.

23. Yerby, MS: Problems and management of the pregnant woman with epilepsy. Epilepsia (suppl 3) 28:S29–S36, 1987.

CHAPTER 9

• •

CAN SEIZURES BE PREVENTED? PROPHYLACTIC USE OF ANTICONVULSANT DRUGS

L. James Willmore, M.D.

Prevention is better than cure, but only if prevention is necessary in the first place. Willmore tackles the vexing question of seizure prophylaxis with emphasis on the nature of the potential epileptogenic process, the likelihood of seizure occurrence, and the systematic review of the indications for prophylactic treatment.

Compliance with medication after a seizure is more likely than when a patient has never experienced one. Thus the difficulties of deciding on prophylaxis are compounded by the lessened likelihood that the prescribed regimen will indeed be followed.

As in so many other fields of neurology, opinions outweigh the evidence. The author's approach is both clear and prudent and can easily accommodate new data.

VCH

Prophylaxis is defined as a process of guarding against the development of a specific disease by a treatment or action that affects pathogenesis. In contrast, *prevention* means to render impossible by an advanced provision, or to keep from happening. A preventive intervention does not imply an effect other than alterations of symptoms, signs, or manifestations of a disease. Prevention may alter some component of a disease, but specificity is not implied, and effect on pathogenesis is not required.

Antiepileptic medications may be administered to patients who are thought to be at risk for tonic-clonic seizures, with the intent to prevent the occurrence of a convulsion. This preventive treatment is often used in selected patients with head trauma of such severity that the hypertension and hypoxia associated with a convulsive seizure would complicate management. Patients with absence seizures may be treated with a broad-spectrum antiepileptic drug prior to occurrence of a tonic-clonic seizure, rather than use a syndrome-specific agent such as ethosuximide. Preventive treatment in these narrow contexts may be successful. However, some patients are given anticonvulsants in an apparent attempt to interfere with the process of epileptogenesis. Examples of this prophylactic use include the routine administration of antiepileptic drugs to patients with head trauma,[17,18] or to patients undergoing neurosurgical procedures requiring incision of the neocortex. Although prevention of seizures is a worthy goal, and may be effective, prophylaxis of epilepsy in the strict sense may not be effective: no data are available to suggest that antiepileptic drug administration has any impact on the process of epileptogenesis. With these definitions in mind, the clinician must decide whether a treatment is preventive or prophylactic for patients with head trauma, stroke, a single seizure, or febrile seizures.

POSTTRAUMATIC EPILEPSY

Injury and Epileptogenesis

Trauma dose, as estimated by factors correlated with severity of head injury, allows a crude prediction of the liability to develop posttraumatic epilepsy (PTE).[4] Classification of head injury based on clinical evidence of severity of trauma reveals a correlation with epilepsy risk.[2] Patients with severe head trauma with cortical injury and neurologic sequelae, but with intact dura mater, have an incidence of epilepsy from 7% to 39%.[2] However, if dural penetration occurred in association with neurologic deficits, then the range of epilepsy incidence was 20% to 57%.[2] Application of weighted risk factors allowing mathematical estimation of liability for development of PTE at the time of injury suggests correlation between severity of injury and subsequent epileptogenesis.[4,29] Brain volume loss reflects trauma intensity and provides a correlation with PTE.[23]

Fifty-seven percent of patients have the first seizure within 1 year of injury.[23] Although specific mechanisms remain unknown, the latency between injury and occurrence of convulsive seizures must represent the process of epileptogenesis. Whether a seizure occurs immediately after injury, within the first week, or beyond the first week may have prognostic significance for development of epilepsy.[7] The occurrence of an immediate seizure, a seizure within hours after trauma, or posttraumatic status epilepticus may complicate management of an injured patient by adding hypoxia and hypertension to the primary processes initiated by trauma. Although an immediate seizure may be a nonspecific reaction, such a symptom may herald the presence of an intracranial hematoma.[7,8] However, if seizures occur within the first week after injury (an early seizure), then an increase in the incidence of late epilepsy has

been observed.[9] Other predictors of risk of late epilepsy include 24 hours of posttraumatic amnesia, the presence of a depressed skull fracture, or an intracranial hematoma.[6]

Prophylaxis of Posttraumatic Epilepsy

Reports of clinical observations indicating efficacy of antiepileptic drugs as prophylactic against the development of posttraumatic epilepsy appeared within a few years of the availability of phenytoin.[18] Rapport and Penry[18] cited reports of observations performed by Hoff and Hoff, by Birkmayer, and by Popek and Musil. These investigators used phenytoin alone or in combination with phenobarbital. Control patients were not treated with anticonvulsant medication. These open studies allowed the investigator to select patients to receive anticonvulsant drugs; blood level measurement was not available. These investigators concluded that prophylactic anticonvulsant administration prevented the development of PTE. Young and colleagues[31] performed an open, prospective, uncontrolled study and reported significant problems with compliance, particularly beyond 1 month of treatment. They compared the observed 6% epilepsy occurrence in their treated group to historical control patients developing posttraumatic seizures and concluded that early administration of anticonvulsant drugs prevented the development of PTE. They recommended prophylactic administration of phenytoin to patients with a 15% or greater risk of developing PTE. Another team[25] treated patients with a combination of phenobarbital and phenytoin. They reported a 25% incidence of PTE in control patients and 2.1% in the treated group. Although blood levels were not measured, this report suggested that remarkably small doses of phenytoin and phenobarbital were effective in preventing PTE.

Rish and Caveness[21] reviewed the incidence of early seizures following head trauma in patients injured in Vietnam. (An early seizure was defined as one occurring during the first 2 days after injury.) They did not detect any difference in early seizure incidence between phenytoin-treated and untreated patients. Wohns and Wyler[30] reviewed records of 62 patients with such severe injury that they were at risk for development of PTE. They selected patients with one or more critical indicators including depressed skull fracture, dural or cortical laceration, or a prolonged period of posttraumatic amnesia. Fifty patients had been treated with phenytoin; 12 patients identified as untreated served as controls. In the phenytoin treatment group, five patients (10%) developed seizures, whereas six patients in the control group (50%) developed seizures. The authors concluded that antiepileptic drug administration prevented the development of PTE. They did, however, identify several problems with their study. The treated and untreated categories contained unequal numbers of patients; retrospective selection of the patients at risk allowed possible bias to enter; and a large number of patients were excluded from the study, raising further questions about selection bias.

Prior reports (Table 9–1) depended on open, uncontrolled, prospective studies, or on retrospective case reviews. Penry and associates[15] administered phenytoin and phenobarbital to head-injured patients in a double-blind fashion, with placebo control.

Their report, in abstract format, indicated a seizure probability of 23% in the treated group, and a probability of 13% in controls. The authors concluded that no significant difference was detected between the treatment and control groups, suggesting that anticonvulsant administration had no effect on the development of PTE in the treated patients.

Young and colleagues[32] reported evidence with 179 head-injured patients treated with phenytoin or with placebo for 18 months in a prospective, double-blind fashion. Patients received loading doses of phenytoin or placebo; anticonvulsant blood levels were measured. Eighty-five patients were included in the treated group; 74 patients were enrolled as placebo control. At the end of the study, seizures had occurred in 12.9% of the treated patients, and in 10.8% of the control patients. Although it appeared that prophylactic anticonvulsant administration did not prevent the development of PTE, the authors recommended that an additional study of patients with phenytoin blood levels maintained at greater than 12 μg/mL was needed before it could be concluded that prophylactic phenytoin is ineffective in preventing posttraumatic epileptogenesis.

Temkin and associates[27] used a double-

TABLE 9–1. **STUDIES ASSESSING THE EFFICACY OF ANTIEPILEPTIC DRUGS AS PROPHYLAXIS OF POSTTRAUMATIC EPILEPSY**

Authors	Drug	PERCENT DEVELOPING EPILEPSY	
		Control	Treated
OPEN STUDIES			
Hoff and Hoff*	Phenytoin	38%	4%
Birkmayer*	Phenytoin	51%	6%
Popek and Musil*	Phenytoin, phenobarbital	21%	0
Young et al[31]	Phenytoin	(1.9%–48%)	6%
Servit and Musil[25]	Phenytoin	25%	2.1%
RETROSPECTIVE STUDIES			
Rish and Caveness[21]	Phenytoin	3.7%	1.6%
Wohns and Wyler[30]	Phenytoin	50%	10%
DOUBLE-BLIND, CONTROLLED STUDIES			
Penry et al[15]	Phenytoin, phenobarbital	13%	23%
Young et al[32]	Phenytoin	10.8%	12.9%
Temkin et al[27]	Phenytoin	15.7%	21.5%

* Cited in Rapport and Penry.[18]

blind, placebo-controlled administration of phenytoin to 404 randomly assigned patients with significant head trauma. Patients received a loading dose intravenously within 24 hours of injury. Monitoring of serum levels was performed on a regular basis for 1 year, with adjustments of phenytoin dose into the therapeutic range. Patients were treated for 1 year and then observed for an additional year.

Following acute drug loading after head injury, only 3.6% of the phenytoin-treated patients had seizures, compared to 14.2% of the placebo patients. However, from the eighth day after injury through the end of the second year, there was no difference in the incidence of seizures between the treated and control groups. Thus, phenytoin appeared to prevent seizures in the time immediately after head trauma, but no prophylactic effect of phenytoin was identified.

ABSENCE EPILEPSY

Patients with absence epilepsy commonly develop generalized convulsive seizures as an additional manifestation of this epilepsy syndrome. Patients with the best prognosis for control of absence seizures have normal intelligence and a negative family history of epilepsy. These patients may have a 90% chance of remission. In contrast, the overall remission rate for all patients with absence epilepsy ranges from 37% to 57%. Patients at high risk for the development of concurrent or subsequent generalized tonic-clonic seizures have late onset of absence epilepsy.[22]

Drugs used for treatment of absence epilepsy include ethosuximide, clonazepam, and valproic acid. Ethosuximide has specific efficacy for nonconvulsive seizures, whereas valproate is effective in controlling both absence and generalized convulsive seizures.[24,28] Ethosuximide used as initial therapy for this seizure syndrome may leave a patient vulnerable to the occurrence of convulsive seizures. Preventive treatment using a broad-spectrum anticonvulsant such as valproic acid would be appropriate for a patient with late-childhood or early-adolescent onset of absence seizures. At the time of writing, there is no published report addressing the specific efficacy of this course of treatment as a preventive for convulsive

seizures, particularly with comparison of ethosuximide and valproate. Clinicians should be aware of the possibility of anticipation and prevention in this context by discussing such problems with parents of patients.

CEREBRAL INFARCTION

Of patients with stroke, 6% to 9% may develop the complication of epilepsy.[10] Precise prediction of development of postinfarction seizures may depend on etiology.[11,20] Not unlike head trauma, a differential liability to develop seizures may depend on acute versus late seizures relative to onset of the infarction.[26] The role of seizures as a so-called precursor to stroke remains controversial.[10] Patients with cerebral infarctions involving the cerebral cortex with persistent paresis have 20% liability to develop seizures.[3] Although the risk of epilepsy following stroke has been recognized, administration of anticonvulsant as a prophylaxis is not a common practice and has not been reported. If medications are to be administered to this group, then specific knowledge of the risks and benefits would be most important before such an action is recommended.

FEBRILE SEIZURES

Children from 3 months to 5 years of age may have convulsive seizures associated with fever or febrile illnesses. Approximately 30% of these patients have an additional febrile seizure; 15% of all with the initial febrile seizure will have a third seizure.[14] Febrile seizures are managed by airway protection, reduction of fever, and, if continuous, the careful use of benzodiazepines, barbiturate, or paraldehyde. Nonfebrile seizures or epilepsy develop in 2% to 6% of patients with febrile seizures.[1,12,13] Risk factors predicting development of epilepsy include the presence of a neurologic abnormality; febrile seizures lasting longer than 15 minutes; a focality to the seizure; recurrent seizures in a single day; onset at less than 1 year of age, but especially during the first 6 months of life; and an immediate family member with epilepsy. Identification of risk factors suggests that fever is a precipitant rather than a cause of epilepsy. Most preventive efforts are directed to the high-risk patients. Management of the acute illness may require pharmacologic interruption of a seizure or prevention of a recurrence during the same febrile illness. Rectal administration of diazepam or valproate is effective, but problems with sedation must be anticipated. Although recurrence can be prevented by chronic use of phenobarbital, behavioral and compliance problems make this approach impractical.[16] Until the issue of epileptogenesis is resolved, chronic prophylactic antiepileptic drug administration should not be used in patients who are without risk factors. Decisions regarding prophylactic drug administration in patients with risk factors for recurrence of febrile seizures or for development of epilepsy must be individualized, insofar as data to guide treatment are not available.

THE SINGLE SEIZURE

The impact of antiepileptic drug therapy on the natural history of the process heralded by a single convulsive seizure is unknown. McLachlan, in Chapter 8, has reviewed the information available and the critical factors involved in deciding when to treat a patient with a single seizure. If the recurrence rate is high, then any risks of antiepileptic drug therapy are justified, and patients should receive chronic preventive treatment. However, if drug administration were to alter the process of epileptogenesis, as signaled by an initial seizure, then prophylactic treatment would be mandatory. None of these admonitions is supported by clinical data.

The risk of recurrence after a single convulsive seizure is 38% to 70%.[5,19] This variability in the reported recurrence occurs because of variation in both the definition of study entry criteria and the pattern of referral and because of possible failure to exclude patients with a history of seizures prior to the observation of the signal seizure. A recurrent seizure will commonly occur within the first 6 months of the initial event. Risk factors for recurrence include a focal seizure, a family history of seizures, a known neurologic injury, an abnormal EEG, and

transient paralysis after the initial seizure. These patients have a recurrence rate of 50% by 3 years after the initial seizure. The recurrence rate at 3 years, in patients without risk factors, is 21.1%.[5] With these data in mind, if a patient has risk factors for recurrence, then treatment should be instituted after an initial seizure. However, if patients are free of risk factors and are willing to anticipate the next seizure, then judicious follow-up may be appropriate. Data to suggest any prophylactic effect in this circumstance do not exist.

CONCLUSIONS

Specific knowledge about the process of epileptogenesis as initiated by trauma, fever, or genetic factors may contain a specific clue about methods of prophylaxis. However, the principal impediment to pharmacologic interruption of the process of epileptogenesis is lack of knowledge of the mechanism that results in the formation or activation of a seizure focus. The clinical problem of a patient with trauma sufficient to initiate epileptogenesis, and with effects of injury that would be worsened by the occurrence of a convulsive seizure, requires practical intervention for protection during his or her acute illness. If an anticonvulsant is to be administered to prevent a seizure after a severe head injury, then that medication should be given intravenously and pharmacologic principles should be followed.

Although literature suggests that prophylactic use of anticonvulsant drugs fails to interrupt epileptogenesis, one question remains. If a therapeutic level of 12 μg/mL or greater is maintained, there may be an effect on the occurrence of a seizure. If phenytoin is used to prevent seizures, then scrupulous attention is required to maintain a therapeutic blood level and to encourage patient compliance. At this time, preventive administration of an anticonvulsant drug should be reserved for the most seriously injured patients in the time immediately following trauma, for patients with absence epilepsy and risk factors associated with development of convulsive seizures, and for patients with a complicated initial convulsive seizure. No evidence is available to suggest that administration of antiepileptic drugs to all head-injured patients will have an impact on the overall incidence of PTE.

REFERENCES

1. Annegers, JF, Hauser, WA, Shirts, SB, and Kurland, LT: Factors prognostic of unprovoked seizures after febrile convulsions. N Engl J Med 316:493–498, 1987.
2. Caveness, WF: Epilepsy, a product of trauma in our time. Epilepsia 17:207–215, 1976.
3. De Carolis, P, D'Alessandro, R, Ferrara, R, Andreoli, A, Sacquegna, T, and Lugaresi, KE: Late seizures in patients with internal carotid and middle cerebral artery occlusive disease following ischaemic events. J Neurol Neurosurg Psychiatry 47:1345–1347, 1984.
4. Feeney, DM and Walker, AE: The prediction of posttraumatic epilepsy. Arch Neurol 36:8–12, 1979.
5. Hauser, WA, Anderson, VE, Loewenson, RB, and McRoberts, SM: Seizure recurrence after a first unprovoked seizure. N Engl J Med 307:522–528, 1982.
6. Jennett, B: Early traumatic epilepsy: Incidence and significance after non-missile injuries. Arch Neurol 30:394–398, 1974.
7. Jennett, B: Epilepsy and acute traumatic intracranial haematoma. J Neurol Neurosurg Psychiatry 38:378–381, 1975.
8. Jennett, B: Epilepsy after nonmissile head injuries. Scott Med J 18:8–13, 1973.
9. Jennett, WB and Lewin, W: Traumatic epilepsy after closed head injuries. J Neurol Neurosurg Psychiatry 23:295–301, 1960.
10. Lesser, RP, Luders, DH, Dinner, KDS, and Morris, HH: Epileptic seizures due to thrombotic and embolic cerebrovascular disease in older patients. Epilepsia 26:622–630, 1985.
11. Louis, S and McDowell, F: Epileptic seizures in non-embolic cerebral infarction. Arch Neurol 17:414–418, 1967.
12. Nelson, KB and Ellenberg, JH: Predictors of epilepsy in children who have experienced febrile seizures. N Engl J Med 295:1029–1033, 1976.
13. Nelson, KB and Ellenberg, JH: Prognosis in children with febrile seizures. Pediatrics 61:720–727, 1978.
14. Nelson, KB and Ellenberg, JH: Febrile sequences. In Dreifuss, FE (ed): Pediatric Epileptology: Classification and Management of Seizures in the Child. John Wright, Boston, 1983, pp 173–198.
15. Penry, JK, White, BG, and Brackett, CE: A controlled prospective study of the pharmacologic prophylaxis of posttraumatic epilepsy. Neurology 29:600–601, 1979.
16. Pilgaard, S, Hanse, FJ, and Paerregaard, P: Prophylaxis against febrile convulsions with phenobarbital: A 3-year prospective investigation. Acta Paediatr Scand 70:67–71, 1981.
17. Rapport, RL and Penry, JK: A survey of attitudes toward the pharmacological prophylaxis of posttraumatic epilepsy. J Neurosurg 38:159–166, 1973.
18. Rapport, RL and Penry, JK: Pharmacologic prophylaxis of post-traumatic epilepsy: A review. Epilepsia (Amst.), 13:295–304, 1972.
19. Reynolds, EH: The early treatment and prognosis of epilepsy. Epilepsia 28:97–106, 1987.
20. Richardson, EP and Dodge, PR: Epilepsy in cerebrovascular disease. Epilepsia 3:49–65, 1954.
21. Rish, BL and Caveness, WF: Relation of prophylactic medication to the occurrence of early seizures following craniocerebral trauma. J Neurosurg 38:155–158, 1973.
22. Rocca, WA, Sharbrough, FW, Hauser, WA, Annegers, JF, and Schoenberg, BS: Risk factors for absence seizures: A population-based case-control study in Rochester, Minnesota. Neurology 37:1309–1314, 1987.
23. Salazar, AM, Jabbari, B, Vance, SC, Grafman, J, Amin, D, and Dillon, JD: Epilepsy after penetrating head injury. I. Clinical correlates: A report of the Vietnam Head Injury Study. Neurology 35:1406–1414, 1985.
24. Sato, S, White, BG, Penry, JK, Dreifuss, FE, Sackellares, JC, and Kupferberg, HJ: Valproic acid versus ethosuximide in the treatment of absence seizures. Neurology 32:157–163, 1982.
25. Servit, Z and Musil, F: Prophylactic treatment of posttraumatic epilepsy: Results of a long-term follow-up in Czechoslovakia. Epilepsia 22:315–320, 1981.
26. Shinton, RA, Gill, JS, Melnick, SC, Gupta, AK, and Beevers, DG: The frequency, characteristics and prognosis of epileptic seizures at the onset of stroke. J Neurol Neurosurg Psychiatry 51:273–276, 1988.
27. Temkin, NR, Dikmen, SS, Wilensky, AJ, Keihm, J, Chabal, S, and Winn, HR: A randomized, double-blind study of phenytoin for the prevention of post-traumatic seizures. N Engl J Med 323:497–502, 1990.
28. Turnbull, DM, Howel, D, Rawlins, MD, and Chadwick, DW: Which drug for the adult epileptic patient: Phenytoin or valproate? Br Med J 290:815–819, 1985.
29. Weiss, GH, Salazar, AM, Vance, SC, Grafman, JH, and Jabbari, B: Predicting posttraumatic epilepsy in penetrating head injury. Arch Neurol 43:771–773, 1986.
30. Wohns, RNW and Wyler, AR: Prophylactic phenytoin in severe head injuries. J Neurosurg 51:507–509, 1979.
31. Young, B, Rapp, R, Brooks, WH, Madauss, W, and Norton, JA: Post-traumatic epilepsy prophylaxis. Epilepsia 20:671–681, 1979.
32. Young, B, Rapp, RP, Norton, JA, Haack, KD, Tibbs, PA, and Bean, JR: Failure of prophylactically administered phenytoin to prevent late post-traumatic seizures. J Neurosurg 58:236–241, 1983.

CHAPTER 10

• •

WHEN TO DISCONTINUE ANTIEPILEPTIC DRUGS: TIMING IS EVERYTHING

Roger J. Porter, M.D.

The question of when to stop antiepileptic drugs is often more difficult than the decision to start them.

Porter distinguishes between stopping a medication to simplify the therapeutic regimen and total discontinuation of drug therapy. In regard to simplifying therapy, Einstein's injunction may well apply: "Make things as simple as possible, but no simpler." The decision to discontinue the last antiepileptic drug may be colored by nonmedical considerations, such as the possibility of losing a driver's license if seizures recur, or the psychologic dependence of the patient on the medication.

The author makes clear that any decision to discontinue antiepileptic drugs depends on patient cooperation.

VCH

Were it not for the adverse effects of antiepileptic drugs, no reason would exist for stopping them in patients who have had seizures, for such patients are almost always at risk of recurrence. Because seizures are very distressing, why not just continue medications indefinitely to prevent their recurrence? Certainly the inconvenience of taking pills is trivial compared with having seizures. Unfortunately, however, the medication may have adverse effects that are not so trivial. These effects may occur suddenly or develop slowly, and they range from annoying to life-threatening. They are to some extent unpredictable, and in certain areas —especially sensitive areas such as cognitive function—insidious or hard to measure, or both.

There are two fundamental concepts in drug discontinuation that are worthy of separate discussion. The first is discontinuation of drugs to simplify the regimen, usually to monotherapy. The second is discontinuation of the "last drug," that is, the achievement of a drug-free state. Patients fall into any of three categories: (1) severely affected patients who require a multidrug regimen, (2) less affected patients who do well on a single medication, and (3) those who no longer need any drugs at all, or for whom the drug effects seem worse than the disorder.

The magnitude of the problem of epilepsy and of epilepsy management is enormous. Of the 2 million persons in the United States with epilepsy, almost 40%—approximately 0.75 million persons—receive regular medical care for their seizures.[3] Many of these patients are not properly categorized into one of the three groups above, and the task is conceptually controversial and difficult to individualize. Yet, such an effort is mandatory for appropriate long-term care of persons with epilepsy.

THE NATURE OF ADVERSE EFFECTS

Because the adverse effects of antiepileptic drugs are the driving force for their discontinuation, a simplified classification of the effects is useful for discussion. Basically, the effects may be dose-related or idiosyncratic, or they may involve drug interactions or teratogenicity.

Dose-Related Adverse Effects

A dose-related side effect of a drug occurs when the patient has received too much of the drug; it is, in effect, the result of a mild overdose. Examples include double vision from carbamazepine, ataxia from phenytoin, sedation from phenobarbital, and tremor from valproate. The appropriate antidote is a lower dose. The single most important reason for maintaining patients on fewer medications is the difficulty of dealing with dose-related adverse effects. When on multiple medications, the patient is more likely to have such effects, for two reasons. First, the control of reasonable, nontoxic drug levels is clearly more difficult with multiple drugs than with a single medication, and physicians vary in their ability to adjust multidrug regimens successfully. Second, some dose-related adverse effects are additive. For example, ataxia may appear sooner with modest doses and plasma levels of carbamazepine combined with phenytoin than with either drug used singly at higher doses and plasma levels.[9]

Idiosyncratic Adverse Effects

Most idiosyncratic side effects of a medication occur within the first few months of therapy; some are severe, and most require complete cessation of the medication. Examples include most skin rashes, bone marrow suppression, and hepatotoxicity. Because of greater patient exposure, the risk of such effects is clearly higher with multiple drugs than with single medications. However, little evidence exists for more than a simple additive effect. The idiosyncratic skin rash of phenobarbital, for example, is not more likely to occur in the presence of ethosuximide, which also may cause a rash. Unlike dose-related side effects (e.g., drowsiness or ataxia), in which the combination of drugs may cumulatively aggravate the toxicity, idiosyncratic reactions are usually related to a single medication.[9]

Patients on multiple drugs who have an idiosyncratic reaction present the difficult problem of identifying which drug is the culprit. Because of the nature of idiosyncratic reactions, however, once a patient tolerates any drug for several months, the likelihood of an idiosyncratic reaction to that drug falls dramatically.[9]

Drug Interactions

The possibility of drug-drug interactions obviously increases with the number of medications prescribed. Furthermore, combinations of antiepileptic drugs may alter the patient's metabolism to produce changes in the levels of active or toxic metabolites. The effects of phenytoin on carbamazepine and of valproate on phenobarbital are representative of this alteration. Monotherapy with carbamazepine, for example, may yield well-tolerated plasma levels in the range of 14 to 16 μg/mL. When phenytoin is added to a multidrug regimen, the maximal tolerated carbamazepine levels may be 8 to 10 μg/mL; although phenytoin increases carbamazepine metabolism, some carbamazepine dose reduction may be required. Likewise, phenytoin levels of 20 to 25 μg/mL or higher may be tolerated with monotherapy, but lower levels (and doses) are often necessary when phenytoin is combined with other drugs. Monotherapy eliminates these difficulties.[9]

Teratogenicity

Little is known about the possible cumulative adverse effects of multiple drugs, either dose-related or idiosyncratic, on the developing fetus. For practical purposes, however, most authorities agree that teratogenic effects are, at least in part, idiosyncratic effects and that women of childbearing potential should take a minimum number of drugs. It has not been proved, however, that high doses of a single drug are safer than moderate doses of multiple drugs. Is a high dose of phenytoin really safer for the fetus than are moderate doses of phenytoin plus carbamazepine? Answers to such questions are not available from controlled studies or current data.[9]

DISCONTINUATION OF DRUGS TO ATTAIN MONOTHERAPY

Monotherapy has received a disproportionate emphasis in the past few years not only because of the overuse of multiple medications but probably also because of the difficulties some physicians have in managing multidrug therapy without toxic side effects. The advantages of monotherapy, however, are considerable and include the following:[9]

1. Adverse drug-drug interactions are much less likely; they obviously do not even occur with monotherapy.
2. Side effects, in general, may be fewer.
3. Compliance may be better, but the physician must pay adequate attention to this issue.
4. Cost of therapy may be lower, but it may also be higher if more expensive drugs are chosen.
5. Seizure control is better in some patients, which may relate to increased compliance because of fewer adverse effects and not to a fundamental alteration in the propensity for seizures.

On the other hand, in certain patients (almost always those with severe, difficult-to-control epilepsy), multiple drugs appear to be more effective than single medications. Some data on this issue are available from the multicenter Veterans Administration study of partial and generalized tonic-clonic seizures.[7] Of 522 patients who were studied in this controlled trial, 82 were considered

failures on monotherapy and were placed on a two-drug regimen. Of these, almost 40% were judged to benefit by such a regimen and nine patients (11%) became seizure-free. Furthermore, in an intensive study of 12 inpatients with intractable partial seizures,[6] a significant improvement—without increased toxicity—was observed when carbamazepine and phenytoin were used together, as compared with each drug used alone. Finally, in a retrospective study,[4] improvement was observed with a combination of carbamazepine and valproate. Thus, although only a minority of patients may respond, the physician should not automatically reject a multidrug regimen as having no potential benefit.[9]

Assuming, however, that the patient warrants a trial of fewer medications, with at least the initial goal of achieving monotherapy, which drugs might be chosen for withdrawal? An increasing number of studies have suggested that certain antiepileptic drugs, notably those with sedative-hypnotic effects, may cause drowsiness and cognitive dysfunction in many patients with epilepsy. If it is accepted that barbiturates and benzodiazepines are, with certain limited exceptions, "second-line" antiepileptic drugs because of their sedating properties, then their removal should be considered first. The manner in which this adjustment can be accomplished is especially dependent on the patient's propensity for generalized tonic-clonic seizures. A patient with absence attacks only, and no history of generalized tonic-clonic seizures, may have drugs withdrawn with relative safety. Even if a generalized tonic-clonic seizure occurs, the likelihood of status epilepticus is minimal, especially if the patient is being treated with valproate. In a patient with frequent complex partial seizures, and with secondary generalized tonic-clonic seizures every month or two, the precautions must be much more vigorous. Clearly it is necessary to protect the patient with appropriate drugs against the occurrence of generalized tonic-clonic seizures during the withdrawal period. The most effective regimen, especially for severely affected patients, is a combination of phenytoin and carbamazepine in maximally tolerated doses, which usually means trough plasma levels of approximately 18 to 20 μg/mL for phenytoin and 6 to 7 μg/mL for carbamazepine. Status epilepticus is uncommon in patients so protected during the withdrawal period, provided that the withdrawal period is reasonably long.[9]

The rate of withdrawal is an important aspect of antiepileptic drug discontinuation. Regardless of the long half-life of both barbiturates and benzodiazepines, a prolonged withdrawal period with careful monitoring and frequent follow-up is the safest way of preventing serious problems. Phenobarbital withdrawal problems are greatest at the lower end of the therapeutic range. Typically, few problems are encountered, for example, in dropping the plasma phenobarbital level from 60 to 30 μg/mL, but generalized tonic-clonic attacks are likely to occur as the level passes through the range of 15 to 20 μg/mL.[13] Antiepileptic drug doses should be decreased over many weeks, especially if barbiturates and benzodiazepines are being withdrawn.[9]

It is also important to distinguish between withdrawal seizures and seizures that occur because of inadequate medication. A common error in the attempt to remove barbiturates occurs when the patient's seizures temporarily worsen and the physician assumes that the worsening indicates a need for the barbiturate rather than a withdrawal phenomenon. The result is continuation of a sedative antiepileptic drug that may not be needed. In many patients, it is important to try to "weather the storm" of withdrawal; the gains may be well worth the effort.[9]

Theodore and Porter[12] successfully withdrew all sedative-hypnotic drugs from 38 outpatients referred for intractable seizures. The patients ranged from 5 to 63 years of age. Withdrawal of the drugs took place over an average of 12 weeks in each patient. Primidone was the most commonly prescribed barbiturate and clonazepam the most common benzodiazepine. Withdrawal was generally well tolerated, with 11 patients reporting a transient increase in seizure frequency during the withdrawal period. Sedative-hypnotic drugs were temporarily restarted in three patients, one of whom was hospitalized for 2 days. Status epilepticus did not occur. At follow-up, averaging 17 months after drug withdrawal, 32 of the patients showed improvement in either seizure frequency or medication toxicity, or both. Six patients showed no change, but no patient's condition was worse. Noteworthy was the increase in the mean plasma phenytoin level from 13.5 to 18.2 μg/mL, and in the mean carbamazepine level from 4.0 to 6.5 μg/mL, after withdrawal of primidone, phenobarbital, and clonazepam (Table 10–1). The largest increases in plasma levels of phenytoin and carbamazepine were accomplished early in the withdrawal period to minimize withdrawal seizures.[9]

In all but the most refractory patients, then, a concerted effort should be made to achieve monotherapy, usually with one of the four major nonsedative drugs: carbamazepine, phenytoin, valproate, or ethosuximide.

TABLE 10–1. MEAN DOSES AND PLASMA LEVELS OF ANTIEPILEPTIC DRUGS TAKEN BY 38 OUTPATIENTS

	BEFORE WITHDRAWAL		AFTER WITHDRAWAL	
Drug	Dose (mg/d)	Plasma Level (μg/mL)	Dose (mg/d)	Plasma Level (μg/mL)
Primidone	808	7.2	0	0
Phenobarbital	115	33.2	0	0
Clonazepam	3	—	0	0
Phenytoin	309	13.5	363	18.2
Carbamazepine	1062	4.0	1144	6.5

Source: Theodore and Porter,[12] with permission.

DISCONTINUATION OF DRUGS TO ATTAIN A DRUG-FREE STATE

Any therapy, including monotherapy, is inferior to a drug-free state when such a state is possible. Some patients with epilepsy prefer to risk an occasional seizure rather than risk toxicity from drug therapy. Others benefit so little from therapy that they may be better off without medication. Such patients are uncommon, but clearly monotherapy is second best to the absence of therapy when none is needed or indicated. Most important, some patients who once required medical therapy may no longer need it and deserve a trial of drug withdrawal. The achievement of a medication-free state, however, is not always possible, as described in the following actual case report:

In 1976 a 27-year-old woman was admitted to the hospital for intractable seizures. The attacks had started at age 13 with generalized tonic-clonic seizures and absence attacks; during the latter she would stare, drop objects, and occasionally slump to the floor. Therapy in the previous 13 years with phenobarbital, primidone, and phenytoin had been largely unsuccessful, and she continued to have one generalized tonic-clonic seizure monthly and one absence attack weekly. The results of her neurologic examination were normal. Her EEG showed 2/s–2/s generalized spike-and-wave activity lasting as long as 45 seconds; these attacks were documented by video-EEG monitoring. She participated in a study of methsuximide and improved on phenytoin (375 mg daily); primidone (750 mg daily); and methsuximide (900 mg daily). Valproate was not yet available. She was discharged home.

The patient continued to have occasional seizures. In 1978 primidone was gradually replaced with valproate, and by May 1979 she was seizure-free on methsuximide, valproate, and phenytoin. In 1982, after she was seizure-free for 3 years, methsuximide was successfully discontinued over a 6-month period; she remained on phenytoin (450 mg daily) and valproate (2000 mg daily). In 1983, after she was seizure-free for 4.5 years, valproate was discontinued over a prolonged period and finally stopped entirely in February 1987, leaving the patient on phenytoin monotherapy. In August 1987 phenytoin was decreased to 400 mg daily. The EEGs over several years had been normal. In March 1988 the patient had a generalized tonic-clonic seizure, and in April the absence attacks returned; these were the first seizures of any type in almost 9 years. Phenytoin was increased and valproate rapidly reinstituted. By June 1988 the patient was again seizure-free on phenytoin and valproate. In June 1989 the phenytoin dose was lowered slightly, with the long-term goal of valproate monotherapy.

Clearly, as shown in the foregoing case report, patients may have drugs withdrawn at the most conservative rate, with the most frequent, benign EEG follow-up, and with meticulous documentation of the seizure-free state during the process of withdrawal, only to crash with a flurry of seizures as the ultimate goal seems within the grasp of the patient and doctor.[9]

VARIABLES AFFECTING DRUG WITHDRAWAL

Many of the variables considered in an attempt to predict the success of antiepileptic drug withdrawal are only of modest benefit in the assessment of an individual patient. The extraordinary heterogeneity of the patients constituting the various clinical series in the literature — patients who are used to create means, medians, and other seemingly important generalizations about drug withdrawal — provides information that is only remotely pragmatic for the patient in the physician's office. This information will continue to be marginally useful until investigators are willing and able to confine their studies to much more homogeneous patient populations. The trend toward large studies that include patients with all kinds of epilepsy will add little to our meager understanding of the prognosis — and potential for drug withdrawal — of the various epilepsies and epileptic syndromes.

An exemplary study of a relatively homogeneous population is that of Sato and colleagues,[11] who conducted a follow-up study of 83 patients with absence seizures. The follow-up period averaged 9.5 years after

TABLE 10–2. PROGNOSTIC VARIABLES IN EPILEPSY REMISSION OR SUCCESSFUL ANTIEPILEPTIC DRUG WITHDRAWAL IN SELECTED STUDIES

Reference	History of Low Seizure Frequency	Less Epileptiform EEG	Normal Neurologic Examination	Childhood Onset of Epilepsy	No Partial Seizures	No Secondary Generalized Seizures	Idiopathic Epilepsy
Annegers et al[1]	+	NE	NE	+	+	?	0
Rowan et al[10]	+	+	+	–	NE	NE	0
Okuma and Kumashiro[8]	+	+	+	+	0	+	+
Emerson et al[5]	+	0	0	NA	0	0	0
Thurston et al[14]	0	0	+	NA	+	NE	NE
Callaghan et al[2]	+	+	NE	NE	0	+	NA

Key: + = positive factor, – = negative factor, 0 = negligible factor, NE = not evaluated, NA = not applicable, ? = unknown.

the initial visit. Multivariate analysis of selected prognostic factors showed that normal or above-average intelligence was the single most important prognostic factor. Other factors suggestive of a favorable outcome were normal results on the neurologic examination, male sex, and absence of hyperventilation-induced spike-and-wave activity on the EEG. Ninety percent of patients with three or four of these criteria had stopped having seizures at the time of follow-up.

In spite of the difficulties in assembling homogeneous populations for appropriate long-term study, a few variables seem to be relevant to most patients. These are summarized in Table 10–2, in which various studies have been (somewhat artificially) categorized in an effort to seek trends in prognostic variables. Although not all of these studies were evaluating drug withdrawal, it is assumed that a good prognosis for epilepsy is the same as having a good prognosis for reduction or withdrawal of antiepileptic drugs.

The data from Table 10–2 suggest the following prognostic signs:

1. Patients with a history of a relatively low seizure frequency usually do better than those who have more frequent attacks; only one of the six studies found no effect of seizure frequency.
2. A mildly abnormal EEG is better than one which is severely abnormal, as concluded in four of five studies that considered this variable.
3. Normal neurologic examination results may be helpful, as concluded by three of four studies that considered this variable.
4. Other factors may be important, but gross generalization from the populations studied are often not useful in an individual patient, as noted earlier.

SUMMARY

A variable but significant percentage of patients can benefit from the reduction of their regimens to either monotherapy or a drug-free state. This effort is important to avoid, as much as possible, the adverse effects of antiepileptic drugs. Individualiza-

tion of the decision process and the withdrawal regimen is required, and only faint guidelines are available for the patients and their physicians. Larger cohorts of more homogeneous patient populations are required to provide more definitive data on this vexing issue.

REFERENCES

1. Annegers, JF, Hauser, WA, and Elveback, LR: Remission of seizures and relapse in patients with epilepsy. Epilepsia 20:729–737, 1979.
2. Callaghan, N, Garrett, A, and Goggin, T: Withdrawal of anticonvulsant drugs in patients free of seizures for two years. N Engl J Med 318:942–946, 1988.
3. Commission for the Control of Epilepsy and Its Consequences: Plan for Nationwide Action on Epilepsy, Vol 1. DHEW Publication No. (NIH) 78-276. US Department of Health, Education and Welfare, Washington, DC, 1978.
4. Dean, JC, Penry, JK, and Smith, LD: When carbamazepine monotherapy fails to control partial seizures. Ann Neurol 24:135, 1988.
5. Emerson, R, D'Souza, BJ, Vining, EP, Holden, KR, Mellits, ED, and Freeman, JM: Stopping medication in children with epilepsy: Predictors of outcome. N Engl J Med 304:1125–1129, 1981.
6. Lorenzo, NY, Bromfield, EB, and Theodore, WH: Phenytoin and carbamazepine: Combination versus single-drug therapy for intractable partial seizures. Ann Neurol 24:136, 1988.
7. Mattson, RH, Cramer, JA, Collins, JF, Smith, DB, Delgado-Escueta, AV, Browne, TR, Williamson, PD, Treiman, DM, McNamara, JO, McCutchen, CB, Homan, RW, Crill, WE, Lubozynski, MF, Rosenthal, NP, and Mayersdorf, A: Comparison of carbamazepine, phenobarbital, phenytoin, and primidone in partial and secondarily generalized tonic-clonic seizures. N Engl J Med 313:145–151, 1985.
8. Okuma, T and Kumashiro, H: Natural history and prognosis of epilepsy: Report of a multi-institutional study in Japan. Epilepsia 22:35–53, 1981.
9. Porter, RJ: Epilepsy: One Hundred Elementary Principles, ed 2. WB Saunders, Philadelphia, 1989.
10. Rowan, AJ, Overweg, J, Sadikoglu, S, Binnie, CD, Nagelkerke, NJD, and Hunteler, E: Seizure prognosis in long-stay mentally subnormal epileptic patients: Interrater EEG and clinical studies. Epilepsia 21:219–226, 1980.
11. Sato, S, Dreifuss, FE, Penry, JK, Kirby, DD, and Palesch, Y: Long-term follow-up of absence seizures. Neurology 33:1590–1595, 1983.
12. Theodore, WH and Porter, RJ: Withdrawal of sedative-hypnotic antiepileptic drugs from outpatients. In Shorvon, S and Birdwood, G (eds):

The Rational Prescription of Antiepileptic Drugs. Hans Huber, Berne, 1983, pp 95–99.

13. Theodore, WH, Porter, RJ, and Raubertas, RF: Seizures during barbiturate withdrawal: Relation to blood level. Ann Neurol 22:644–647, 1987.

14. Thurston, JH, Thurston, DL, Hixon, BB, and Keller, AJ: Prognosis in childhood epilepsy: Additional follow-up of 148 children 15 to 23 years after withdrawal of anticonvulsant therapy. N Engl J Med 306:831–836, 1982.

CHAPTER 11

• •

MANAGING INTRACTABLE SEIZURE DISORDERS

Warren T. Blume, M.D., F.R.C.P(C)

Intractable seizures are a question of definition, since almost any seizure can be controlled if one is willing to live with the side effects. Blume is willing to accept "a reasonable compromise between seizure control and mild drug toxicity" and quotes Troupin[53] approvingly to the effect that therapeutic ranges should not be considered as "immutable confines into which given patients must be crammed."

The author emphasizes establishing an objective and a plan for each patient that will take into account all relevant factors such as the number of epileptic foci and the likely nature of the underlying process.

*In dealing with intractable seizures, the physician can become as impatient as the patient and change to a new regimen before the prescribed one has had a chance to work. It may be worth keeping an ancient aphorism in mind: "If you apply all the regular treatments without getting the regular result, do not therefore change the treatment so long as your original diagnosis remains unchanged." ***

VCH

DEFINITION

For every patient with a chronic seizure disorder, the physician should set a goal of management. For almost all patients this objective would be complete seizure control without symptoms or signs of medication toxicity. The physician will encounter the rare situation where this has not been attained, and a reasonable compromise between seizure control and mild drug toxicity might have to be accepted.

Intractable epilepsy can therefore be defined as either (1) persistent seizures de-

spite adequate medical management or (2) seizure control bought at the expense of drug toxicity. As suggested above, two situations in managing epilepsy may pertain: (1) the goal of full seizure control without toxicity is deemed attainable or (2) a compromise must be reached. This chapter discusses recognition and management of each circumstance.

DIAGNOSIS AND ETIOLOGY

Four fundamental circumstances can lead to an apparently intractable seizure disorder: (1) seizures originate from a particularly epileptogenic region; (2) multiple or widespread seizure foci exist in the setting

---

*Lloyd, GER (ed): *Hippocratic Writings*. Penguin, Harmondsworth, Middlesex, England, 1978, p. 212.

of a diffuse encephalopathy; (3) the etiology is a progressive focal or diffuse disorder; and (4) some or all of the patient's attacks are not epileptic.

Epileptogenic Regions

Clinical[37] and experimental[22,31] data indicate that the hippocampi have a low threshold for partial seizures and therefore tend to be therapy-resistant. Excluding benign epilepsy of childhood with Rolandic spikes (BECRS), which is not lesion-based, seizures arising from a lesion in the Rolandic area likewise may present a therapeutic challenge. Seizures arising from some other locations may resist therapy, as they are commonly associated with other epileptogenic foci. Thus occipital seizures may be associated with anterior temporal foci.[26,55] Frontal seizures, unless arising from a single discrete lesion, commonly involve interaction of multiple foci bilaterally. Such multiple foci enhance the likelihood of secondary generalization, that is, to a grand mal attack.[6]

Several experimental data support clinical experience that the seizure tendency augments disproportionately with the number of epileptogenic foci. When Chusid and colleagues[14,15] applied twice as much of the chronic epileptogenic agent alumina cream to the Rolandic cortex of monkeys, the seizure tendency increased threefold to fourfold. Epileptogenic foci give rise to inhibitory postsynaptic potentials, either locally[33] or in the contralateral homotopic region.[16,43] Presumably such inhibition can be less easily generated in patients with multifocal diffuse encephalopathies.

Progressive Central Nervous System Lesions

Progressive lesions, such as slowly growing tumors or chronic regionally accentuated encephalitis of Rasmussen, commonly present as intractable partial seizure disorders.[4,34] Hamartomas and cortical dysplasias may do likewise. Therefore, suspect such conditions when a partial seizure disorder becomes unexpectedly difficult to control. Diffuse degenerative conditions such as Lafora's disease or neuronal ceroid lipofuscinosis should be considered in the setting of refractory generalized epilepsies, especially if dementia, ataxia, and/or visual impairment accrues.[3]

Whereas nearly every type of neurologic condition can create epileptic seizures at any age, their relative incidences vary with age of seizure onset. Table 11–1 lists common causes of refractory seizure disorders by age of onset.

TABLE 11–1. CENTRAL NERVOUS SYSTEM DISORDERS PRESENTING PRIMARILY AS INTRACTABLE SEIZURES BY AGE OF ONSET

3–10 Years

Partial
    Mesial temporal sclerosis from febrile convulsions
    Cortical dysplasia
    Hamartoma
    Glial tumor
    Phakoma
    Perinatal asphyxia
    Meningoencephalitis
    Trauma
    Landau-Kleffner

Generalized
    Lennox-Gastaut syndrome
    Infantile spasms
    Absence
    Degenerative CNS disorders
    CNS poisoning (e.g., lead encephalopathy)

11–20 Years
    Trauma
    Arteriovenous malformation
    Glial tumor

21–40 Years
    Trauma
    Glial tumor
    Arteriovenous malformation
    Alcoholism

41–60 Years
    Glial tumor
    Alcoholism
    Stroke

Above 60 Years
    Stroke
    Brain tumor, primary or secondary
    Senile dementia (rapidly advancing)

* Disorders which are rarely intractable, such as benign epilepsy of childhood with Rolandic spikes and syndrome of Janz, are omitted.

Conditions External to the Central Nervous System

Because general medical conditions may present as a seizure disorder or augment an inherent seizure tendency, the physician should be aware of any disorder outside the nervous system. Conditions as diverse as hypoglycemia, hypoparathyroidism, uremia, vasculitis, embolic strokes, and porphyria may all produce or aggravate epileptic seizures. Coexisting disorders and their therapies may aggravate a seizure tendency. For example, asthma affects this in two ways: (1) asthmatic attacks curtail sleep and (2) theophylline, an effective antiasthmatic, may lower the seizure threshold.

Medication for another illness may alter the pharmacology of anticonvulsant therapy. For example, cimetidine and isoniazid each increase phenytoin serum concentrations.

Precipitating and Augmenting Factors

Psychologic stress and sleep loss are the most common factors that augment a seizure tendency, and these factors operate at every age. Therefore a thorough lifestyle review may reduce seizures as effectively as would treatment with another anticonvulsant.

Precipitating factors should be probed for and avoided. Sudden changes in illumination or a flickering light can provoke generalized or occipitally originating seizures. Startle (very difficult to avoid) can produce mesial frontal motor attacks with falling. Less common factors are listed by Niedermeyer.[30]

Pseudoseizures

The physician should also consider whether some or all of a patient's attacks do not represent epilepsy, as its differential diagnosis includes many diverse conditions.[8] For example, a neurologically intact adult who recently develops refractory, apparently partial and/or generalized tonic-clonic attacks and whose EEGs and magnetic resonance imaging (MRI) scans show no focal or epileptiform abnormality may have pseudoseizures.

MANAGEMENT

Assessment

The Seizure History

Determination of seizure type(s), duration, incidence, and cause is the first step in assessing any patient with epilepsy, and particularly an apparently refractory case. Principles of distinguishing partial, primary generalized and secondary generalized seizures have been outlined elsewhere.[7,17] The seizures of almost all patients can be accurately classified from the patient's and witnesses' seizure description, the neurologic examination, and interictal EEGs. A detailed sequential description of one or two attacks is far more helpful than are generalities. Resort to the latter only if patients simply cannot adequately describe any particular attack.

This sequential description should begin with the first symptom or sign of the ictus and follow step by step through the attack until its termination. This description should be obtained first from the patient and then from witnesses. The latter would describe events for which the patient is amnesic, that is, when consciousness is partially or completely lost. (See Blume[7] for further guides to history taking.)

Rarely, EEG monitoring by telemetry may be required to categorize attacks.

Overall seizure incidence and timing of seizures during the day or month can help to evaluate the effectiveness of management and determine the timing and variation of any dosage adjustment. Histograms with annotation of significant events, exacerbations of concurrent illnesses, and dosage adjustments are useful.

Patients vary, however, in their record-keeping diligence. Because an inaccurate daily record is less helpful than an overall summation, I suggest, but do not require, this effort.

Neurologic Examination and Functional Inquiry

The neurologic examination may reveal many conditions causing epilepsy, among which are the following: (1) abnormal or changing mental status, suggesting a frontal or diffuse progressive lesion or a degenerative process; (2) unilateral corticospinal dysfunction, suggesting that grand mal seizures are secondarily generalized or that complex partial seizures are consequent to the hemiconvulsions, hemiplegia, epilepsy (HHE) syndrome of Gastaut[21]; (3) visual impairment and cerebellar dysfunction, raising the possibility that myoclonus and grand mal seizures represent one of the progressive myoclonic epileptic conditions.[3]

The general and neurologic examination should include a search for unwanted effects of chronic anticonvulsant therapy. These are discussed by McLachlan in Chapter 8.

Neuroimaging

Neuroimaging (computed tomography [CT] or MRI) is not mandatory but can be helpful when the etiology is uncertain and when epilepsy surgery is being considered. A focal cortical lesion would strongly suggest that seizures emanate from it, but confirmation of this is required from the seizure history and EEG.

Anticonvulsants Used

A next step is taking the anticonvulsant medication history. This is best done simply by discussing each antiepileptic drug individually, as a chronology of each attempted combination of medications will become mired in complexities. For each drug, tabulate the following: current daily dose, maximum dose ever taken, patient's and associates' estimation of effectiveness, and side effects. You may wish to make a table of these assessments as follows:

Drug	Current Dose	Maximum Dose	Effect on Seizures $(+, -, \pm)$	Side Effects

Obtain descriptions of side effects to classify them as dose-related (e.g., cognitive impairment, ataxia); hypersensitive (e.g., rash, exfoliative dermatitis); and idiosyncratic (e.g., leukopenia, thrombocytopenia, hepatic failure). Some patients may classify all side effects as "allergic." Of course, drugs causing only dose-related side effects might be tried again, especially if the side effects result from drug interactions (see below). If the patient has more than one type of seizure (as distinct from varying severity of the same type), assess the performance of each drug for each type. Patients may be unable to assess a single anticonvulsant's performance if polypharmacy (multiple drugs) was used. Scrutinize particularly any negative assessment of a drug's performance to assure that adequate blood levels were obtained and that significant drug interactions or intercurrent illnesses were not present. Because the number of effective anticonvulsants is limited, one cannot afford to discard potentially helpful therapeutic options.

Planning Medical Management

To effectively plan medical therapy in refractory cases, three topics should be understood: basic pharmacology of commonly used anticonvulsants, the therapeutic range, and drug interactions. The first of these is discussed in Chapter 8.

Therapeutic Range

Ability to measure serum levels of anticonvulsants has enhanced our ability to use them. In seizure management, one tries to balance the therapeutic efficacy of a drug against its side effects. The "therapeutic range" therefore refers to that distribution of serum values in which the drug will be most effective with minimal or no unwanted effects. The lower end is that level needed by most patients for the drug to show some therapeutic effect; the high end is that point beyond which most patients show side effects. A low serum level suggests that a dose increase will give greater efficacy with little chance of side effects. Several studies have shown a positive correlation between seizure control and antiepileptic drug concentrations.[27,41] At a high serum level, a dosage increase is more likely to produce side effects than increased seizure control.

Patients' reactions to medications differ, however, as do strengths of seizure disorders. Moreover, the range for all commonly used antiepileptic drugs has been determined empirically in a nonsystematic manner and represents at best a statistical probability regarding the likelihood of efficacy and toxicity. It is important that this range should not be considered as "immutable confines into which given patients must be crammed. . . ."[53] The therapeutic range must be determined for each patient, using the laboratory range as an initial guide. For example, a 26-year-old patient with difficult-to-control grand mal attacks experiences sequential seizures if her phenytoin level drops below 80 μmol/L and side effects if her level exceeds 110 μmol/L. Therefore her therapeutic range varies from 80 to 110 μmol/L, whereas the usual laboratory therapeutic range is 20 to 80 μmol/L.[53] Unfortunately, other anticonvulsants had either failed to control these attacks or given side effects.

As outlined in Chapter 8, trough serum levels are more reliable than levels obtained after dosing unless identification of the agent producing midday toxicity is needed. Although total drug levels usually suffice, free fractions would be helpful when protein binding alterations are suspected, as in renal disease or from drug interaction. Toxicity and efficacy relate more precisely to the free fraction than to total levels.[9]

Several pharmacokinetic and practical factors may alter serum anticonvulsant levels. Those relating to pharmacokinetics[13] include rates of absorption, distribution, biotransformation, and excretion, as well as drug interactions and protein binding. Poor compliance is the main practical factor that lowers serum levels.[25] Serum sampling at different hours of the day will also disclose spurious varying levels that in fact reflect normal fluctuations.

Clinical Medication Toxicity

Reflecting our excessive reliance on laboratory tests to determine drug toxicity and side effects, clinical signs of toxicity can be overlooked. Not all the signs in Table 11–2

TABLE 11–2. SYMPTOMS AND SIGNS OF POSSIBLE DRUG EXCESS

Impaired cognition, manifested by:
  Lower school, job performance
Forgetfulness due to:
  Impaired memory or inattention
Irritability due to:
  Disrupted wake-sleep cycle
  Drug-induced anemia
  Direct side effect
Lethargy
Daytime sleepiness
Nystagmus
Incoordination
Ataxia

can automatically be attributed to medication excess, but the relationship should be considered. Intermittent signs may be absent in the morning on arising but may begin at midmorning, coinciding with excessive peak serum levels from early morning dosing if the trough is relatively high.

Drug Interactions

Simultaneous use of two or more drugs, antiepileptic or other, creates the possibility of clinically significant drug interactions, elevating or depressing their serum levels. Such interactions can therefore produce either toxicity or decreased effectiveness. How drugs interact on a cellular level is insufficiently known, so the following statements apply to effects on pharmacokinetics by drug interaction.

The addition of a second anticonvulsant may increase the rate of metabolism of both drugs. Consequently the serum level of each drug is lower than if given alone and both drugs' half-lives would be shorter.[53] For example, the addition of phenobarbital may lower phenytoin serum levels, because phenobarbital is a potent inducer of hepatic metabolism (Table 11–3).

Troupin[53] gives the following example of this. A patient's seizures are originally well controlled on phenytoin for a few weeks, but they recur. Not realizing that this may result from autoinduction of phenytoin metabolism, the physician adds phenobarbital. Seizures worsen as phenobarbital, a potent

TABLE 11–3. ANTIEPILEPTIC DRUG INTERACTIONS*†

MAY AFFECT SERUM LEVELS OF:

Adding This Drug	Phenobarbital	Carbamazepine	Carbamazepine Epoxide	Phenytoin	Primidone	Phenobarbital Metabolite of Primidone	Valproate
Carbamazepine	↓			↑↓		↑	↓
Phenobarbital		↓		↑↓	↓		↓
Phenytoin	↑	↓	↑	— or ↓↑	↑	↑	↓
Primidone	↑	↓	↑				↓
Valproate		—	↑	↓↑		↑	↓↓↓

↑ = increase; ↓ = decrease; — = no effect; ↑↓ = variable effect.
* Double vertical lines separate drugs. Single vertical lines separate a drug and its metabolite.
† Total concentration reduced but unbound concentrations may be higher because of enzyme inhibition. Toxicity with a total phenytoin serum level within therapeutic range could result. Carbamazepine may reduce ethosuximide levels; little else is known about ethosuximide interactions.
Source: Adapted from Taylor and Caviness,[55] Welty et al,[54] and Bourgeois.[10]

inducer of hepatic metabolism, lowers phenytoin levels further.

Increased metabolism can sometimes paradoxically result in toxicity through accumulation of metabolites. Phenytoin, primidone, and phenobarbital decrease carbamazepine concentrations through enzyme induction, but carbamazepine epoxide concentrations consequentially increase.[28]

On the other hand, metabolism of drugs can be inhibited by competition for enzyme sites. In this instance the addition of a second drug could reduce the rate of metabolism of the original drug, thereby increasing its serum level and prolonging its half-life. Carbamazepine may increase phenytoin levels in this manner.

Table 11–3 presents some common drug interactions.

On a practical level, reduced compliance or patient confusion about instructions also can alter serum levels when multiple medications are taken.

Monotherapy

Most practicing epileptologists agree that the seizure control achieved for most patients with one drug can be as good as that achieved with two or more. Several studies[29,35,39,40] have shown that only 13% to 39% of patients will have significantly fewer seizures when a second drug is added, including 11% to 22% of patients with partial seizures.[42] In one study,[40] 30 of 36 patients (83%) with uncontrolled partial seizures had the same or fewer seizures when transferred from multiple to single drug therapy: Thirteen (36%) improved, 17 (47%) did not change, and 6 (17%) worsened. Thus, total antiepileptic medication can be reduced or the regimen simplified even when seizures are not controlled!

For several reasons, monotherapy is more effective for intractable epilepsy. First, the effectiveness of each medication can be assessed more accurately. A greater quantity of a single medication can be taken before toxic symptoms accrue. When multiple medications are given, neither the patient nor the physician can determine which drug plays the major role in seizure control.

Secondly, drug interactions are complex and vary considerably among patients. As noted in the previous section, a second drug can alter not only the original drug serum level but also its metabolite, which also may produce toxicity.

Thirdly, multiple drugs, although all in the "therapeutic range," can produce clinical toxicity, particularly cognitive and behavioral side effects. Finally, compliance may deteriorate when the patient must swallow many kinds of pills a day.

If a patient is currently on a single medication that has had some — but an incomplete — effect, be sure that its level is high within the patient's therapeutic range before deciding that a second drug is needed. If the added second drug effectively stops the attacks, you can cautiously attempt to withdraw the initial drug (e.g., at one pill per 2 to 4 weeks' reduction). If the patient is already taking multiple medications, cautiously withdraw the one deemed least effective or the one at the lowest relative dose.

Attempts at attaining monotherapy can be risky if the patient has prolonged seizures or commonly falls during the attacks. Dosage adjustments should be slow (once per 4 to 8 weeks) and involve one medication at a time. Watch serum levels of all medications carefully. Furthermore, overzealous efforts at monotherapy may increase seizures. Some disorders are so severe that 2 or 3 drugs are necessary.[51] Other patients benefit from "one-and-a-half" therapy: a full dose of one drug plus a subtherapeutic range of another, such as valproate with a low-dose benzodiazepine, phenytoin, or carbamazepine. Phenytoin plus subtherapeutic primidone is another possibility, particularly for complex partial seizures. Several such combinations are possible.

Thus there remains a role for two-drug therapy in some severely intractable patients. This is justified when monotherapy has clearly failed or when an attempt at reaching monotherapy entails excessive risk.

Planning the Antiepileptic Medication Regimen

Choice of Antiepileptic Medication. The following suggestions assume that the intractable patient has already tried several anticonvulsants and currently takes one or more without seizure control. Almost always, at least one potentially helpful medication has a less-than-optimum serum level. The initial step is to determine which drug to increase and which to reduce. As outlined earlier, inquiry into the anticonvulsant drug history will usually determine the relative performance of each drug and identify which drugs have been adequately tried. If drug performances correspond closely with the rank order preferences for the seizure disorder in question, the sequence of drugs to emphasize is straightforward (Table 11–4). For example, if a patient with complex partial seizures takes low-to-average doses of carbamazepine and phenobarbital and feels that carbamazepine has been more helpful, gradually increasing it along with stepwise phenobarbital reduction seems indicated.

Rarely, a patient's (or relative's) preference may not correspond to that usually recommended for the seizure disorder. If the drug is clearly not indicated, establish (1) that your classification of seizure type is accurate; (2) whether its "good" performance was due to drug-induced elevation of

another, more appropriate drug (drug interaction); or (3) whether factors external to the seizure disorder could have improved it, such as a lessening of stress. An example would be apparent improvement of absence attacks by carbamazepine or phenobarbital.

A more common situation occurs when the patient's medication preference would be most epileptologists' third or fourth choice for a given seizure disorder (e.g., primidone or clonazepam for complex partial seizures). After establishing (preferably from a well-kept seizure and medication diary) that the data are factually correct and that items two and three (above) do not apply, it is usually best to accept the patient's preference and reduce the other medications gradually. Compliance may be better, and the patient may be right!

Dosage Adjustment. In adjusting or distributing doses, remember some simple suggestions.

1. Determine compliance with the current regimen. If the patient actually takes only 400 mg of a prescribed 600-mg dose of drug X, increasing it to 800 mg only adds to the confusion.
2. Make one, or at most two, adjustments at a time. It is all right to increase primidone while lowering carbamazepine, but do not alter phenytoin at the same time.
3. Often small dosage adjustments suffice to markedly improve seizure control or to eliminate toxicity. Large dosage changes risk releasing the seizure–then toxicity–then seizure pendulum, as serum levels swing wildly out of control. This principle is particularly important when dealing with drugs exhibiting nonlinear kinetics, such as phenytoin.
4. Watch for effects of drug interaction on any unaltered medication during such adjustments by checking serum levels every month until stable.
5. Alternating dosages (e.g., phenytoin 300 mg one day, 400 mg the next) is less satisfactory than prescribing the same dose (350 mg) every day.
6. Twice-daily dosing is best for most patients: often enough to prevent significant serum fluctuations, yet convenient enough to assure compliance. Once-a-

TABLE 11–4. PREFERRED ANTIEPILEPTIC MEDICATIONS

Partial Seizures (Simple and Complex)
1. Carbamazepine
2. Phenytoin
3. Primidone
4. Valproate
5. Benzodiazepines

Primary Generalized Seizures
Grand mal
1. Valproate
2. Carbamazepine
3. Phenytoin
4. Benzodiazepines
Absence
1. Valproate
2. Ethosuximide
3. Benzodiazepines

Secondarily Generalized Seizures
1. Carbamazepine
2. Valproate
3. Phenytoin
4. Primidone
5. Benzodiazepines

day dosing is insufficient for intractable patients.

7. If required by the severity of the seizure disorder and/or the number of pills per day, multiple dosing may be essential. To avoid toxicity, take advantage of the extremes of the day as follows:

Pills/Day	Morning	Noon	Supper	Bedtime
3	1	—	1	1
4	1	1	1	1
5	1	1	1	2
6	2	1	1	2

8. Consider altering time of dosing if seizures or toxicity tend to occur at a certain part of the day.
9. Varying the dosage according to need allows a lower dose most of the time. This helps women with more seizures around menses and anyone before sporadic periods of increased stress. Such a variation should be maintained for at least 2 to 3 days and its rationale well founded. Effects of such variation should be precisely monitored.

Changing Medication. Before changing to another antiepileptic medication, be sure that the original drug attained serum levels high in the therapeutic range and failed to adequately control the seizures.

To change from one drug to another, add an initial dose of the new drug (one sixth to one tenth of the ultimate "plateau") to the existing regimen. Four to seven days later, the dose of the new drug can be slowly increased while the old drug is decreased proportionately. Initial increases are usually smaller than later ones. About six to seven steps (24 to 42 days) are required. The initial dose plateau of the new drug depends on your estimation of the severity of the seizure disorder, but it usually ranges between one half to two thirds of the usual maximum. Thus, for primidone, whose maximum in adults is usually about 1000 mg/d, the plateau would be 500 to 625 mg/d. Always write out the changeover schedule precisely for the patient. An example for a patient on carbamazepine 1200 mg/d changing to Primidone 625 mg/d is shown in Table 11–5.

Warn patients that seizure control may deteriorate slightly during a changeover and that mild transient toxicity may occur. De-

TABLE 11–5. **SAMPLE SCHEDULE FOR CHANGEOVER FROM CARBAMAZEPINE TO PRIMIDONE**

Day	Carbamazepine (Old Drug)	Primidone (New Drug)
1–4	1200 mg*	62.5 mg*
5–9	1000 mg	125 mg
10–14	800 mg	250 mg
15–19	600 mg	375 mg
20–24	400 mg	500 mg
25–29	200 mg	625 mg
30–33	0 mg	625 mg

* Total daily dose.

cember is the worst month for major medication changes, because the "festive season" may augment seizures through anxiety, depression, sleep loss, and alcohol-related changes in drug biotransformation.

Other suggestions:

1. Monitor the patient's lifestyle to avoid fatigue and stress.
2. Monitor any other ills and their management. Watch for drug interactions.
3. Equip relatives with fast-acting medication for patients with prolonged or repetitive seizures. Examples are liquid diazepam, 5 to 10 mg, given rectally by syringe and pentobarbital suppositories, 50 to 100 mg.

Establishing a Plan. Whatever the situation, adopt a plan according to principles outlined in the above paragraphs and in Table 11–6. Include within it several "if" statements covering the possible range of drug performance in the areas of seizure control and drug toxicity. Communicate this plan to the patient and his or her relatives more than once. Keep the primary physician informed of your steps and their rationale. Primary physicians can become competent practical epileptologists through active participation in the care of only one refractory patient.

Surgery. Patients with medically refractive partial seizures may be candidates for epilepsy surgery. See Chapter 12.

TABLE 11–6. **PLANNING ANTIEPILEPTIC MANAGEMENT**

1. Assure that most or all attacks are epileptic.
2. Classify the attacks:
    Partial
    Primary generalized
    Secondarily generalized
3. Assess relative merits of current and past medical therapy.
4. Emphasize favored medication(s):
    De-emphasize others
    Evolve toward monotherapy
5. Monitor effects of #4:
    Seizure control
    Drug side effects
        Clinical signs
        Trough serum levels
        Hematologic changes
6. Monitor lifestyle:
    Adequate sleep
    Diminish stress
    Assess other conditions and their therapy
7. Consider surgery:
    Partial seizure origin
    Appropriate center available

MANAGEMENT OF SOME SPECIAL SITUATIONS

Full descriptions of these entities can be found in textbooks such as *Epilepsy in Children*.[1] Only some aspects of their management will be discussed here.

Infantile Spasms

Infantile spasms usually begin in the first year of life. They are accompanied by an arrest or regression of development or follow already delayed milestones. Hypsarhythmia is the usual EEG correlate. Etiologies and prognosis will not be discussed here. Because infantile spasms often resist initial medical management, the physician must be equipped with alternate strategies. A suggested sequence of therapy appears in Table 11–7.

Conventional antiepileptic drugs are ineffective. Corticotropin (adrenocorticotropic hormone, ACTH), benzodiazepines, valproate, and corticosteroids each may be effective.

TABLE 11–7. **A RECOMMENDED SEQUENCE OF INFANTILE SPASMS THERAPY**

1. Pyridoxine: 50–100 mg orally for 2–4 d
2. Corticotropin: regimens outlined in Riikonen[36] or Sneed[48]
3. Benzodiazepines
    Nitrazepam: 0.2 mg/kg per day to start
    Clonazepam: 0.025 mg/kg per day to start
4. Valproate/valproic acid: 20 mg/kg per day to start

Corticotropin (ACTH) and Steroids

Agreement on whether corticotropin or steroids is more effective has not been reached, as several factors have influenced results of clinical trials. Several studies indicate that steroids are as effective as corticotropin, whereas others find corticotropin more effective.[1]

A popular and effective protocol for corticotropin has been that outlined by Snead and colleagues[48] as follows:

75 IU/m² IM twice daily for 1 week
75 IU/m² IM once daily for 1 week
75 IU/m² IM every other day for 1 week
Gradual further reductions over 9 weeks
(m² = per meter squared body surface)

The possibility of unwanted effects such as hypertension and glucosuria are monitored daily, especially in the first week of therapy. Snead's group[48] reported control of spasms in 14 of 15 children using this protocol. However, Riikonen[36] has found that smaller doses (20 to 40 IU/d for 4 weeks) can be equally effective.

Corticosteroids may also be effective. Regimens such as prednisolone (2 to 10 mg/kg per day); hydrocortisone (5 to 20 mg/kg per day); and dexamethasone (0.3 to 0.5 mg/kg per day) have been advocated.[1] Corticosteroids can be given orally, avoiding the inconvenience of injections and the possibility of injection-related abscesses.

Duration of such therapy has varied considerably among investigators, from 3 to 8 weeks to 6 to 10 months.

Both corticotropin and corticosteroids have produced serious side effects. Increased incidence of infections is probably the most significant: the majority of deaths in large series have resulted from infection.[1] Arterial hypertension may occur but seldom produces serious consequences. Hyperglycemia, glucosuria, and electrolyte imbalances may occur. Irritability may be evident.

Spasms disappear in 46% to 83% of infants on corticotropins or steroids.[1] Such results have indicated to Bourgeois[11] that corticotropin is the treatment of first choice. Cryptogenic cases usually fare better than symptomatic ones. The effect is usually apparent in the first week of therapy.

The relapse rate after corticotropin therapy is about 30% to 33%, higher among patients whose infantile spasms have complicated a preexisting encephalopathy.[1,19] A second course will improve 75% of patients in whom the first corticotropin course reduced or stopped the spasms.[19] Aicardi[1] also advocates a second course of hormone therapy, although his experience with this is less favorable.

Benzodiazepines

Benzodiazepines, particularly nitrazepam, may be effective, but there are doubts that they are as helpful as corticotropin or steroids.[1] However, Fenichel[19] has found corticotropin ineffective for spasms related to prenatal or perinatal cerebral abnormalities and believes that nitrazepam or clonazepam should be tried first in this situation.

Valproate

Valproic acid/valproate also may control infantile spasms, but its use has been curtailed by fear of hepatotoxicity. However, the risk is low, even for children less than 2 years old. Dreifuss[18] found one hepatic fatality in 7025 infants on valproate. Such data will likely increase the use of valproate in young patients.

Pyridoxine Hydrochloride

Because pyridoxine-dependent seizures do not always begin in the neonatal period, pyridoxine HCl (vitamin B_6) 50 to 100 mg orally could be tried for 2 to 4 days first.

Lennox-Gastaut Syndrome and Early Myoclonic Seizures

Because these disorders commonly resist the most thoughtful and ingenious medical management, goals of therapy should be realistically assessed and reassessed. Although full seizure control remains ideal, occasional attacks may have to be accepted.

Most authors favor valproate and benzodiazepines, either alone or in combination.[1,12,19,23] These drugs, particularly valproate, can control all types of seizures of the Lennox-Gastaut syndrome, alone or in combination. Although our experience is limited, clobazam may become the most useful of currently available benzodiazepines because it sedates less than do nitrazepam and clonazepam for equivalent therapeutic effectiveness. Nonetheless, nitrazepam and clonazepam remain useful adjuncts with valproate or other drugs.

Most anticonvulsants other than benzodiazepines significantly lower valproate serum levels. Moreover, valproate may increase blood levels of other anticonvulsants or their metabolites (see section on drug interactions p. 139. These two facts commonly lead the patient's family and the physician to conclude that valproate not only is ineffective but also sedates the patient. In that circumstance, try to withdraw the second anticonvulsant gradually to allow valproate a freer rein.

Phenytoin may help tonic and myoclonic attacks even when valproate clearly fails. A small amount (150 to 200 mg) of phenytoin with a full valproate dose may help. Carbamazepine may help control grand mal attacks, but some evidence suggests that myoclonic, atonic, and absence attacks may worsen with carbamazepine.[44,47]

Primidone and phenobarbital may occasionally control grand mal and tonic seizures within the Lennox-Gastaut syndrome, but absence seizures and myoclonic attacks may increase, perhaps because of the drugs' sedation effect.

Ethosuximide improves atonic, absence, and myoclonic seizures only in a minority of

1. Valproate
2. Benzodiazepines
   Clobazam
   Nitrazepam
   Clonazepam
3. Phenytoin
4. Ethosuximide
5. Primidone
6. Phenobarbital

* In order of preference.

patients.[1] However, it is worth trying because of its occasional effectiveness, low degree of toxicity, and lack of drug interactions.[1,12] Combining ethosuximide with valproate is therefore practical and may be effective.

Table 11–8 lists the approximate order of preference of these medications.

Although corticotropin or corticosteroids can transiently control the seizures of many patients with Lennox-Gastaut Syndrome, the relapse rate is high.[1,12]

Corpus callosotomy may control seizures in which the patient falls, but it has no effect on other types of attacks.[1,5,49]

The ketogenic diet is impractical to implement and can no longer be seriously considered.

Progressive Myoclonus Epilepsies

Valproate and benzodiazepines most effectively control the myoclonus of these disorders.[3] Administration of 5-hydroxytryptophan with carbidopa also may help.

Absence

Ethosuximide and/or valproate are considered the most effective medications against absence.[1,38] Adolescent-onset absences have a higher incidence of grand mal than do those beginning earlier.[1] Therefore, ethosuximide, which does not prevent grand mal, would be less favored in this group. Ethosuximide is probably the drug of choice for absence in the younger age group

because of its lower incidence of side effects and lower cost.

Combining valproate with ethosuximide may help where each alone has failed. When this combination fails, benzodiazepines should be tried. Although nitrazepam and clonazepam may control absence, they sedate at higher doses. The antiabsence effect may diminish with time.

Complex Partial Seizures of Temporal Origin

This is the most common medically refractory seizure disorder among children and adults, particularly among patients who are not otherwise neurologically handicapped.

As with other forms of epilepsy, monotherapy is preferred. Carbamazepine and phenytoin are the two most commonly used drugs and the most effective against complex partial seizures (CPS). When these have been compared in crossover trials, half the patients have done better on one and half on the other.[24,45,52] Carbamazepine is usually tried first, because it impairs memory less than does phenytoin,[2] an important consideration among such temporal lobe epilepsy patients with a propensity for memory difficulty.

A third effective drug is primidone, which is less favored because of its sedative properties. It has been suggested, however, that its toxicity is lowered considerably when used alone because the biotransformation to the sedating phenobarbital occurs less readily.[20,46] Moreover, if primidone more effectively controls CPS than did carbamazepine or phenytoin, its dose can be relatively less. My patients in this circumstance feel more alert on primidone than on carbamazepine.

Any two of these three drugs can be used in combination for particularly refractive cases in whom each alone at high-therapeutic-range doses has failed. However, after failure with monotherapy, the chances of success with such combinations is low.

Penry and Dean[32] controlled or improved the condition of a majority of patients with CPS using valproate monotherapy. Such data suggest that valproate's role in this situation will grow.

Temporal lobectomy should always be considered in patients with complex partial seizures originating in the temporal lobe. If the clinical seizure history, ictal and interictal EEGs, neuropsychologic tests of memory, and neuroimaging indicate that most or all of the seizures arise from one temporal lobe, then epilepsy surgery should not be deemed a measure of last resort. Thus, if the aforementioned data are congruent and unifocal, I proceed to strong consideration of temporal lobectomy after failure of two anticonvulsants given sequentially. The chance of controlling CPS with a third choice is low. Epilepsy surgery is more conservative therapy than long-term polypharmacy for temporal lobe epilepsy in this situation. When clinical and laboratory data indicate bilateral temporal epileptogenesis, however, then a more complete medication trial is warranted.

SUMMARY

Despite the plethora of neurologic laboratory investigations today, an accurate history is still the most reliable guide to management of seizure disorders of any severity. A thorough neurologic and psychiatric history will provide clues to the etiology of the disorder in question. A step-by-step history of the attack sequences will determine whether the events in question represent a seizure disorder and its type.

Anti-epileptic management should follow a plan, even though this plan must be replete with "if" statements. Long-term goals usually should take precedence over short-term exigencies.

REFERENCES

1. Aicardi, J: Epilepsy in Children. Raven Press, New York, 1986.
2. Andrewes, DG, Tomlinson, L, Elwes, RDC, and Reynolds, EH: The influence of carbamazepine and phenytoin on memory and other aspects of cognitive function in new referrals with epilepsy. Acta Neurol Scand 99:23–30, 1984.
3. Berkovic, SF, Andermann, F, Carpenter, S, and Wolfe, LS: Progressive myoclonus epilepsies: Specific causes and diagnosis. N Engl J Med 315:296–305, 1986.
4. Blume, WT, Girvin, JP, and Kaufmann, JCE: Childhood brain tumors presenting as chronic uncontrolled focal seizure disorders. Ann Neurol 12:538–541, 1982.
5. Blume, WT: Corpus callosum section for seizure control: Rationale and review of experimental and clinical data. Cleve Clin Q 51:319–332, 1984.
6. Blume, WT and Pillay, N: Electrographic and clinical correlates of secondary bilateral synchrony. Epilepsia 26:636–641, 1985.
7. Blume, WT: Epileptic seizure disorders. Am J EEG Tech 28:165–184, 1988.
8. Blume, WT: Differential diagnosis of epileptic seizures. In Wada, J and Ellingson, RJ (eds): Handbook of Electroencephalography and Clinical Neurophysiology. Elsevier, New York, 1989.
9. Booker, HE and Darcey, B: Serum concentrations of free diphenylhydantoin and their relationship to clinical intoxications. Clin Chem 17:607–611, 1973.
10. Bourgeois, B: Pharmacologic interactions between valproate and other drugs. Am J Med (Suppl 1A)84:29–33, 1988.
11. Bourgeois, BFD: The rational use of antiepileptic drugs in children. Clev Clin J Med (Suppl) 56:5248–5253, 1989.
12. Brett, EM: The Lennox-Gastaut syndrome: Therapeutic aspects. In Niedermeyer, E and Degen, R (eds): The Lennox-Gastaut Syndrome. Alan R Liss, New York, 1988, pp 329–339.
13. Browne, TR: Pharmacokinetics of antiepileptic drugs. Merritt Putnam Quarterly 4:3–13, 1987.
14. Chusid, JG, Pacella, BL, Kopeloff, LM, and Kopeloff, N: Chronic epilepsy in the monkey following multiple intracerebral injections of alumina cream. Proc Soc Exp Biol Med 78:53–54, 1951.
15. Chusid, JG, Kopeloff, LM, and Kopeloff, N: Experimental epilepsy in the monkey following multiple intracerebral injections of alumina cream. Bull NY Acad Med 29:898–904, 1953.
16. Crowell, RM: Distant effects of a focal epileptogenic process. Brain Res 18:137–154, 1970.
17. Delgado-Escueta, AV, Trieman, DM, and Walsh, GO: The treatable epilepsies (first of two parts). N Engl J Med 308:1508–1514, 1983.
18. Dreifuss, FE, Santilli, N, Langer, DH, Sweeney, KP, Moline, KA, and Menander, KB: Valproic acid hepatic fatalities: A retrospective review. Neurology 37:379–385, 1987.
19. Fenichel, GM: Clinical Pediatric Neurology. WB Saunders, Philadelphia, 1988.
20. Fincham, RW and Schottelius, DD: Primidone: Interactions with other drugs. In Levy, R, Mattson, R, Meldrum, B, Penry, JK, and Dreifuss, FE (eds): Antiepileptic Drugs, ed 3. Raven Press, New York, 1989, pp 413–422.
21. Gastaut, H, Poirier, F, Payan, H, Salamon, G, Toga, M, and Vigouroux, M: HHE syndrome: Hemiconvulsions, hemiplegia, epilepsy. Epilepsia 1:442, 1960.

22. Green, JD: The hippocampus. Physiol Rev 44:561–608, 1964.

23. Jeavons, PM, Clarke, JE, and Maheshwari, MC: Treatment of generalised epilepsies of childhood and adolescence with sodium valproate. Dev Med Child Neurol 19:9–25, 1977.

24. Kosteljanetz, M, Christiensen, J, Dam, AM, Hansen, BS, Lyon, BB, Pedersen, H, and Dam, M: Carbamazepine vs phenytoin. Arch Neurol 36:22–24, 1979.

25. Kutt, H and Penry, JK: Usefulness of blood levels of antiepileptic drugs. Arch Neurol 31:283–288, 1974.

26. Ludwig, B and Ajmone Marsan, C: Clinical ictal patterns in epileptic patients with occipital electroencephalographic foci. Neurology 25:463–471, 1975.

27. Lund, L: Anticonvulsant effect of diphenylhydantoin relative to plasma levels. Arch Neurol 31:289–294, 1974.

28. MacKichan, JJ: Carbamazepine. In Taylor, WJ and Caviness, MHD (eds): A Textbook for the Clinical Application of Therapeutic Drug Monitoring. Abbott Laboratories, TX, 1986, pp 211–224.

29. Mattson, RH, Cramer, JA, Collins, JF, Smith, DB, Delgado-Escueta, AV, Browne, TR, Williamson, PD, Treiman, DM, McNamara, JO, McCutchen, CB, Homan, RW, Crill, WE, Lubozynski, MF, Rosenthal, NP, and Mayersdorf, A: Comparison of carbamazepine, phenobarbital, phenytoin, and primidone in partial and secondarily generalized tonic-clonic seizures. N Engl J Med 313:145–151, 1985.

30. Niedermeyer, E: Epilepsy Guide: Diagnosis and Treatment of Epileptic Seizure Disorders. Urban & Schwarzenberg, Baltimore and Munich, 1983.

31. Olney, JW, Collins, RC, and Sloviter, RS: Excitotoxic mechanisms of epileptic brain damage. In Delgado-Escueta, AV, Ward, AA, Woodbury, DM, and Porter, RJ (eds): Advances in Neurology, Vol 44. Raven Press, New York, 1986, pp 857–877.

32. Penry, JK and Dean, JC: Valproate monotherapy in partial seizures. Am J Med 84:14–16, 1988.

33. Prince, DA and Wilder, BJ: Control mechanisms in cortical epileptogenic foci "surround inhibition." Arch Neurol 16:194–202, 1967.

34. Rasmussen, T, Olszewski, J, and Lloyd-Smith, D: Focal seizures due to chronic localised encephalitis. Neurology 8:435, 1958.

35. Reynolds, EH and Shorvon, SD: Monotherapy or polytherapy for epilepsy. Epilepsia 22:1–10, 1981.

36. Riikonen, R: Infantile spasms: Modern practical aspects. Acta Paediatr Scand 73:1, 1984.

37. Rodin, EA: The Prognosis of Patients with Epilepsy. Charles C Thomas, Springfield, IL, 1968, p 202.

38. Sato, S: Medical management of absence, atonic, and myoclonic seizures. In Porter, RJ and Morselli, PL (eds): The Epilepsies. Butterworths, London, 1985, pp 191–205.

39. Schmidt, D: Two antiepileptic drugs for intractable epilepsy with complex-partial seizures. J Neurol Neurosurg Psychiatry 45:1119–1124, 1982.

40. Schmidt, D: Reduction of two-drug therapy in intractable epilepsy. Epilepsia 24:368–376, 1983.

41. Schmidt, D: Single drug therapy for intractable epilepsy. J Neurol 229:221–226, 1983.

42. Schmidt, D: Adverse effects of antiepileptic drugs in children. Cleve Clin J Med (Suppl) 56:S132–S139, 1989.

43. Schwartzkroin, PA, Mutani, R, and Prince, DA: Orthodromic and antidromic effects of a cortical epileptiform focus on ventrolateral nucleus of the cat. J Neurophysiol 38:795–811, 1975.

44. Shields, WD and Saslow, E: Myoclonic, atonic and absence seizures following institution of carbamazepine therapy in children. Neurology 33:1487–1489, 1983.

45. Simonsen, N, Olsen, PZ, Kuhl, V, Lund, M, and Wendelboe, J: A comparative controlled study between carbamazepine and diphenylhydantoin in psychomotor epilepsy. Epilepsia 17:169–176, 1976.

46. Smith, DB: Primidone: Clinical use. In Levy, R, Mattson, R, Meldrum, B, Penry, JK, and Dreifuss, FE (eds): Antiepileptic Drugs, ed 3. Raven Press, New York, 1989, pp 423–438.

47. Snead, OC and Hosey, LC: Exacerbation of seizures in children by carbamazepine. N Engl J Med 313:916–921, 1985.

48. Snead, OC, Benton, JW, Hosey, LC, Swann, JW, Spink, D, Martin, D, and Rej, R: Treatment of infantile spasms with high-dose ACTH: Efficacy and plasma levels of ACTH and cortisol. Neurology 39:1027–1031, 1989.

49. Spencer, SS: Corpus callosum section in children: Indications and issues. II. Epileptic physiology and rationale. J Epilepsy (Suppl)3:197–204, 1990.

50. Taylor, WJ and Caviness, MHD: A Textbook for the Clinical Application of Therapeutic Drug Monitoring. Abbott Laboratories, TX, 1986.

51. Treiman, DM: Medical management of intractable epilepsy. Epilepsy Forum 88, Scottsdale, Arizona, 1988.

52. Troupin, AS, Ojemann, LM, Halpern, L, Dodrill, C, Wilkus, R, Friel, P, and Feigl, P: Carbamazepine: A double-blind comparison with phenytoin. Neurology 27:511–519, 1977.

53. Troupin, AS: Practical pharmacokinetics. In Robb, JP (ed): Epilepsy Updated: Causes and Treatment. Year Book Medical Publishers, Chicago, 1980, pp 101–117.

54. Welty, TE, Graves, NM, and Cloyd, JC: Antiepileptic drug therapy. Postgrad Med 74:287–305, 1983.

55. Whiting, SE, Blume, WT, and Girvin, JP: Epilepsy surgery in the posterior cortex (abstr). Ann Neurol 29:638–645, 1991.

CHAPTER 12

• •

CURRENT INDICATIONS FOR SURGICAL MANAGEMENT OF EPILEPSY

John P. Girvin, M.D., Ph.D., F.R.C.S(C)

Not since the days of Wilder Penfield has epilepsy surgery commanded such attention. Many factors have contributed to this, but among them are the realization that not only clinically manifest but subclinical seizure activity and kindling can lead to clinical deterioration, that some epilepsies are progressive, and that epilepsy surgery is becoming increasingly precise and safe.

Further factors are the close collaboration between physicians and surgeons in choosing the most appropriate treatment. Long gone are the days when Bacon* performed castrations for epilepsy due to masturbation in adult insane patients and Gowers† advocated circumcision for epileptic boys "in which there is reason to associate the disease with masturbation."

Epilepsy surgery has gained its advances by careful steps that, on the available evidence, appear justified.

VCH

The rationale on which the surgery of epilepsy is based is threefold: That the epilepsy is truly focal, that the focus is one that can be removed without the production of an unwanted neurologic deficit, and that the removal of the focus will lead to abolition of the seizure disorder. The surgical management of epilepsy involves basically two types of surgery: (1) resective and (2) interruption of conducting (spread) pathways. In candidates for resective surgery, the focus of the epilepsy must be in an area that can be removed without producing a significant

deficit (such a cortical area hereinafter will be referred to as "noneloquent"). Thus, by further extension, in normal individuals only the partial epilepsies would be amenable to surgical resection. The second type of surgical management, interruption of conducting pathways involved in the spread of the seizure, is very definitely second best in my opinion. It is less frequently carried out and lacks the beneficial results of resective surgery.

EXTENT OF THE PROBLEM

The extent of the problem of surgical management includes a consideration of the incidence and prevalence of epilepsy, the

---

*Journal of Mental Science, October 1880, p. 470.
†Gowers, WR: Epilepsy. Dover Publications, New York, 1964, p. 236.

proportion of cases within the categories of "partial" versus "primary generalized" epilepsy, the criteria for the determination of intractability, the proportion of cases amenable to surgical therapy in the various classification categories of epilepsy, and the changing attitudes toward the surgery of epilepsy in recent years.

Incidence and Prevalence

Epidemiologic studies have disclosed the incidence of epilepsy to be 5 per 10,000 and the prevalence 650 per 100,000.[24,25,30,31,49,75] Thus at any time, 650 individuals out of every 100,000 will be afflicted with epileptic seizures. With respect to neurologic illness, this prevalence is exceeded only by that of headaches and perhaps by brain injuries of one type or another.

Intractability

The medical treatment of the primary generalized epilepsies is more satisfactory than that of the partial epilepsies. One study found that 80% to 85% of patients with such seizures were free from epilepsy 20 years following diagnosis.[1] Partial seizures represent about two thirds of all seizures,[25] and traditionally it was considered that only about two thirds of patients with partial seizures were controlled by medication.[1,5] Thus partial seizures are more common than primary generalized seizures and are less likely to be controlled by medication.

The major criterion for the consideration of surgical treatment of an epileptic patient is medical intractability. That is to say, the patient has been tried on the major anticonvulsants and these have failed to control the seizures satisfactorily. From the type of information that has been available, it has been estimated that about 5% to 10% of all patients with epilepsy are candidates for surgical treatment.[56,69]

There has been more concern recently, however, as to whether the outlook for the partial epilepsies is as optimistic as has been traditionally accepted (e.g., see Currie et al.[6]). Rodin[57,58] has consistently considered the figure of 20% to 30% intractability in the partial epilepsies to be an underestimate of the problem. Reynolds[55] shared the concern of Rodin about the "widespread misconception that 70% to 80% of epileptics are controlled by drugs." In fact, he believed that only about 10% of patients, if observed for 10 years, had complete control of their seizures by medication. Thus, for this and other reasons (see below), there has been an increasingly widespread acceptance of the view that many more patients are potential candidates for the surgical relief of their epilepsy than had been considered until the early 1980s.

Changing Attitude Toward Epilepsy Surgery

The 1980s saw a remarkable increase in interest in the surgical treatment of epilepsy, with a corresponding proliferation of centers performing this surgery. This changing attitude toward epilepsy surgery has resulted from a number of factors that are worth considering as a preamble to a discussion of the surgery itself. The time-honored criteria for the selection of patients for surgery have included (1) intractability, (2) disability, (3) the establishment of a true cortical focus, (4) the absence of significant psychopathy/sociopathy, and (5) potential usefulness of the procedure to the patient. Thus the prototype patient considered for surgical treatment would have intractable seizures producing significant disability; the epilepsy would be demonstrated as arising from a specific cortical focus; the patient would not show any significant sociopathy or psychopathy; and there would be reason to believe that the individual would have an enhanced potential in the community if the seizures were abolished. Of these rather traditional criteria, perhaps only the second continues to command rigid adherence. To varying degrees there have been some modifications in the other criteria. For example, experience has taught me that even if a focus may appear on surface encephalography (EEG) to be centered over eloquent cortex, in all probability it does not involve that cortex, or that cortical function has been "transferred," if there is not a clinical or neuropsychologic deficit of the function served by the cortical area. With respect to psychopathy and sociopathy, there is no doubt that behavior can be altered by cortical resection — particularly temporal lobectomy — and although this change is neither uniform nor predictable, the presence of behavioral abnormalities should not in itself represent a contraindication to surgical treatment. Finally, if control of seizures might: (1) preclude institutionalization (2) allow institutionalized management on a "chronic" rather than an "acute" ward (3) significantly reduce the requirements for nursing or custodial care, then such patients may be considered for surgery even though they may not necessarily be able to take a more independent place in community life.

What changes have occurred in the philosophy of treatment of epilepsy, and why has there been an increased interest in surgical treatment? Many factors have given rise to this recent change, some of which are (1) the failure of recently introduced pharmacotherapy, (2) the increasing notion that some forms of epilepsy represent a progressive disorder, (3) a change in attitude of referring physicians, (4) the tendency to operate at earlier ages, and (5) the view that earlier surgery provides improved results of surgical therapy.

Failure of Medical Therapy

The disappointment in pharmacologic control of seizure disorders has already been noted.[55,57,58] The last 10 to 15 years have seen no change in this, unfortunately. Although the newer drugs have provided a wider armamentarium with respect to choice and perhaps even better specificity for use, they have failed to control the larger proportion of patients, especially those with temporal lobe epilepsy. There has been an increasing move to monotherapy, as opposed to polypharmacy, over the past decade. Recently Porter and Ferendelli concluded independently that if patients remain intractable after a year of having tried two or three of the major medications, then it is unlikely that they will benefit from other medication, and at that point they

should be considered for investigation as candidate for surgical therapy.[14,48] This stand contrasts markedly with the traditional stance of neurologists.

Epilepsy: A Progressive Disorder?

Is epilepsy a progressive disorder? This question has been pondered for some time, but the last two decades have disclosed compelling evidence that at least some cases of limbic, or temporal lobe, epilepsy indeed may be progressive. Whether the so-called kindling phenomenon of Goddard and colleagues[22,23] can be implicated in the human disorder still remains controversial, but certainly increasing evidence suggests that this may be so (see Morrell[36]). Furthermore, a substantial body of evidence from the experimental epileptic literature suggests that the excitatory neurotoxicity of Olney[41] may produce marked ongoing damage in experimental seizure models.

Attitudes of Referring Physicians

The dynamic, changing attitude of referring physicians has perhaps been the factor most responsible for the increased acceptance of surgery in treatment of epilepsy. The reasons for this acceptance include (1) increased public awareness and understanding of epilepsy and the various modes of treatment; (2) increased public education as a result of the International League Against Epilepsy and its branch organizations; (3) improved electrographic and neuroimaging technology in the localization of structural lesions; (4) increasing aggressivity of epileptologists in particular in requests for surgical treatment; (5) frustration arising from the failure of new drugs to provide substantial improvement in the relief of intractable seizures; (6) increasing awareness of subtle toxicity from antiepileptic drugs, especially when used in combination; (7) increasing awareness of the fact that certain cases of epilepsy may be progressive; (8) the notion that earlier operations frequently provide better results and better-adapted adolescents and young adults if the seizures are brought under control; and (9) the clear demonstration that surgery significantly benefits a majority of patients whose epileptic foci have been properly localized.

Earlier Operations

Toward the end of his career, Falconer[8,10-13] continually stressed the advantages of early operation in young children. His main concern at that time was not the question of a progressive disorder but the fact that if young children are left long enough without operation, many of them, because of their epilepsy, fail to develop the proper social skills during adolescence. He felt that operations in their twenties that might succeed in abolishing the seizures might still leave them socially wanting as young adults. Thus he advised that children should be operated on earlier rather than later.

Other observations have suggested that earlier operation, with a shorter duration of the habitual seizure pattern, improves outcome,[27] a suggestion that had been made a number of years earlier.[47] Whereas these types of observations have pointed to the efficacy of the surgical treatment of epilepsy, perhaps the most important impetus to such efficacy is provided by the nearly uniform view held by medical and surgical epileptologists that operative treatment is highly beneficial for a large proportion of patients with medically intractable epilepsy.

PATHOPHYSIOLOGY

Epilepsy is a symptom that may result from any of a number of etiologic causes. With the passage of time, it has emerged that an increasingly smaller proportion of cases can be labeled "idiopathic." The most important reason for this reduction probably relates to the increasing acceptance of the association between complicated febrile seizures and sclerosis of inferomesial temporal structures as a cause of subsequent seizures. Perhaps just as important has been the demonstration of this sclerosis by newer neuroimaging technology. Computed tomography (CT) was a remarkable advance in neurologic diagnosis, and patients with epilepsy shared the benefits of the enhanced quality of the resulting images. Perhaps only the area of demyelinating disease has shared with epilepsy the overwhelming diagnostic importance of magnetic resonance imaging (MRI). In those units possessing an MRI unit with a field strength of at least 1.5 T, MRI now represents the only necessary diagnostic imaging investigation.

Neurophysiologically the actual structural "lesion" producing the epilepsy does not necessarily give rise *within* its structure to epileptic discharge. Rather, the alteration in some manner of the normal discharge of populations of neurons that are disturbed by the lesion may be what gives rise to the offending discharge. Whether this discharge is due to neuronal membrane abnormalities, some type of primary excessive excitation, a lack of inhibition, or defective modulation of a critical population of neurons, remains unknown. What is known, however, is that, whatever the neurophysiologic disturbance, there is a rhythmic, synchronous discharge of neurons that then, by a cascading vicious cycle, recruits increasing numbers of neurons until a self-sustained electrographic seizure occurs. If this electrographic seizure is unchecked, it will spread by recruitment to involve a sufficient amount of the brain, or all of the brain, such that the areas involved in the production of clinical symptomatology become apparent and the typical clinical seizure occurs.

Thus, from the pathophysiologic point of view, the lesion per se is usually removed, but the surrounding parenchyma, which may be in physiologic disarray, may represent the true epileptic focus and must be removed as well.

PRACTICAL MANAGEMENT AND ITS RATIONALE

As already stated, the practical management of seizure disorders is that of medical, or conservative, therapy with the appropriate anticonvulsant medication and behavioral modification, where the latter is required. This statement obviously must be modified for those cases where there is a lesion that on its own merits provides clear indications for surgical intervention. Such lesions would include abscesses, some vascular malformations, and tumors and various other lesions for which it is believed that histologic diagnosis might alter management. This chapter does not address the issue of these particular cases, but the rationale and surgical technique may well apply to such cases. For example, it is my practice to watch patients who display hypodensities on the CT scan (or with increased T_2-weighted signal on the MRI scan) who have had single seizures or only a few seizures, with one of the indications for intervention being the development of intractable seizures.

SURGICAL MANAGEMENT

Resection

An insult to the brain, including any surgical procedure no matter how carefully the procedure might be carried out, will leave a lesion that is thus capable of giving rise to an area of epileptogenicity. How then can surgery be used as a treatment for epilepsy? There have been criticisms of the surgery of epilepsy,[2] especially common two or three decades ago. Many of these criticisms were

justified, but certainly many were not, at least not in the light of present knowledge.

Technique

Subpial dissection is used for the removal of epileptogenic tissue.[26,44,46,60,64] This technique allows selective cortical removal, the minimization of the potential scar from the surgery, and the preservation of normal blood supply to the remaining cortex. Figure 12–1 illustrates a cortical sulcus with its included vasculature. Anatomically, therefore, subpial dissection implies the preservation of the leptomeninges (pial and arachnoid membranes) and the pertinent vasculature contained within the subarachnoid space in the sulcus. Such a removal is illustrated in Figure 12–2. Figure 12–2A depicts the same diagram as Figure 12–1, but in fact the densely stippled area on the right side of the sulcus represents the "epileptic cortical lesion." Figure 12–2B depicts the resulting scar from an optimal subpial resection of the epileptogenic lesion. In this case the only scar left behind is the small, darkly stippled area in the cortex at the bottom of the sulcus, corresponding to the cortical resection line. In this case the

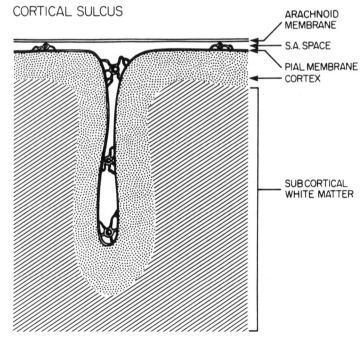

FIGURE 12–1. Diagram of the anatomy of the cortical sulcus. S.A. = subarachnoid.

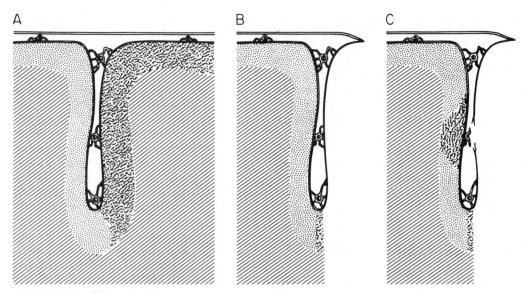

A

B

C

FIGURE 12–2. *A*, Diagram of the cortical sulcus as outlined in Figure 12–1, but the right half of which is darkly stippled to represent the epileptogenic lesion. *B*, The presumed result of an optimal subpial removal of the epileptogenic lesion. The small surgical scar left behind is represented by the irregularly densely stippled area at the resection line within the cortex at the depth of the sulcus. The leptomeninges are left intact, and the vessels in the subarachnoid space supplying the cortex on either side of the sulcus are similarly left intact. *C*, In this subpial resection of epileptogenic cortex, a vessel has been damaged in the middle of the sulcus, with a resulting lesion produced in the "preserved" cortex. Thus in this case the same minimal surgical lesion is present at the base of the sulcus on the resection line, but there is a further lesion in the cortex to the left of the sulcus represented by the dark, irregularly stippled area adjacent to the destroyed vessel.

small sulcal vessels have not been injured. This very small cortical lesion at the bottom of the sulcus may be larger, at least in theory, as a result of interference with the afferent supply to the cortex through removal of white matter underlying the anatomically preserved gray matter. (This resulting partial deafferentation was considered by Ward[70] to be perhaps the important pathophysiologic basis for the epileptogenicity of the focus.) In Figure 12–2C, the vessel halfway between the bottom of the sulcus and the subarachnoid space has been injured and coagulated. This in turn has resulted in the production of a lesion, on the basis of focal ischemic necrosis, in the "preserved" gray matter of the remaining side of the sulcus. Therefore, an additional scar is produced, which increases the potential epileptogenicity produced by the resection. Thus meticulous attention must be paid to the technique of subpial removal of cortex to achieve the objectives outlined above.

When a "cortical incision" is made, in the general neurosurgical sense, it is usually made down the center of a gyrus, in which case there may be left behind on either side of the incision, within the nearest sulci, cortex that is denervated, ischemic, or contused. This type of damaged cortex must be avoided in epilepsy surgery. Hence, if subpial dissection is performed in making such incisions, the scar will be minimized. A comparison of Figures 12–2A and 12–2B best depicts the rationale for the use of subpial dissection and why the resulting surgical scar may be much smaller and less epileptogenic than the removed epileptic lesion.

When operating in the sylvian fissure, and more particularly when removing the superior temporal gyrus, both of the leptomeningeal layers (pial and arachnoid) will provide a barrier to potential injury to the underlying middle cerebral artery and there will be a further similar layer between the latter and the insular cortex.

In keeping with the tenets of subpial dissection, sulcal boundaries are followed wherever possible. However, part of the resection line must be carried across gyri, relatively perpendicular to the sulci. In this instance the scar is minimized by a restricted use of coagulation and by preservation of as much white matter as possible beneath the scar so as to decrease the possibility of denervation of the neurons left at the resection line.

General Principles

The philosophy of the Montréal school, which pioneered epilepsy surgery in the Western world, gradually underwent an evolution with respect to the size of the removals. Initially the removals were relatively restricted, some being restricted to the lesion itself. With increasing experience this practice changed to the resection of larger amounts of cortex. Whereas many of the small resections gave good results, the results could be improved by increasing the size of the removal during the initial operation or by secondary operations.[50,53] This gave rise to the philosophy that a critical amount of cortex must be removed to achieve abolition of the seizure disorder. Others have similarly supported this view.[59] The potential exception to this philosophy is the recently adopted practice in some centers of carrying out a relatively limited amygdalohippocampectomy for some selected cases of temporal lobe seizures (see Wieser and Yasargil[71]). The rationale for this limited removal arose from analyses of the results of temporal lobectomy, which have disclosed that one of the factors strongly correlated with favorable outcome is the extent of the removal of the hippocampus.[3,21]

An epileptic focus is generally identified by scalp and/or invasive electrography. Following this, my own practice is to then more narrowly localize it with the use of intraoperative electrocorticography (ECoG). In this way each operation involving resection of a focus is individualized. In addition to electrographic tailoring, the resection is also tailored functionally. That is, either by a knowledge of the safe limits of removal of a certain cortical area or by intraoperative cortical mapping of functional areas by electrical stimulation, unwanted surgical encroachment on important functional, or eloquent, cortex is avoided. There is some controversy as to whether operations for epilepsy should be carried out under general anesthesia, or local anesthesia with neurolept analgesia. To carry out cortical mapping, of course, local anesthesia must be used. Details regarding the use of local anesthesia may be found elsewhere.[18,43,45]

Types of Resective Surgery

Resective surgery is that associated with removal of cerebral cortex, and hence properly comes under the term *corticectomy*. This term includes gyrectomy, topectomy, lobectomy, and even hemispherectomy cited in the literature. The most common resective operation carried out for epilepsy is that of lobectomy, with the commonest site being the temporal lobe. Temporal lobectomy comprises approximately 50% to 100% of the operations for seizures carried out at any given center. This proportion usually decreases with the increasing sophistication and expertise of the center in question, the more experienced centers usually dealing additionally with more cases of extratemporal epilepsy.

Most of the literature on the surgery of epilepsy deals with the temporal lobe, not only because temporal lobectomy is the commonest operation for epilepsy, but also because of the special functional significance of the inferomesial structures of the temporal lobe involved with anterograde memory, in other words, the laying down ("learning") of new material and the recall of this material at will. The description of temporal lobectomy is not pertinent to this discussion, and the reader is referred to other sources.[46,68] Quite briefly, the typical temporal lobectomy consists of an anterior lobectomy, the neocortical removal being limited in the dominant hemisphere by the cortical temporal speech zone, which may be as anterior as 5 cm behind the tip of the temporal pole, and on the nondominant side by the subcortical visual radiation fibers serving the contralateral upper homonymous visual quadrant, situated as far forward as 6 to 6.5 cm behind the temporal pole. As more experience is gained with cortical mapping, the sophistication of the tailoring of the dominant lobectomy is improved.[37-40]

The most predictably efficacious surgical treatment of epilepsy is that of hemispherectomy in very specialized cases of the infantile hemiplegic patient with intractable epilepsy. Such a patient typically has a spastic motor hemiplegia with all loss of individual finger movements and the retained motor ability only to use the arm for "trapping" objects against the body. There is a sensory deficit that is disproportionately much less than would be anticipated from the lack of contralateral cortical sensory integrity, and there is usually an accompanying homonymous hemianopia. This condition classically results from a febrile illness of infancy,[15,16,66] although it may occur spontaneously without any ostensible cause in infancy or even earlier at the time of birth or in intrauterine life.

Although hemispherectomy had been performed for tumors,[7,33] McKenzie[35] first performed the operation for intractable seizures and infantile hemiplegia on a young girl in 1938, but it was really Krynauw[29] in 1950 who brought the operation to prominence. In a series of 12 patients, he showed the remarkable beneficial effects of the operation on the hemiplegia, the seizures, and, interestingly, the episodic outbursts of behavioral aggression.

Initially the operation of "hemispherectomy" consisted not of a true hemispherectomy but rather a hemidecortication with preservation of the deep gray matter of the hemisphere. Unfortunately, this remarkably consistently excellent operation, which usually results in a drug-free, seizure-free patient, may be associated with a peculiar type of late hemorrhage.[32,42] Over the ensuing years it was realized that this hemorrhagic complication (called superficial hemosiderosis, or superficial cerebral hemosiderosis) occurred many years following operation in about 25% of patients, of whom approximately 50% died. Rasmussen[51] compared the results of large multilobe removals with those of complete hemispherectomies and noted the lack of complications in the former group. Consequently the operation has been modified: a subtotal hemispherectomy is carried out, in which a part of the hemisphere is left in place.[52] In 1981 I modified the operation

such that only the temporal lobe and the rolandic cortex are removed, with a disconnection of the remaining parts of the hemispheric cortex from the deep gray matter.[17] This "functional" hemispherectomy has provided similarly beneficial results while attempting to preclude the complications of anatomic hemispherectomy.

Operations Interrupting Pathways of Propagation

Many operations ostensibly have been directed either at decreasing the excitability of the epileptogenic focus or the whole brain or at interrupting the pathways of propagation. Many of the operations in the former category have been stereotaxic procedures, none of which has survived as a popular method of treatment. However, the operation of corpus callosum section (CCS), or corpus callosotomy, which interrupts the large interhemispheric commissure, has been of proven value.

The operation of corpus callosotomy is based on a large body of experimental evidence that has accrued over the last 50 years.[9,28,67] Because of experimental evidence disclosing propagation of epileptic discharge across the corpus callosum, the suggestion arose that if this commissural pathway were incised, the subsequent interruption of the propagated discharge would lead to an alleviation or beneficial alteration of the seizures resulting from such discharge.

Sporadic reports appeared in the clinical literature, in which the corpus callosum was damaged either by a disease process and/or surgery, with beneficial effects on preexisting seizures. However, Van Wagenen and Herren[65] made the initial foray into the specific use of the CCS for patients with generalized epilepsy. They reported on the varied success of a series of 10 patients in whom the corpus callosum had been divided. The operations in these patients could not be considered as pure corpus callosotomies, because in some patients other pathways of propagation, and particularly other interhemispheric commissural pathways, were interrupted as well. In recent years the operation of interhemispheric commissurotomy was reintroduced by Wilson and colleagues.[72-74] The operation itself was initially that of complete division of the corpus callosum, but because of the neuropsychologic complications of separating the right and left hemispheres that occurred in some patients (i.e., "disconnection" syndromes), the operation has since been revised and in most centers consists of a subtotal CCS. Usually in this operation a varying amount of splenium is left intact. With the CCS, however, the hippocampal commissure, which is attached to the undersurface of the posterior portion of the corpus callosum is divided as well.

The indications for CCS vary to some degree between different centers. The prime indications for its use involve patients with various types of primary generalized epilepsy and those types with multiple foci, especially where secondary generalization occurs. Nearly immediate abolition of akinetic seizures follows the operation; and Spencer and her colleagues[61,63] have shown that the pattern of secondarily generalized seizures is usually altered and frequently abolished. The operation has been used for focally originating cortical seizures or as an alternative to hemispherectomy in patients with infantile hemiplegia and intractable seizures, but its use in these cases is much more controversial and less generally accepted.

The results of CCS are varied, and it is very difficult to get an accurate picture from the literature. The one point that is absolutely clear is that the so-called akinetic, or atonic, primary generalized seizures are usually dramatically relieved in much the same way as they are relieved in the infantile hemiplegic patient by hemispherectomy. The physiologic mechanism underlying these seizures remains just as poorly understood as the reason for their abolition by CCS or hemispherectomy. My view is that most patients are helped in the immediate postoperative period but that results should not be considered for any kind of public scrutiny before a postoperative period of at least 36 to 48 months has elapsed. In our unit many patients who at first have shown rather dramatic improvement have shown after 2 or 4 years a loss of some of the improvement that was initially seen.

Many other points are pertinent to a discussion of CCS, including (1) long-term follow-up, (2) the use of the operation in left-handers with left cerebral dominance, (3) the question of the neuropsychologic deficits following operation, (4) its use in the infantile hemiplegic with intractable seizures as an alternative to subtotal hemispherectomy, (5) its potential efficacy in sorting out unilateral foci with rapid secondary bilateral synchrony from bilateral frontal foci, (6) its use in the pediatric age groups, (7) the effect of the operation on the EEG, and (8) the questionable efficacy of tailoring selective section of various parts of the corpus callosum to the type of epilepsy in question. Detailed discussion of these points is beyond the scope of this chapter, but the reader is referred to a recent symposium touching on many of these aspects.[4,62]

RESEARCH QUESTIONS THAT ARE LIKELY TO YIELD ANSWERS

Analyses of the Intracarotid Amytal Procedure

The intracarotid amytal test, which involves transient (a few minutes') narcotization of a hemisphere, was originally used to determine the lateralization of speech. For the last 25 years it has been used, more importantly, for the preoperative assessment of memory. Narcotization of the hemisphere supplied by the carotid artery, which includes the temporal lobe, allows assessment of the contribution to memory of each of the temporal lobes. The use and method of the intracarotid amytal procedure for the evaluation of memory (ICAP-M) vary markedly from one center to another.[54] In some centers, every temporal lobectomy has as part of the preoperative investigation bilateral intracarotid amytal procedures; at the other end of the scale are centers in which only 20% to 30% of such patients are investigated with the use of the ICAP-M. The validity[20] and reliability[34] of this test for memory are only now beginning to be questioned and investigated. The difficulties in addressing this issue scientifically are obvious to those familiar with the process. However, the next decade will produce much more information. It is my view that not all patients require the test. Through collation of results, epileptologists and neuropsychologists should be able to reach a consensus on indications for the use of the procedure. Further, there must be some vehicle by which any untoward complications with respect to memory in patients who have had temporal lobectomy are recorded, employing a bank of observations in which some degree of anonymity is maintained.

The Interictal EEG in Localization

The use of interictal spikes as the definitive localization for epileptic foci is controversial. In at least one center, for as many as 75% of the patients considered for temporal lobectomy the interictal spike is the primary electrographic investigation for localization. Other centers indicate that the interictal spike cannot be used in localization. If in fact the results from those centers that do use interictal spike localization are similar to those who demand electrographic recording of seizures, either by scalp or invasive recording, then it would be hard to justify the notion that the interictal spike is of no value in this regard. If, of course, the interictal spike were to be shown to be of equal value to the more sophisticated methods of recording, then it would cut down tremendously the economic burden of investigation.

The Extent of the Use of Invasive Electrography

Some centers have required invasive electrography (e.g., depth electrode, subdural recording) in all patients with temporal lobe epilepsy. If one looks historically at those centers that have taken this stance, the view is usually very much modified with the passage of time. It is my view that invasive electrography is required only in the minority of patients, perhaps as many as 20% to 30%.

Economic Benefit of Surgical Treatment

The burgeoning field of epilepsy surgery demands some kind of accountability with respect to the benefits of surgical treatment, including economic benefits. In countries with universal health care systems, such economic analyses could be carried out more easily. Thus it is incumbent on those in the field to demonstrate the economic benefit of the procedure, which is particularly important to those centers who receive large investigative or research support from granting foundations. Such an investigation undoubtedly would provide valuable data about benefit and cost, provided that good, quantifiable criteria for the analyses were set out.

Intraoperative Assessment of Memory

One of the great concerns in temporal lobectomy is the question of altered memory following surgery. Reference has already been made to the use of the ICAP-M for preoperative assessment. However, further evidence exists that some patients with failed memory may still undergo a temporal lobectomy without undergoing a permanent loss of recent memory.[20] One of the problems facing the epilepsy surgeon has always been the difficulty of determining any type of memory impairment intraoperatively. In other words, if memory could be assessed intraoperatively, then one could determine at that time, perhaps in conjunction with a preoperative ICAP-M, how much, if any, hippocampus could be removed with impunity.

Preliminary results with intraoperative stimulation of the hippocampus have suggested that in fact this technique may be used for such assessment, but only the accumulation of more observational data will allow this to be determined with certainty.[19]

Standardization of the Results of Epilepsy Surgery

One problem in assessing the results of surgery for epilepsy is the great difficulty in comparing results of different surgical approaches, preoperative investigations, and selection criteria between different centers. There must be some standard by which both input and outcome in particular can be assessed. Only in this way will true scientific accountability and comparison in the assessment of outcome be achieved.

SUMMARY

Epilepsy has been treated surgically for more than a century. The criteria for surgery in medically intractable epilepsy have been altered over the years, particularly because of recent changes in attitude. Surgical management may be resective (corticectomy, lobectomy, hemispherectomy) or may be directed toward controlling the spread of seizures (various stereotactic lesions, corpus callosotomy).

Resective surgery has been the most beneficial, with a proven track record. The objective of such surgery is to remove the area, or focus, of the brain giving rise to seizures, leaving behind minimal surgical scar. Although surgeons cannot guarantee that any procedure will permanently abolish seizures, the beneficial effects of operative intervention nevertheless far outweigh the potential costs. It is predicted that sophistication with respect to the investigation of epilepsy and the standardization of results will increase greatly over the next decade, allowing better comparisons and almost certainly clearing up some of the controversies between various centers.

ACKNOWLEDGMENT

Becky Bannerman ably provided secretarial assistance in the preparation of this chapter.

REFERENCES

1. Annegers, JF, Hauser, WA, and Elveback, LR: Remission of seizures and relapse in patients with epilepsy. Epilepsia 20:729–737, 1979.
2. Bates, JAV: The surgery of epilepsy. In Williams, D (ed): Modern Trends in Neurology, Vol 3. Butterworth Publishers, Stoneham, MA, 1962, pp 125–137.
3. Bengzon, ARA, Rasmussen, T, Gloor, P, Dussault, J, and Stephens, M: Prognostic factors in the surgical treatment of temporal lobe epileptics. Neurology 18:717–731, 1986.
4. Blume, WT: Normal anatomy and physiology of the corpus callosum. J Epilepsy 3(Suppl):187–196, 1991.
5. Boshes, LD and Kienast, HW: Community aspects of epilepsy. Ill Med J 138:140–146, 1970.
6. Currie, S, Heathfield, KWG, Henson, RA, and Scott, DF: Clinical course and prognosis of temporal lobe epilepsy: A survey of 666 patients. Brain 94:173–190, 1971.
7. Dandy, WE: Removal of right cerebral hemisphere for certain tumors with hemiplegia. JAMA 90:823–825, 1928.
8. Davidson, S, Falconer, MA, and Stroud, CE: The place of surgery in the treatment of epilepsy in childhood and adolescence: A preliminary report in 13 cases. Dev Med Child Neurol 14:796–803, 1972.
9. Erickson, TC: Spread of the epileptic discharge. Arch Neurol Psychiatry 43:429–452, 1940.
10. Falconer, MA: Significance of surgery for temporal lobe epilepsy in children and adolescents. J Neurosurg 33:233–252, 1970.
11. Falconer, MA: The place of surgery in epileptic children and adolescents with mesial temporal (Ammon's horn) sclerosis. Ir J Med Sci 141:147–161, 1972a.
12. Falconer, MA: Place of surgery for temporal lobe epilepsy during childhood. Br Med J 2:631–635, 1972b.
13. Falconer, MA and Davidson, S: The rationale of surgical treatment of temporal lobe epilepsy with particular reference to childhood and adolescence. In Harvis, P and Mawdsley, C (eds): Epilepsy: Proceedings of the Hans Berger Centenary Symposium. Churchill Livingstone, Edinburgh, 1974, pp 209–214.
14. Ferendelli, J: Personal communication, October 1989.
15. Gastaut, H, Poirier, F, Payan, H, Salamon, G, Toga, M, and Vigouroux, M: H.H.E.S. syndrome: Hemiconvulsions, hemiplegia, epilepsy. Epilepsia 1:418–447, 1960.
16. Gastaut, H, Vigouroux, M, Trevisan, C, and Regis, H: Le Syndrome: Hémiconvulsion–Hémiplegie–epilepsie (syndrome) H.H.E. Rev Neurol (Paris) 97:37–52, 1957.
17. Girvin, JP: Unpublished observations, 1981.
18. Girvin, JP: Resection of intracranial lesions under local anaesthesia. Int Anesthesiol Clin 24:133–155, 1986.
19. Girvin, JP and Gorecki, J: Intraoperative memory assessment by hippocampal stimulation. (to be submitted for publication), 1990.
20. Girvin, JP, McGlone, J, McLachlan, RS, and Blume, WT: On the validity of the intracarotid amytal test for memory. (Submitted for publication.) Presented at the American Epilepsy Society Mtg, Baltimore, Dec 1987.
21. Glaser, GH: Treatment of intractable temporal lobe–limbic epilepsy (complex partial seizures) by temporal lobectomy. Ann Neurol 8:455–459, 1980.
22. Goddard, GV: Development of epileptic seizures through brain stimulation at low intensity. Nature 214:1020–1021, 1967.
23. Goddard, GV, McIntyre, DC, and Leech, CK: A permanent change in brain function resulting from daily electrical stimulation. Exp Neurol 25:295–330, 1969.
24. Hauser, WA and Kurland, LP: Incidence, preva-

lence, time trends of convulsive disorders in Rochester, Minnesota: A community survey. In Alter, M and Hauser, WA (eds): The Epidemiology of Epilepsy: A Workshop DHEW Publication No. 73-390, pp 41–44, 1972.

25. Hauser, WA and Kurland, LP: The epidemiology of epilepsy in Rochester, Minnesota, 1935 through 1967. Epilepsia 16:1–66, 1975.

26. Horsley, V: Brain-surgery, Br Med J 2:670–675, 1886.

27. Jensen, I: Temporal lobe epilepsy: Type of seizures, age, and surgical results. Acta Neurol Scand 53:335–357, 1976.

28. Kopeloff, N, Kennard, MA, Pacella, BL, Kopeloff, LM, and Chusid, JG: Section of corpus callosum in experimental epilepsy in the monkey. Arch Neurol Psychiatry 63:719–727, 1950.

29. Krynauw, RA: Infantile hemiplegia treated by removing one cerebral hemisphere. J Neurol Neurosurg Psychiatry 13:243–267, 1950.

30. Kurtzke, JF: The current neurological burden of illness and injury in the United States. Neurology 32:1207–1214, 1982.

31. Kurtzke, JF: Neuroepidemiology. Ann Neurol 16:265–277, 1984.

32. Laine, E, Pruvet, P, and Ossen, D: Résultats élloignés de l'hémisphérectomie dans les cas d'hémiatrophie cérbrale infantile génératrice d'epilepsie. Neurochirurgie 10:507–522, 1964.

33. L'Hermitte, J: L'ablation complète de l'hémisphère droit dans les cas de tumeur cérébrale localisée compliquée d'hémiplègie: la décérébration supra-thalamique unilatérale chez l'homme. Encephale 23:314–322, 1928.

34. McGlone, J and MacDonald, BH: Reliability of sodium amobarbital test for memory. J Epilepsy 2:31–39, 1989.

35. McKenzie, KG: The present status of a patient who had the right cerebral hemisphere removed. Proceedings of the American Medical Association 111:168, 1938.

36. Morrell, F: Secondary epileptogenesis in man. Arch Neurol 42:318–335, 1985.

37. Ojemann, G: Organization of short-term verbal memory in language areas of human cortex: Evidence from electrical stimulation. Brain Lang 5:331–340, 1978.

38. Ojemann, GA: Mapping of neuropsychological language parameters at surgery. Int Anesthesiol Clin 24:115–131, 1986.

39. Ojemann, GA and Dodrill, C: Reducing the verbal memory deficit after left temporal lobectomy for epilepsy: Role of lateral cortical memory mechanisms. Epilepsia 25:664, 1984.

40. Ojemann, G, Ojemann, J, Lettich, E, and Berger, M: Cortical language localization in left dominant hemisphere: An electrical stimulation mapping investigation in 117 patients. J Neurosurg 71:316–326, 1989.

41. Olney, JW: Neurotoxicity of excitatory amino acids. In McGeer, Olney, JW, and McGeer, P (eds): Kainic Acid as a Tool in Neurobiology. Raven Press, New York, 1978, p 95.

42. Oppenheimer, DR and Griffith, HB: Persistent intracranial bleeding as a complication of

hemispherectomy. J Neurol Neurosurg Psychiatry 29:229–240, 1966.

43. Pasquet, A: Combined regional and general anesthesia for craniotomy and cortical exploration. Part II. Anesthetic considerations. Current Research in Anesthesia and Analgesia 33:156–164, 1954.

44. Penfield, W: The epilepsies: With a note on radical therapy. N Engl J Med 221:209–218, 1939.

45. Penfield, W: Combined regional and general anesthesia for craniotomy and cortical exploration. Part I. Neurosurgical considerations. Current Research in Anesthesia and Analgesia 33:145–155, 1954.

46. Penfield, W and Baldwin, M: Temporal lobe seizures and the technique of subtotal temporal lobectomy. Ann Surg 136:625–634, 1952.

47. Penfield, W and Flanigin, H: Surgical therapy of temporal lobe seizures. Arch Neurol Psychiatry 64:491–500, 1950.

48. Porter, R: Personal communication, April, 1989.

49. Poskanzer, DC: House-to-house survey of a community for epilepsy. In Alter, M and Hauser, WA (eds): The Epidemiology of Epilepsy: A Workshop. DHEW Publication No. 73-390, pp 45–46, 1972.

50. Rasmussen, T: Surgical therapy of frontal lobe epilepsy. Epilepsia 4:181–190, 1963.

51. Rasmussen, T: Postoperative superficial haemosiderosis of the brain: Its diagnosis, treatment and prevention. Transactions of the American Neurological Association 98:133–137, 1973.

52. Rasmussen, T: Hemispherectomy for seizures revisited. Can J Neurol Sci 10:71–78, 1983.

53. Rasmussen, T and Gossman, H: Epilepsy due to gross destructive brain lesions: Results of surgical therapy. Neurology 13:659–669, 1963.

54. Rausch, R: Psychological evaluation. In Engel, J Jr (ed): Surgical Treatment of the Epilepsies. Raven Press, New York, 1987, pp 181–195.

55. Reynolds, EH: Unsatisfactory aspects of the drug treatment of epilepsy. Epilepsia 17, 3:xii–xv, 1976.

56. Robb, P: Focal epilepsy: The problem, prevalence, and contributing factors. In Purpura, DP, Penry, JK, and Walter, RD (eds): Raven Press, New York, 1975, pp 11–22.

57. Rodin, EA: The Prognosis of Patients With Epilepsy. Charles C Thomas, Springfield, IL, 1968.

58. Rodin, EA, Klutke, G, and Chayasirisobohn, S: Epileptic patients who are refractory to anticonvulsant medications. Neurology 32:1382–1384, 1982.

59. Rossi, GF: Considerations on the principles of surgical treatment of partial epilepsies. Brain Res 95:395–402, 1975.

60. Sachs, E: The subpial resection of the cortex in the treatment of Jacksonian epilepsy (Horsley operation) with observation on Areas 4 and 6. Brain 58:492–503, 1935.

61. Spencer, SS: Corpus callosotomy in the treatment of intractable seizures. In Pedley, TA, Meldrum, BS (eds): Recent Advances in Epilepsy,

Vol 4. Churchill Livingstone, Edinburgh, 1988, pp 181–204.

62. Spencer, SS: Corpus callosum section in children: Indications and issues. II. Epileptic physiology and rationale. J Epilepsy 3 (Suppl 1):197–204, 1991.

63. Spencer, SS, Gates, JR, Reeves, AR, Spencer, DD, Maxwell, RE, and Roberts, D: Corpus callosum section. In Engel, J (ed): Surgical Treatment of the Epilepsies. Raven Press, New York, 1987, pp 425–444.

64. Steelman, HF: Technique of cortical excision: An experimental study of postoperative cicatrization. Archives of Neurology and Psychiatry 62:479–492, 1949.

65. Van Wagenen, WP and Herren, RY: Surgical division of commissural pathways in the corpus callosum: Relation to spread of an epileptic attack. Archives of Neurology and Psychiatry 44:740–759, 1940.

66. Vigouroux, M: Etude electroencephalographique des hémiconvulsions suivies d'hémiplégie (syndrome H.H.) et de ses séquelles épileptiques (syndrome H.H.E.) Rev Neurol (Paris) 99:39–53, 1958.

67. Wada, JA and Komai, S: Effective anterior two-thirds callosal bisection upon bisymmetrical and bisynchronous generalized convulsions kindled from amygdala in epileptic baboon, Papio papio. In Reeves, AG (ed): Epilepsy and the Corpus Callosum. Plenum Press, New York, 1985, pp 75–97.

68. Walker, AE: Temporal lobectomy. J Neurosurg 26:642–649, 1967.

69. Ward, AA: Surgery of epilepsy: Overview. Presented at the 15th Epilepsy International Symposium. Washington, DC, September 26–30, 1983.

70. Ward, AA Jr: The epileptic neuron: Chronic foci in animals and man. In Jasper, HH, Ward, AA, and Pope A (eds): Basic Mechanisms of the Epilepsies. Little, Brown & Co, Boston, 1969, pp 263–288.

71. Wieser, HJ and Yasargil, MG: Die to >> selektive Amygdala-Hippokampektomie << als chirurgische Behandlungsmethode der mediobasal-limbischen Epilepsie. Neurochirurgia (Stuttg) 25:39–50, 1982.

72. Wilson, DH, Culder, C, Waddington, M, and Gazzaniga, M: Disconnection of the cerebral hemispheres: An alternative to hemispherectomy for the control of intractable seizures. Neurology 25:1149–1153, 1975.

73. Wilson, DH, Reeves, A, and Gazzaniga, M: Division of a corpus callosum for uncontrolled epilepsy. Neurology 28:649–653, 1978.

74. Wilson, DH, Reeves, A, Gazzaniga, M, and Culver, C: Cerebral commissurotomy for control of intractable seizures. Neurology 27:708–715, 1977.

75. Zielinski, JJ: Epidemiology of epilepsy in Poland on the basis of visits to physicians. (In Polish.) Przegl Epidemiol 29:123, 1975.

MOVEMENT DISORDERS

EDITOR'S COMMENTARY

Progress in movement disorders has not been smooth. After a century and a half of acceptance of Parkinson's disease as a classic "degenerative" disorder, a dopamine deficiency in the basal ganglia was recognized. Early attempts to replace the deficit with levodopa failed because the dose was not high enough. After George C. Cotzias* showed a therapeutic effect at higher doses, there followed convincing positive studies and dramatic individual reports captured in an article called "L-DOPA Set Me Free" in the Reader's Digest† *and the moving classic of medical literature,* Awakenings, *by Oliver Sacks.‡ Disappointment followed elation with the realization that L-DOPA helped the symptoms but did not halt the disease and that improvement came at the price of serious side effects.*

Then came the report of Madrazo and colleagues[68] in 1987 of the successful open microsurgical autograft of adrenal medulla to the right caudate nucleus in two patients with intractable Parkinson's disease. Worldwide reports of similar surgery followed with hyperkinetic disregard for patient selection, evaluation, and follow-up. Predictably, several conferences and meetings of experts have called for restraints and retrenchment. And yet the scientific bases for transplantation are sound, as Drucker-Colín and García-Hernández document in their chapter. Tessler provides a rationale for transplantation not only in Parkinson's disease but also in spinal cord injury.

As enthusiasm for surgical treatment retreated to the laboratories, the DATATOP study confirmed earlier reports that deprenyl may slow the progression of Parkinson's disease. Before unqualified enthusiasm crashes on some hard realities, we may well heed the balanced approach to the treatment of the refractory parkinsonian patient advocated by Stoessl.

VCH

---

* Cotzias, GC, Papavasilious, and Gellene R: Modification of parkinsonism: Chronic treatment with L-dopa. N Engl J Med 280:337–345, 1969.
† L-DOPA set me free. *Reader's Digest.*
‡ Sacks, O: *Awakenings.* Summit Books, New York, 1987.

CHAPTER 13

• •

Can We Treat Parkinson's Disease Using Adrenal Transplants?

René Drucker-Colín, M.D., Ph.D. and Fernando García-Hernández, Ph.D.

Contrary to some predictions from the 1960s, Parkinson's disease is not disappearing but rather may well be on the rise. More disturbingly, the impression of physicians managing large numbers of parkinsonian patients is that the mean age of onset of the disease is younger than it used to be.

Even with the addition of deprenyl to the treatment repertoire, with its promise of slowing the disease, the need to explore other treatments remains great.

Drucker-Colín and García-Hernández provide a good scientific rationale for transplantation treatment but at the same time caution that the mechanisms of how transplants may work are not necessarily the obvious ones, such as dopamine replacement. They emphasize the potential role of trophic factors.

Although transplant treatment of Parkinson's disease thus far has been more impressive for its daring than for its results, it remains an avenue of promise and worthy of further exploration.

VCH

CURRENT PRINCIPLES OF TREATMENT

Present-day treatment of Parkinson's disease relies considerably on the concept that the primary biochemical abnormality is a decrease in the availability of dopamine in the nigrostriatal pathway. The severity of symptoms relates to the degree of this defect,[54] and the mechanism by which symptoms are produced results from a disturbance of dopaminergic relationships with other neurotransmitters, particularly acetylcholine.

During the past 15 years significant advances have been made in controlling the devastating effects of Parkinson's disease.

Not only are symptoms more effectively controlled and the quality of life of those affected improved, but the mortality rate that markedly shortened life expectancy has been substantially reduced.[4,106,108]

Drug Treatment

All drugs presently in use are directed toward reestablishing normal neurotransmitter function to the affected brain region; their primary pharmacologic effects are to either increase dopaminergic activity or decrease cholinergic activity. Since the introduction of high-dosage levodopa therapy by Cotzias and colleagues in 1967,[21] levodopa,

165

given in combination with a peripheral dopa-decarboxylase inhibitor such as carbidopa, is the most potent and commonly used treatment. Thus, levodopa therapy can be considered a replacement for the missing dopamine normally present. Such replacement depends on the presence of remaining dopa-decarboxylase activity in the striatum. Direct-acting dopamine receptor agonists are the next most efficient agents.[17,46,65,66,83] Although apomorphine and N-propyl-*nor*-apomorphine were the first dopamine agonists to be employed in the treatment of Parkinson's disease,[21,92] these drugs never achieved a sufficiently high therapeutic index for acceptance. On the other hand, bromocriptine has become of quite frequent use in the early treatment phase, as an alternative to a continuously increasing dosage of levodopa, as symptoms increase in severity.

Anticholinergics and amantadine, a group of weaker antiparkinsonian drugs, are given in the early stages of the disease, when symptoms are mild; however, their usage is not recommended in patients over age 70, in whom they can cause confusion and hallucinations.

The introduction of levodopa, a dopamine receptor agonist, and other drugs capable of altering storage catabolism of dopamine, have significantly contributed to the relief of Parkinson's symptoms, occasionally for extended periods of time. However, after long-term use of levodopa, usually after 5 years, various problems develop, and only a small minority of patients have no complications.[34,72] Most patients have either clinical fluctuations, inadequate responses, or toxicity even at a subtherapeutic dosage of levodopa. The most common type of clinical fluctuation is the "wearing-off" effect, also known as "end-of-dose deterioration."[73] A summary of the action of these drugs in a dopaminergic synapse is illustrated in Figure 13–1.

Surgical Treatment

Because none of these pharmacologic agents are capable of reestablishing normal neurotransmitter function, eliminating the cause of the disease, or halting the underlying progressive neuronal loss, all such treatments and therapies must be regarded as mere palliatives. As investigators have searched for more long-lasting and nonpharmacologic treatments for Parkinson's disease, and based on a large experimental background, dopamine-rich tissues have been grafted into the striatum of Parkinson's patients.[2,27,67–69] In what follows we provide a description of the experimental knowledge that led to the practice of this procedure, as well as an account of the results.

EXPERIMENTAL MODELS IN PARKINSON'S DISEASE

Since the discovery that the main features causing Parkinson's disease were the loss of the neuronal population in the substantia nigra[102] and the subsequent deficiency of dopaminergic transmission in the striatum,[33] several models were developed to achieve the same clinical features in animals. The subsequent discovery that 6-hydroxydopamine (6-OHDA) selectively destroys central dopaminergic and noradrenergic neurons,[10,12,47,103] causing caudate dopamine postsynaptic supersensitivity,[104] made this neurotoxin an extremely valuable tool in neurobiologic research. Specifically, 6-OHDA has been widely used to produce lesions of central catecholaminergic neurons, in particular the nigrostriatal system, which produces well-defined and stable behavioral deficits. Although exogenous 6-OHDA has not been implicated as an etiologic agent in Parkinson's disease because of its inability to cross the blood-brain barrier (although it causes selective destruction of peripheral noradrenergic sympathetic nerve endings),[101] it has been extensively used to study this disorder. The selectivity of 6-OHDA is believed to be due to its accumulation by dopaminergic and noradrenergic neurons through their high-affinity uptake systems. Indeed, compounds interfering with catecholamine uptake protect against its neurotoxic action.[59,98] The mechanism of action of 6-OHDA has never been fully elucidated. Although it is known that 6-OHDA must first gain entry into dopaminergic and noradrenergic neurons and at-

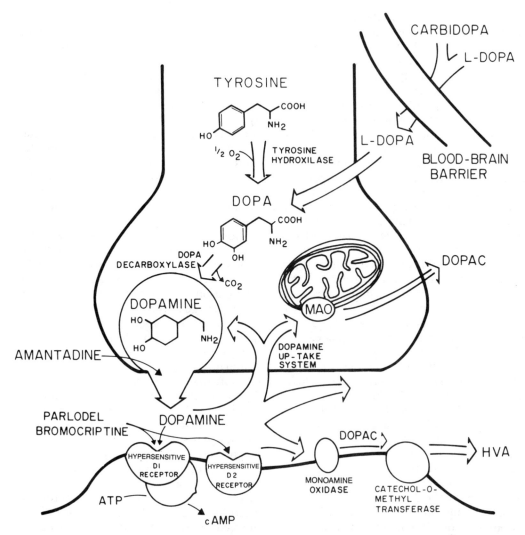

FIGURE 13-1. Schematic representation of a dopaminergic synapse. In the terminal, tyrosine is converted to dopa via tyrosine hydroxylase and finally to dopamine by dopadecarboxylase. Vesiculated dopamine is released into the synaptic cleft, where it binds to D_1 and D_2 dopamine receptors. Dopamine is then converted to dihydroxyphenylacetic acid (DOPAC) by monoamine oxidase (MAO) and aldehyde oxidase and finally to homovanillic acid (HVA) via catechol-O-methyltransferase (COMT). Reuptake systems introduce dopamine into the presynaptic terminal, where it may be revesiculated or converted to DOPAC by mitochondrial MAO. Common Parkinson's treatment utilizes L-DOPA, which enters the biosynthetic dopamine pathway in combination with a peripheral dopa-decarboxylase inhibitor, carbidopa. Also used are amantadine, which facilitates dopamine release, and Parlodel and bromocriptine, which bind and stimulate the hypersensitive dopamine receptor.

tain a critical toxic concentration,[59] the exact molecular series of events by which 6-OHDA produces cell death remains incompletely understood. Possible explanations include the production of free radicals and covalent bonding of quinone oxidation products.[45,49,89] In primates, bilateral intra-

nigral administration of 6-OHDA has been shown to produce a behavioral syndrome reminiscent of parkinsonism.[60,84] In rats, unilateral complete 6-OHDA lesions cause asymmetric posture; sensory inattention (toward stimuli applied to the side of the body contralateral to the lesion); impaired initiation of movement in the direction contralateral to the lesion; and, most evident, asymmetric motor behavior or turning behavior both spontaneously and in response to dopamine-releasing drugs such as amphetamine and dopamine receptor agonists such as apomorphine. All this is believed to be due to denervation supersensitivity. Bilateral lesions result in a state of profound behavioral unresponsiveness including akinesia, bilateral sensory inattention, hunched posture, aphagia, and adipsia.

First sold as a narcotic substitute to heroin addicts,[61] the recently discovered 1-methyl-4- phenyl-1,2,3,6- tetrahidropyridine (MPTP) has also been considered as a parkinsonian etiologic agent.[3,25] Nontoxic systemically, MPTP crosses the blood-brain barrier, destroying in a most selective way the dopaminergic neurons in the substantia nigra pars compacta.[16,25,35,62] For MPTP to exert its neurotoxic action, a series of biochemical reactions must take place. It is known that MPTP is rapidly converted to 1-methyl-4-phenylpyridinium ion, or MPP⁺. The reaction takes place via an intermediate, 1-methyl-4-phenyl-2,3-dihidripyridine, or MPDP⁺.[20] The reaction MPTP to MPDP⁺ appears to be mediated by monoamine oxidase B.[19,50,88] The utilization of MAO B inhibitors prevents dopamine depletion in rodents[51,71] and nigral cell death and parkinsonism in primates.[62,71] MPP⁺ but not MPTP is taken up by the dopamine uptake system with the same affinity as dopamine.[20,56] The cytotoxicity of MPTP is yet to be explained, although several theories have been postulated.[63] The clinical analogy between Parkinson's disease and MPTP-induced parkinsonism in humans is nearly complete, and it is considered the best agent so far discovered for its ability to produce consistent and unalloyed parkinsonism.[3] Because of its unique properties, MPTP has been extensively used to induce a parkinsonianlike state in primates and rodents.

NEURAL TRANSPLANTS: EXPERIMENTAL MODELS

During the 1980s neural transplant technique rapidly developed into a versatile research tool in neurobiology. Although the first attempt at neural transplantation was published by Thompson[99] in 1890, it was only around 1970 that widespread research using neural transplant techniques began. These attempts were based on earlier reports indicating that transplanted nervous tissue survived quite adequately.[22,28,64,74,82,100] The next few reports were basically morphologic and included the first monoaminergic neuronal transplant to the brain of mammals.[9,94]

Several methodologic considerations had to be solved to achieve good and consistent results. From early reports it was established that the age of the donor tissue was a very important feature. The best survival and integration of the transplant was achieved when fetal nervous tissue was used; adult tissue was rarely used because of its poor integration and survival. To a lesser degree, the age of the recipient was an important factor for good survival of neural grafts,[23,24,77,93] although, as we will see, this was not the case in Parkinson patients with adrenal transplants.

Graft placement also was of critical importance for the long-term survival and integration of the transplanted tissue. Neural grafts are placed in two main ways: either as a block of tissue or as a cell suspension, with slight variations according to the experimental protocol. In block transplants, high survival rates are achieved when the tissue is placed in contact with the cerebrospinal fluid in the cerebral ventricles or in a preformed cavity in the cortex. In both cases, a profuse vascularization of the grafted tissue can be observed shortly after grafting. Unlike block transplants, cell suspension transplants can be placed into discrete regions of the host brain. However, the graft survival rates range from 01.% to 1% only.[13,14] Increased survival of intrastriatal adrenal medulla grafts may be achieved by free-radical scavengers and calcium channel blockers.[43]

Not until both the animal 6-OHDA–induced parkinsonian model and the transplant methods were completely developed did the first report of recovery of motor functions by dopaminergic neuron transplants appear,[79] confirmed shortly after by an independent study.[7] In fact, those were the first reports of an induced recovery of a lost function elicited by neural transplants, opening such transplantation as a potential tool for use in the therapy of neurodegenerative diseases. What these early studies demonstrated is that fetal mesencephalic tissue containing dopamine neurons, placed either in the lateral ventricle[79] or in a cortical cavity[7] of a 6-OHDA–denervated striatum, reduced both spontaneous and apomorphine- or amphetamine-induced turning behavior. A particularly interesting aspect of these studies was that they demonstrated that the grafted dopamine neurons not only survived, as revealed by fluorescence histochemical techniques, but also extended dopamine-containing process into the host brain.[7,30–32,79] Furthermore, the extent of the transplant-derived reinnervation of the previously denervated neostriatum was related to the degree of striatal denervation and behavioral recovery.[6,7,79] It has since been postulated that these transplants produced behavioral changes by means of a diffuse release mechanism, whereby dopamine released from the transplant activates the supersensitive dopamine receptor in the denervated striatum.[36–38,40] More recently, Becker and Freed[5] have suggested that the bloodstream is the vehicle of dopamine transport.

The importance of the continued presence of the transplant for the persistence of behavioral effects was demonstrated when it was found that the amphetamine-induced rotational response recorded prior to grafting could be reinstated by surgical removal of the graft.[6] For this experimental procedure to induce functional recovery, the dopamine-containing transplant must be placed in contact with the denervated striatum; otherwise, no behavioral effects are observed. To date, the only features that dopamine grafts have not been able to affect in a major way are the aphagia and adipsia induced by bilateral 6-OHDA lesions.[6,8,29,31]

Shortly after the functional effects of fetal mesencephalic dopamine-containing neurons on the 6-OHDA lesion deficiencies were reported, the possibility of transplanting other catecholaminergic tissues was rapidly explored. Adrenal medulla chromaffin cells were the first to be reported as capable of reducing 6-OHDA lesion deficiencies,[11,36–38,52,75,78,80,87,96,97] followed by PC-12 pheochromocytoma cells,[39,48,55]

sympathetic ganglion cells,[57] and cross-species grafting of dopamine neurons.[15,57,58,80,95] Biochemical studies have revealed that behaviorally effective substantia nigra grafts that reinnervate the host's denervated striatum maintain metabolic rates characteristic of the intact nigrostriatal system, as assessed by the ^{14}C-2-deoxy-D-glucose autoradiography.[90,91] Dopamine synthesis by the transplanted tissue has also been demonstrated.[36] The general observation is that adrenal-medulla and nigral catecholaminergic transplants not only synthesize but also release their neurotransmitters including dopamine, restoring the level to as much as 80% of normal conditions. Consequently, dopamine turnover and release rates approach normal levels.[36,91,96,107] Furthermore, nigral transplants placed in the contralateral ventricle of animals unilaterally lesioned with 6-OHDA are also capable of reducing the apomorphine-induced turning behavior.[26] Figure 13–2 illustrates that regardless of whether the transplant is placed ipsilateral or contralateral to the 6-OHDA–lesioned side, it will produce decreases in apomorphine-induced rotation and in dopamine receptor binding.

This finding is particularly important when using adrenal medulla grafts, because of their poor reinnervating properties.[36,37] Also, solid nigral grafts will release dopamine as a response to potassium-induced depolarization.[53,85] Interestingly, dopamine infusion with an osmotic minipump directly into the dopamine-denervated striatum over a 2-week period can produce a reduction of apomorphine-induced rotational behavior similar to that observed in adrenal medullary grafts.[97] Using electrophysiologic techniques, it has been possible to demonstrate that intraventricular nigral grafts contain dopamine neurons with firing patterns resembling those found in the substantia nigra pars compacta in situ.[105] Nigral grafts are not entirely devoid of afferent host inputs. Grafted neurons, identified by antidromic activation, have been shown to be responsive to stimulation in a variety of host sites, including striatum, prefrontal cortex, locus ceruleus, and dorsal raphe nucleus.[1] This suggests a regulated release model for nigral graft function. Anatomic examination of grafted animals has revealed not only the

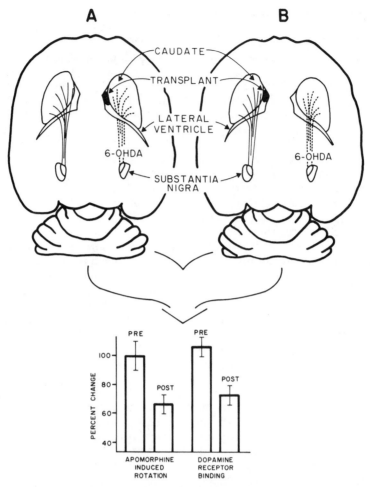

FIGURE 13-2. Schematic horizontal sections of rat brain showing the 6-hydroxydopamine–lesioned nigrostriatal pathway. *A,* Ipsilateral and *B,* contralateral catecholaminergic transplants reduce apomorphine-induced rotation as well as dopamine receptor binding. This suggests that dopamine release is definitely involved in reducing motor asymmetries following nigral lesions.

presence of catecholamine-containing neurons within the transplant but also the actual establishment of normal synaptic contacts between transplant and host neurons.[41,70]

In spite of an extensive experimental background for catecholaminergic brain transplants, not everything is clear about their mechanism of action. Most recently the role of trophic factors and dopamine-releasing factors is being investigated. The discovery of a putative dopamine-releasing factor partially purified from rat adrenal gland,[18] and the possibility that adrenal medulla grafts exert a neurotrophic action in the host brain to enhance recovery of MPTP-lesioned

dopaminergic neurons[11] have suggested new possible mechanisms of action of catecholaminergic transplants. Furthermore, the reduction of turning behavior in aged rats by a combination of nerve growth factor and adipose tissue[81] gives added support to the notion that the participation of trophic factors is essential for recovery of function following induction of lesions of the nigrostriatal pathway. Moreover, adrenal medulla grafts induce the recovery of motor deficits evaluated by swimming behavior and increase tyrosine hydroxylase immunoreactivity in both ipsilateral and contralateral nigrostriatal pathways in aged rats.[42]

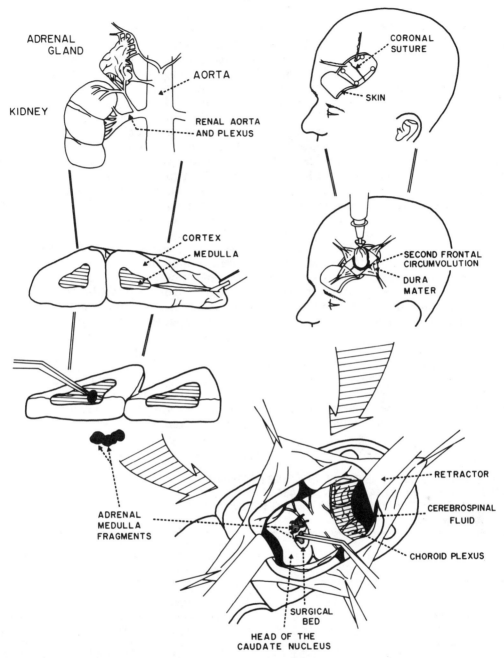

FIGURE 13-3. Schematic representation of medullary transplant surgery on Parkinson's patients. The adrenal gland is extracted and opened, exposing the medullary tissue. Several fragments are then separated. Simultaneously, the caudate nucleus is approached when exposing the lateral ventricle, which is arrived at through a nontraumatic transcortical (second frontal circumvolution) craniotomy. After caudate nucleus identification, a surgical bed is made on its head and the medullary fragments are implanted within the bed and secured to the ependyma by stainless steel miniature staples. The graft is placed in such way that it is embedded within the caudate nucleus but still in contact with the cerebrospinal fluid.

ADRENAL AUTOTRANSPLANTS: HUMAN TRIALS

Based on the extensive experimental background, the adrenal medulla autotransplant in Parkinson patients was first reported by Backlund and associates in 1985.[2] However, they described rather modest improvements during very short periods. The autotransplant procedure in these cases involved stereotaxic placement within the caudate nucleus of a stainless steel spiral that contained the adrenal medullary tissue. It is quite possible that the grafted tissue soon degenerated as a result of being encapsulated. Because adrenal medulla grafts in animals also seemed to survive more adequately when placed in the ventricles rather than directly within the caudate,[38] it is possible that absence of contact with the cerebrospinal fluid (CSF) was also a negative factor.

In view of these possibilities it was decided to attempt a different approach, illustrated in Figure 13 – 3. The objective of this procedure was to maintain the adrenal medulla fragments in direct contact with both the CSF and the caudate nucleus.

The first results were published after a relatively short follow-up period.[27,68,69] The effects of these transplants in a larger group of patients and for a follow-up period ranging from 12 to 27 months (median 16.7) are described below.

Table 13 – 1 shows the percent change in score from pretransplant to post-transplant in the Unified Rating Scale for Parkinsonism during both the "on" and the "off" period of levodopa administration. As can be seen from this table, the younger patients show more substantial improvements, particularly during the on period. It is important to note that the percent improvements in this table merely reflect the percent change in the score of the scale and by no means are meant to indicate an absolute degree of improvement of the disease. It is also evident from this table that neither evolution in years of the disease nor levodopa dosage has any predictive value in determining the type of patient most suitable for a transplant. Age, however, definitely seems to play a major role.

In an effort to quantify changes induced by the transplant in at least some of the Parkinson's symptoms, electromyographic (EMG) recordings were carried out. By such

TABLE 13–1. RESULTS OBTAINED FROM 22 PATIENTS WITH ADRENAL AUTOTRANSPLANTS BASED ON PERCENT CHANGE IN THE UNIFIED RATING SCALE FOR PARKINSONISM*

	No.	Age	Evolution PD (Years)	L-DOPA (mg) Pre	L-DOPA (mg) Post
On					
Good (100–70%)	9	44.7 ± 9.1	8.8 ± 3.2	1194 ± 349	186 ± 195
Regular (70–40%)	7	48.6 ± 10	7.3 ± 3.1	1089 ± 614	410 ± 208
Poor (40–0%)	2	53.5 ± 1.5	9 ± 3	1875 ± 125	750 ± 750
Worse†	4	59.7 ± 4.3	11.2 ± 0.8	1812 ± 207	375 ± 375
Off					
Good (100–70%)	2	34 ± 1	12.5 ± 2.5	1125 ± 2.5	125 ± 125
Regular (70–40%)	12	48.3 ± 8.6	7.9 ± 2.9	1239 ± 416	233 ± 219
Poor (40–0%)	4	50.5 ± 8.7	7.2 ± 2.8	1250 ± 770	468 ± 162
Worse	4	59.7 ± 4.3	11.2 ± 0.8	1812 ± 207	750

* Of the nine good patients in on, seven become regular in off. Of the seven regular patients in on, two become poor in off.
† Of this group of patients, the worsening range in on was from 61% to 105% and in off from 18% to 42%.
All patients in the "worse" category died.

TABLE 13–2. TREMOR FREQUENCY UNDER DIFFERENT CONDITIONS

Subject	RESTING TREMOR PREOP L	R	POSTOP (X 7.7 mo) L	R	TREMOR WITH EXTENSION PREOP L	R	POSTOP (X 7.7 mo) L	R	TREMOR WITH FLEXION PREOP L	R	POSTOP (X 7.7 mo) L	R
1	0	6	0	0	5	5	0	0	5	0	0	0
2	0	5	0	0	7	7	0	0	0	0	0	0
3	5	4	0	0	0	0	0	7	0	10	6	7
4	11	0	0	0	11	11	10	10	0	0	11	11
5	5	0	10	8	5	0	8	0	5	0	0	8
6	5	8	5	0	0	5	0	8	6	0	6	6
7	6	0	4	0	7	0	6	0	4	0	5	0
8	5	4	0	6	6	0	0	0	0	0	0	0
	4.6	3.4	2.4	1.7	5.1	3.5	3.1	3.1	2.5	1.2	3.5	4.0
	±3.2	±2.9	±3.5	±3.1	±3.4	±3.9	±4.1	±4.1	±2.5	±3.3	±3.9	±4.2

	RESTING TREMOR SUCCESSFUL (N = 4) L	R	NON-SUCCESSFUL (N = 4) L	R	TREMOR WITH EXTENSION SUCCESSFUL (N = 4) L	R	NON-SUCCESSFUL (N = 4) L	R
Preop	4 ±4.5	3.7 ±2.3	5.2 ±0.4	3 ±3.3	5.7 ±0.8	3 ±3.0	4.5 ±4.7	4 ±4.5
Postop	0	0	4.7 ±3.6	3.5 ±3.6	0	0	4.0 ±4.2	6.2 ±3.8

L = left extremity; R = right extremity.

173

recordings it is possible to determine the exact tremor frequency per second. It should be pointed out, however, that not all patients exhibit tremor, and of those who do, not all are "good" electromyographically. Of the 22 patients in Table 13–1, we were able to obtain good EMGs from 8. We recorded tremor in resting position, with extension and with flexion. Table 13–2 shows that only four of the eight patients showed a significant change in resting tremor and in tremor with extension. Tremor with flexion was unchanged. In Table 13–3 the pharmacologic treatment of these eight patients clearly indicates that their medication was substantially decreased, as was that of patients shown in Table 13–1. Therefore, even if the transplant did not significantly modify their symptomatology, at least their medication level was diminished, which in any event could be useful in long-term pharmacologic treatment.

Another interesting observation pertains to the EEG activity. Many Parkinson's patients showed an important slowing of the EEG, giving off 2- to 4-Hz frequency under conditions in which normally they should present to 8 to 12 Hz. After the transplant, however, the EEG did show the latter frequencies in the seven patients in whom this abnormality was present. Some patients had normal EEGs preoperatively, and no changes emerged as a result of the transplant (Fig. 13–4).

From the results of adrenal autotransplants it is evident that the procedure induces some important clinical improvements in about 50% of patients and that the improvement seems to benefit preferentially patients below the age of 50.

A recent multicenter study of 19 patients[44] found some significant improvements in motor function and an increase in the on time during the day, but the investigators were unable to reduce medication

TABLE 13-3. PHARMACOLOGIC TREATMENT IN PARKINSON PATIENTS BEFORE AND AFTER TRANSPLANT

DAILY DOSES (in mg)			
Preoperative		Postoperative	
1. Levodopa	1250–1500	Levodopa	1250
Biperiden	4	Biperiden	6
Diazepam	30	Amitriptyline	25
2. Untreated		Levodopa	375
		Amantadine	150
3. Levodopa	750–1000	Levodopa	375
Bromocriptine	7.5	Amantadine	100
		Amitriptyline	50
4. Levodopa	750	Levodopa	375
Trihexyphenidyl	2.5	Biperiden	2
5. Levodopa	750	Amantadine	150
Amitriptyline	25	Amitriptyline	25
6. Levodopa	750	Amantadine	100
Amantadine	300	Levodopa (occasional)	30
Biperiden	3		
Lorazepam	1		
7. Levodopa	2000	Levodopa	250
8. Levodopa	750	Levodopa	375
Biperiden	3	Biperiden	3
Propranolol	120		
Bornaprine	12		
Amitriptyline	25		

X ± SD 937.5 ± 555.5   378.7 ± 360.7
Levodopa doses

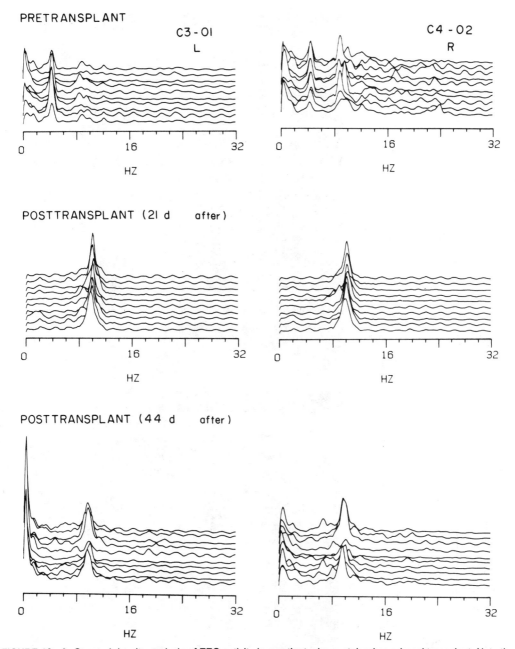

FIGURE 13-4. Spectral density analysis of EEG activity in a patient who sustained an adrenal transplant. Note the slowing of the EEG prior to the graft and recovery of normal EEG activity a few weeks after the graft.

dosage without producing untoward effects. Although this is in sharp contrast with our results, no explanation can presently be put forward to explain these discrepancies. Moreover, in view of such differences, an attempt should be made to determine as efficiently as possible the similarities and differences between surgical procedures, evaluations, and so on, so as to get a clearer idea as to which patients can be ideal for a trans-

YOUNG
(4 mo)

AGED
(22 mo)

APOMORPHINE
(2 mg / kg)

A
D
R
E
N
A
L

G
R
A
F
T

10 D

50 D

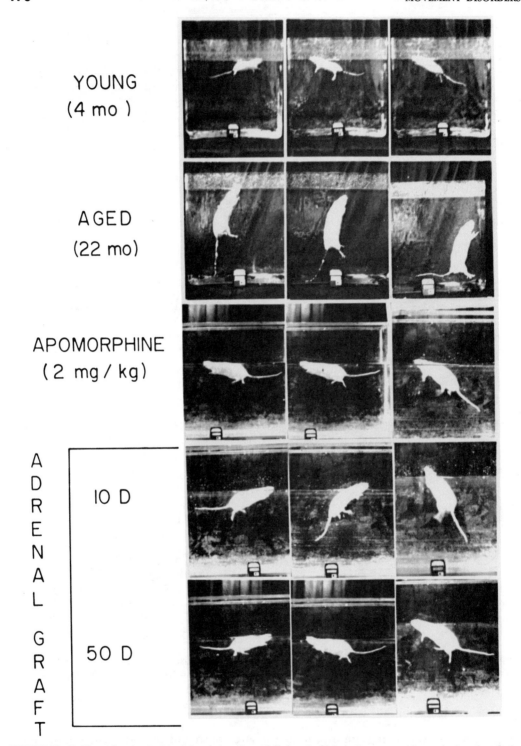

FIGURE 13-5. The swimming test to determine motor activity in rats. Note how apomorphine and adrenal grafts in-duce in aged rats a swimming behavior resembling that seen in young rats.

plant. Certainly, general use of the procedure should not be recommended until such analysis is clearly made.

CONCLUSIONS

Regardless of the controversies, the results obtained with patients have certainly stimulated research in the area of transplants to the brain and have produced more questions than answers. The most interesting aspect for neurology is the relationship of transplanted tissue to trophic factors. The 1987 article of Bohn and colleagues,[11] and more recently of Rosenberg and associates,[86] have certainly suggested that it is possible to create conditions under which regeneration can be induced or degeneration prevented. Also, the fact that adrenal medullary cells can be phenotypically modified and induce recovery of motor disturbances[76] certainly suggests that in the future, cultured cells whose phenotype has been modified can provide the basis for transplantation techniques. Experiments in our laboratory have suggested that in the aged rat, transplants of adrenal tissue induce a significant recovery from motor dysfunctions that in aged rats occur naturally. Figure 13–5 shows how the transplant has been capable of inducing good motor recovery of swimming behavior. Tyrosine hydroxylase immunoreactivity was improved in such aged rats, thus indicating that the transplanted tissue somehow (perhaps through growth factors) improved enzymatic activity of the nigrostriatal pathway (Fig. 13–6). This also agrees with the recent observations[81] that adipose tissue with nerve growth factor is capable of inducing recovery of turning behavior in lesioned rats.

In sum, therefore, although clinical trials should continue with caution and with careful analysis of patient inclusion, research should go hand in hand with such trials, particularly in relation to growth factors and genetically engineered cells.

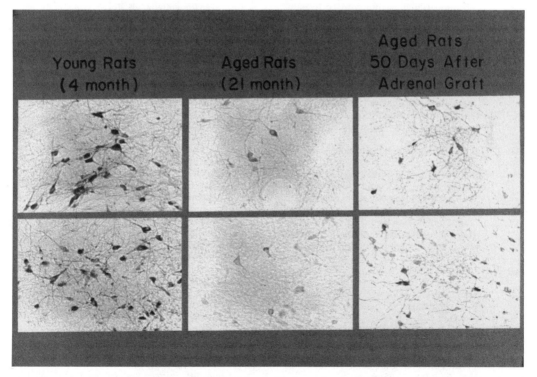

FIGURE 13–6. TH-immunoreactivity of substantia nigra cells in young and aged rats and aged rats with adrenal transplants. Note how the graft induced quite a significant recovery of TH-immunoreactivity.

REFERENCES

1. Arbuthnott, G, Dunnett, SB, and MacLeod, N: Electrophysiological recording from nigral transplants in the rat. Neurosci Lett 57:205–210, 1985.
2. Backlund, EO, Grandberg, PO, Hamberger, B, Sedvall, G, Sieger, A, and Olson, L: Transplantation of adrenal medullary tissue to striatum in parkinsonism: First clinical trials. J Neurosurg 62:169–173, 1985.
3. Ballard, PA, Langston, JW, and Tetrud, JW: Permanent human parkinsonism due to 1-methyl-4-phenyl-1,2,3,6-tetrahydropyridine (MPTP): Seven cases. Neurology 35:946–956, 1985.
4. Bauer, RB, Stevens, C, Reveno, WS, and Rosenbaum, H: L-dopa treatment of Parkinson's disease: A ten year follow-up study. J Am Geriatr Soc 322–326, 1980.
5. Becker, JB and Freed, JW: Adrenal medulla grafts enhance functional activity of the striatal dopamine system following substantia nigra lesions. Brain Res 462:401–406, 1988.
6. Bjorklund, A, Dunnett, SB, Stenevi, U, Lewie, ME, and Iversen, SD: Reinnervation of the denervated neostriatum by substantia nigra transplants: Functional consequences as revealed by pharmacological and sensorimotor testing. Brain Res 199:307–333, 1980.
7. Bjorklund, A and Stenevi, U: Reconstruction of the nigrostriatal dopamine pathway by intracerebral nigral transplants. Brain Res 177:555–560, 1979.
8. Bjorklund, A, Stenevi, U, Dunnett, SB, and Iversen, SD: Functional reactivation of the deafferented neostriatum by nigral transplants. Nature 289:497–499, 1981.
9. Bjorklund, A, Stenevi, U, and Svendgaard, NA: Growth of transplanted monoaminergic neurons into the adult hippocampus along the perforant path. Nature 262:787–790, 1976.
10. Bloom, FE: Fine structural changes in brain after intracisternal injection of 6-hydroxydopamine. In Malforms, R and Thoenen, H (eds): 6-Hydroxydopamine and Catecholamine Neurons. North Holland, Amsterdam, 1971, p 135.
11. Bohn, CM, Cupit, L, Marciano, F, and Gash, D: Adrenal medulla grafts enhance recovery of striatal dopaminergic fibers. Science 237:913–916, 1987.
12. Breese, GR and Taylor, TD: Effect of 6-hydroxydopamine on brain norepinephrine and dopamine: Evidence for selective degeneration of catecholaminergic neurons. J Pharmacol Exp Ther 174:413–420, 1970.
13. Brundin, P, Isacson, O, and Bjorklund, A: Monitoring of cell viability in suspensions of embryonic CNS tissue and its use as a criterion for intracerebral graft survival. Brain Res 331:251–259, 1985.
14. Brundin, P, Isacson, O, Gage, FH, and Bjorklund, A: Intrastriatal grafting of dopamine-containing neuron cell suspensions: Effects of mixing with target or non-target cells. Dev Brain Res 24:77–84, 1986.
15. Brundin, P, Nilsson, GO, Gage, FH, and Bjorklund, A: Cyclosporin A increases survival of cross-species intrastriatal grafts of embryonic dopamine-containing neurons. Exp Brain Res 60:204–208, 1985.
16. Burns, RS, Chiueh, C, Markey, SP, Ebert, MH, Jacobwitz, DM, and Kopin, IJ: A primate model of parkinsonism: Selective destruction of dopaminergic neurons in pars compacta of the substantia nigra by MPTP. Proc Natl Acad Sci U S A 80:4546–4550, 1983.
17. Burton, K and Clane, DB: Pharmacology of Parkinson's disease. Neurol Clin 2:461–472, 1984.
18. Chang, GD and Ramirez, VD: A potent dopamine-releasing factor is present in high concentrations in the rat adrenal gland. Brain Res 463:385–389, 1988.
19. Chiva, K, Trevor, AJ, and Castagnoli, N: Metabolism of the neurotoxic tertiary amine, MPTP, by brain monoamine oxidase. Biochem Biophys Res Commun 1209:574–578, 1984.
20. Chiva, K, Trevor, AJ, and Castagnoli, N: Active uptake of MPP$^+$, a metabolite of MPTP, by brain synaptosomes. Biochem Biophys Res Commun 128:1229–1232, 1985.
21. Cotzias, GC, Van Woert, MH, and Schiffer, LM: Aromatic aminoacids and modification of Parkinsonism. N Engl J Med 276:374–379, 1967.
22. Das, GD and Altman, J: Transplanted precursors of nerve cells: Their fate in the cerebellum of young rats. Science 173:637–638, 1971.
23. Das, GD and Hallas, BH: Transplantation of brain tissue in the brain of adult rats. Experientia 34:1304–1306, 1978.
24. Das, GD, Hallas, BH, and Das, KG: Transplantation of brain tissue in the brain of rat. I. Growth characteristics of neocortical transplants from embryos of different ages. Am J Anat 158:135–145, 1980.
25. Davis, GC, Williams, AC, Markey, SP, Ebert, MH, Caine, ED, Reichert, CM, and Kopin, IJ: Chronic parkinsonism secondary to intravenous injection of meperidine analogues. Psychiatry Res 1:249–254, 1979.
26. Drucker-Colín, R: Grafts placed contralateral to the nigrostriatal lesioned side induce a decrease in motor disturbances. Unpublished material, 1989.
27. Drucker-Colín, R, Madrazo, I, Ostrosky-Solís, F, Shkurovich, M, Franco, R, and Torres, C: Adrenal medullary tissue transplants in the caudate nucleus of Parkinson's patients. In Gash, DM and Sladek, JR (eds): Transplantation into the mammalian CNS. Prog Brain Res 78:567–574, 1988.
28. Dunn, EH: Primary and secondary findings in a series of attempts to transplant cerebral cor-

tex in albino rat. J Comp Neurol 27:565–582, 1917.

29. Dunnett, SB, Bjorklund, A, Schmidt, RH, Stenevi, U, and Iversen, SD: Intracerebral grafting of neuronal cell suspensions: V. Behavioral recovery in rats with bilateral 6-OHDA lesions following implantation of nigral cell suspensions. Acta Physiol Scand (Suppl)522:39–47, 1983.

30. Dunnett, BS, Bjorklund, A, Stenevi, U, and Iversen, SD: Behavioral recovery following transplantation of substantia nigra in rats subjected to 6-OHDA lesions of the nigrostriatal pathway. Brain Res 229:209–217, 1981a.

31. Dunnett, BS, Bjorklund, A, Stenevi, U, and Iversen, SD: Behavioural recovery following transplantation of substantia nigra in rats subjected to 6-OHDA lesions of the nigrostriatal pathway. I. Unilateral lesions. Brain Res 215:147–161, 1981b.

32. Dunnett, BS, Bjorklund, A, Stenevi, U, and Iversen, SD: Behavioral recovery following transplantation of substantia nigra in rats subjected to 6-OHDA lesions of the nigrostriatal pathway. II. Bilateral lesions. Brain Res 229:457–470, 1981c.

33. Ehringer, H and Hornykiewics, O: Verteilung von Noradrenalin und Dopamin (3-hydroxytyramin) im Gehin des Menschen und ihr Verhalten bei Erkankungen des extrapyramidalen Systems. Klin Wocheschr 38:1236–1239, 1960.

34. Fahn, S and Calne, DB: Considerations in the management of parkinsonism. Neurology 28:5–7, 1978.

35. Forno, LS, DeLanney, LE, Irwin, I, and Langston, JW: Neuropathology of MPTP-treated monkeys: Comparison with neuropathology of human idiopathic Parkinson's disease. In Markey, SP, Castagnoli, N, Trevor, A, and Kopin, IJ (eds): MPTP: A neurotoxin Producing a Parkinsonian Syndrome. Academic Press, New York, 1986, p 119.

36. Freed, W, Karoum, F, Spoor, EH, Morihisa, JM, Olson, L, and Wyatt, R: Catecholamine content of intracerebral adrenal medulla grafts. Brain Res 269:184–189, 1983.

37. Freed, W, Morihisa, JM, Spoor, E, Hoffer, BJ, Olson, L, Sieger, A, and Wyatt, RJ: Transplanted adrenal chromaffin cells in rat brain reduce lesion-induced rotational behavior. Nature 229:351–351, 1981.

38. Freed, WJ, Olson, L, Ko, GN, Morisha, JM, Niehoff, D, Stromberg, I, Kuhar, M, Hoffer, BJ, and Wyatt, RJ: Intraventricular substantia nigra and adrenal medulla grafts: Mechanisms of action and (3-H)spiroperidol autoradiography. In Bjorklund, A, and Stenevi, U (eds): Neural Grafting in the Mammalian CNS. Elsevier, Amsterdam, 1985, p 471.

39. Freed, WJ, Patel, VU, and Geller, MH: Properties of PC-12 pheochromocytoma cells transplanted to the adult rat brain. Exp Brain Res 63:557–566, 1986.

40. Freed, W, Perlow, MJ, Karoum, F, Sieger, A,

Olson, L, Hoffer, BJ, and Wyatt, R: Restoration of dopaminergic function by grafting of fetal rat sustantia nigra to the caudate nucleus: Long-term behavioral, biochemical and histochemical studies. Ann Nuerol 8:510–519, 1980.

41. Freund, TF, Bolam, JP, Bjorklund, A, Stenevi, U, Dunnett, SB, Powel, JF, and Schmidt, AD: Efferent synaptic connections of grafted dopaminergic neurons reinnervating the host neostriatum: A tyrosine-hydroxylase immunocytochemical study. J Neurosci 5:603–616, 1985.

42. García-Hernández, F, and Drucker-Colín, R: Recovery of motor impairments and TH-IR in aged rats with intraventricular adrenal transplants. Unpublished material, 1989.

43. García-Hernández, F, Drucker-Colín, R, and Azmitia, EC: Increased survival of adrenal medulla transplants by free radical scavengers and calcium channel blockers. Unpublished material, 1989.

44. Goetz, CG, Olanow, CW, Koller, WC, Penn, RD, Cahill, D, Morantz, R, Srebbing, G, Tanner, CM, Klawans, HL, Shannon, MK, Comella, CL, Witt, T, Cox, C, Waxman, M, and Gauger, L: Multicenter study of autologous adrenal medullary transplantation to the corpus striatum in patients with advanced Parkinson disease. N Engl J Med 320:337–341, 1989.

45. Graham, DG: Oxidative pathways for catecholamines in the genesis of neuromelanin and cytotoxic quinones. Mol Pharmacol 14:663–634, 1978.

46. Grimes, JD: Bromocriptine in Parkinson's disease: Results obtained with high and low dose therapy. Can J Neurol Sci (Suppl) 11(1):125–128, 1984.

47. Hedreen, JS and Chalmers, MP: Neuronal degeneration in rat brain induced by 6-hydroxydopamine: A historical and biochemical study. Brain Res 47:1–36, 1972.

48. Hefti, F, Hartikka, J, and Schlumpf, M: Implantation of PC-12 cells into the corpus striatum of rats with lesions of the dopaminergic nigrostriatal neurons. Brain Res 348:283–288, 1985.

49. Heikkila, R and Cohen, G: Inhibition of amine uptake by hydrogen peroxide: A mechanism for the toxic effects of 6-hydroxydopamine. Science 172:1257–1258, 1971.

50. Heikkila, RE, Hess, A, and Duvoisin, RC: Dopaminergic neurotoxicity of 1-methyl-4-phenyl-1,2,3,6-tetrahydropyridine (MPTP) in the mouse: Relationship between monoamine oxidase, MPTP metabolism and neurotoxicity. Life Sci 36:231–236, 1985.

51. Heikkila, RE, Manzino, L, Cabbat, FS, and Duvoisin, RC: Protection against the neurotoxicity of 1-methyl-4-phenyl-1,2,3,6-tetrahydropyridine by monoamine-oxidase inhibitors. Nature 311:467–469, 1984.

52. Herrera-Marschitz, M, Stromberg, I, Olson, D, Ungerstedt, U, and Olson, L: Adrenal medullary implants in the dopamine-denervated rat

striatum. II. Acute behavior as a function of graft amount and localization and its modulation by neuroleptics. Brain Res 297:53–61, 1984.

53. Hoffer, B, Rose, G, Stromberg, I, and Olson, L: Demonstration of monoamine release from transplant-reinnervated caudate-nucleus by in vivo electrochemical detection. In Bjorklund, A and Stenevi, U (eds): Neural Grafting in the Mammalian CNS. Elsevier, Amsterdam, 1985, p 437.

54. Hornykiewics, O: Brain neurotransmitter changes in Parkinson's disease. In Marsden, CH and Fahn, S (eds): Movement Disorders. Butterworth Scientific, London, 1982, p 41.

55. Jaeger, CB: Immunocytochemical study of PC-12 cells grafted to the brain of immature rats. Exp Brain Res 59:615–624, 1985.

56. Javitch, JA, D'Amato, RJ, Strittmatter, SM, and Snyder, SH: Parkinsonism-inducing neurotoxin, N-methyl-4-phenyl-1,2,3,6-tetrahydropyridine: Uptake of the metabolite N-methyl-4-phenylpyridine by dopamine neurons explains selective toxicity. Proc Natl Acad Sci U S A 82:2173–2177, 1985.

57. Kamo, H, Kim, SU, McGeer, PL, and Shin, DH: Functional recovery in rat model of Parkinson's disease following transplantation of cultured human sympathetic neurons. Brain Res 397:372–376, 1986.

58. Kamo, H, Kim, SU, McGeer, PL, Tago, H, and Shin, DH: Transplantation of cultured human adrenal chromaffin cells into 6-OHDA lesioned rat brain. Synapse 1:324–328, 1987.

59. Kostrzewa, R and Jacobwitz, D: Pharmacological actions of 6-hydroxydopamine. Pharmacol Rev 26:199–287, 1974.

60. Kramer, G, Breese, G, Prange, A, Moran, E, Lewis, J, Kemmitz, J, Bushnell, P, Howard, J, and McKinney, W: Use of 6-hydroxydopamine to deplete brain catecholamines in the rhesus monkey: Effects on urinary metabolites and behavior. Psychopharmacology (Berl) 7:1–11, 1981.

61. Langston, JW, Ballard, PA, Tetrud, JW, and Irwin, I: Chronic parkinsonism in humans due to a product of meperidine-analog synthesis. Science 219:979–980, 1983.

62. Langston, JW, Forno, LS, Rebert, CS, and Irwin, I: Selective nigral toxicity after systemic administration of MPTP in the squirrel monkey. Brain Res 292:390–394, 1984.

63. Langston, JW, Irwin, I, and Ricaute, GA: Neurotoxins, parkinsonism and Parkinson's disease. Pharm Ther 32:19–49, 1987.

64. LeGros-Clark, WE: Neuronal differentiation in implanted fetal cortical tissue. J Neurol Neurosurg Psychiatry 3:264–284, 1940.

65. LeWitt, PA, Ward, CD, Larsen, TA, Raphaelson, MI, Newman, RP, Foster, N, Dambrosia, JM, and Clane, DB: Comparison of pergolide and bromocriptine therapy in parkinsonism. Neurology 33:1009–1014, 1983.

66. Lieberman, A, Gopinathan, G, Hassouri, A, Neophytides, A, and Goldstein, M: Should dopamine agonists be given early or late? A review of nine years experience with bromocriptine. Can J Neurol Sci (Suppl)11(1):233–237, 1984.

67. Lindvall, O, Baklund, EO, Sieger, A, Freedman, R, Sedvall, G, Farde, L, and Olson, L: Transplantation of adrenal medulla in the putamen of patients with Parkinson's disease: Report of two cases. Ann Neurol 22:457–468, 1987.

68. Madrazo, IM, Drucker-Colín, R, Díaz, V, Martínez-Mata, J, Torres, C, and Becerril, JJ: Open microsurgical autograft of adrenal medulla to the right caudate nucleus in two patients with intractable Parkinson's disease. New Engl J Med 316:831–834, 1987.

69. Madrazo, I, Leon, V, Torres, C, Aguilera, MA, Varela, G, Alvarez, F, Fraga, A, Drucker-Colín, R, Ostrosky, F, Shkurovich, M, and Franco, R: Transplantation of fetal substantia nigra and adrenal medulla to the caudate nucleus in two patients with Parkinson's disease. New Engl J Med 318:51, 1987.

70. Mahalik, TJ, Finger, TE, Stromberg, I, and Olson, L: Substantia nigra transplants into the denervated striatum of the rat: Ultrastructure of graft and host interconnections. J Comp Neurol 240:60–70, 1985.

71. Markey, SP, Johannessen, JN, Chiueh, CC, Burns, RS, and Herkenham, MA: Intraneuronal generation of a piridinium metabolite may cause drug-induced parkinsonism. Nature 311:464–467, 1984.

72. Marsden, CD and Parkes, JD: Success and problems of long-term levodopa therapy in Parkinson's disease. Lancet 1:345–348, 1977.

73. Marsden, CD, Parkes, JD, and Quinn, N: Fluctuations in Parkinson's disease: Clinical aspects. In Marsden, CD and Fahn, S (eds): Movement Disorders. London, Butterworth Scientific, 1982, p 96.

74. May, RM: Regeneration cérébale provoquée par la greffe intraoculaire simultanée de tissue cérébral de nouveau-né et de nerf sciatique chez la souris. Bulletin de Biologie Franco Belge 79:151, 1945.

75. Morisha, JM, Nakamura, RK, Freed, WJ, Mishkin, M. and Wayatt, RJ: Adrenal medulla grafts survive and exhibit catecholamine-specific fluorescence in the primate brain. Exp Neurol 84:643–653, 1984.

76. Nishino, H, Ono, T, Shibata, R, Kawamota, S, Watanabe, H, Shiosaka, S, Tohyama, M, and Karradi, Z: Adrenal medullary cells transmitted into dopaminergic neurons in dopamine-depleted rat caudate ameliorate motor disturbances. Brain Res 445:325–337, 1988.

77. Olson, L, Sieger, A, and Stromberg, I: Intraocular transplantation in rodents: A detailed account of the procedure and example of its use in neurobiology with special reference to brain tissue grafting. In Federoff, S (ed): Advances in Cellular Neurobiology. Academic Press, New York, 1982, p 4.

78. Patel-Vaidya, U, Wells, MR, and Freed, WJ: Survival of dissociated adrenal chromaffin cells

of rat and monkey transplanted into the rat brain. Cell Tissue Res 240:281–285, 1985.

79. Perlow, MJ, Freed, WJ, Hoffer, BJ, Seiger, A, Olson, L, and Wyatt, RJ: Brain grafts reduce motor abnormalities produced by destruction of nigrostriatal dopamine system. Science 204:643–647, 1979.

80. Perlow, MJ, Kumakura, K, and Guidotti, A: Prolonged survival of bovine adrenal chromaffin cells in rat cerebral ventricles. Proc Natl Acad Sci U S A 77:5278–5281, 1980.

81. Pezzoli, G, Fahn, S, Dwork, A, Tmoung, DD, Yabenes, JG, Jackson-Lewis, V, Herbert, J, and Codet, JL: Non-chromaffin tissue plus nerve growth factor reduce experimental parkinsonism in aged rats. Brain Res 459:398–403, 1988.

82. Ranson, SW: Transplantation of the spinal ganglion, with observations on the significance of the complex types of spinal ganglion cells. J Comp Neurol 24:547–558, 1914.

83. Rascol, A, Montastruc, JL, and Rascol, O: Should dopamine agonist be given early or late in the treatment of Parkinson's disease? Can J Neurol Sci (Suppl)11(1):229–232, 1984.

84. Redmond, DE, Heindrichs, RL, Maas, JW, and Kling, A: Behavior of free-ranging macaques after intraventricular administration of 6-hydroxydopamine. Science 181:1257–1259, 1973.

85. Rose, G, Gerhardt, G, Stromberg, L, Olson, L, and Hoffer, B: Monoamine release from dopamine-depleted rat caudate nucleus reinnervated by substantia nigra transplants: An in vivo electrochemical study. Brain Res 341:92–100, 1985.

86. Rosenberg, MB, Frienmann, T, Robertson, RC, Tvszynski, M, Wolff, JA, Breakefield, YO, and Gage, FH: Grafting genetically modified cells to the damaged brain: Restorative effects of NGF expression. Science 242:1575–1578, 1988.

87. Rosenstein, JM: Adrenal medulla grafts produce blood-brain barrier dysfunction. Brain Res 414:192–196, 1987.

88. Salach, JI, Singer, TP, Castagnoli, N, and Trevor, A: Oxidation amine 1-methyl-4-phenyl-1,2,3,6-tetrahydropyridine (MPTP) by monoamine oxidase A and B and suicide inactivation of the enzymes by MPTP. Biochem Biophys Res Commun 125:831–835, 1984.

89. Saner, A and Thoenen, H: Model experiments on the molecular mechanism of action of 6-hydroxydopamine. Mol Pharmacol 7:147–154, 1971.

90. Schmidt, HR, Bjorklund, A, Stenevi, U, Dunnett, SB, and Gage, FH: Activity of intrastriatal nigral suspension implants as assessed by measurements of dopamine synthesis and metabolism. Acta Physiol Scand (Suppl)522:9–18, 1983.

91. Schmidt, HR, Ingvar, M, Lindvall, O, Stenevi, U, and Bjorklund, A: Functional activity of substantia nigra grafts reinnervating the striatum: Neurotransmitter metabolism and

(C-14)-deoxy-D-glucose autoradiography. J Neurochem 38(3):737–748, 1982.

92. Schwab, RS and England, AC: Projection technique for evaluating surgery in Parkinson's disease. In Gillingham, FJ and Donaldson, MC (eds): Third Symposium on Parkinson's Disease. Churchill Livingstone, Edinburgh, 1969, p 152.

93. Sieger, A and Olson, L: Quantitation of fiber growth in transplanted central monoamine neurons. Cell Tissue Res 179:285–316, 1977.

94. Stenevi, U, Bjorklund, A, and Svendgaard, NA: Transplantation of central and peripheral monoamine neurons to the adult rat brain: Techniques and conditions for survival. Brain Res 114:1–20, 1976.

95. Stromberg, I, Bygdeman, M, Goldstein, M, Sieger, A, and Olson, L: Human fetal substantia nigra grafted to the dopamine-denervated striatum of immunosuppressed rats: Evidence for functional reinnervation. Neurosci Lett 71:271–276, 1986.

96. Stromberg, I, Herrera-Marschitz, M, Hultgren, L, Ungerstedt, U, and Olson, L: Adrenal medullary implants in the dopamine-denervated rat striatum. I. Acute catecholamine levels in grafts and host caudate as determined by HPLC-electrochemistry and fluorescence histochemical image analysis. Brain Res 297:41–51, 1984.

97. Stromberg, I, Herrera-Marschitz, M, Ungerstedt, U, Ebendal, T, and Olson, L: Chronic implants of chromaffin tissue into the dopamine-denervated striatum. Effects of NGF on graft survival, fiber growth and rotational behavior. Exp Brain Res 60:335–349, 1985.

98. Thoenen, H and Tranzer, JP: The pharmacology of 6-hydroxydopamine. Annu Rev Pharmacol Toxicol 132:169–180, 1973.

99. Thompson, WG: Successful brain grafting. NY Med J 51:701–702, 1890.

100. Tidd, CW: The transplantation of spinal ganglia in the white rat: A study of the morphological changes in surviving cells. J Comp Neurol 55:531–543, 1932.

101. Tranzer, JP, and Thoenen, H: An electron microscopic study of selective acute degeneration of sympathetic nerve terminals after administration of 6-hydroxydopamine. Experientia 24:155–156, 1968.

102. Tretiakoff, C: Contribution a l'étude de l'anatomie pathologique du locus niger de Soemmering avec quelques deductions relatives à la pathogenie des troubles due tonus musculaire et de la maladie de Parkinson. Université de Paris These de Paris, 1919.

103. Undgerstedt, U: 6-Hydroxydopamine induced degeneration of central monoaminergic neurons. Eur J Pharmacol 5:107–110, 1968.

104. Undgerstedt, U: Postsynaptic supersensitivity after 6-OHDA induced degeneration of the nigro-striatal dopamine system. Acta Physiol Scand (Suppl)367:69–93, 1971.

105. Wuerthele, SM, Olson, L, Freed, W, Wyatt, R, and
     Hoffer, B: Electrophysiology of substantia
     nigra transplants. In Usdin, E, Carlsson, A,
     Dahlstrom, A, and Engel, J (eds): Catechol-
     amines: Part B. Neuropharmacology and
     Central Nervous System: Theoretical
     Aspects. New York, Alan R Liss 1984, p 333.
106. Yahr, MD: Evaluation of long term therapy in Par-
     kinson's disease: Mortality and therapeutic
     efficacy. In Birkmayer, W and Hornykiewicz,
     O (eds): Advances in Parkinsonism. Edi-
     tiones Roches, Basel, 1975, p 435.

107. Zetterstrom, T, Brundin, P, Gage, FH, Sharp, T,
     Isacson, O, Dunnett, SB, Ungerstedt, Y, and
     Bjorklund, A: In vivo measurement of sponta-
     neous release and metabolism of dopamine
     from intrastriatal nigral grafts using intrace-
     rebral dialysis. Brain Res 362:344–349,
     1986.
108. Zumstein, H and Siegfried, J: Mortality among
     Parkinson's patients treated with L-dopa
     combined with decarboxylase inhibitor. Eur
     Neurol 14:321–327, 1979.

CHAPTER 14

• •

DOES NEURAL TRANSPLANTATION AID THE RECOVERY OF CNS FUNCTION?

Alan R. Tessler, M.D.

When Sir Peter Medawar was asked about the application of his work on experimental transplantation he responded, "nothing." Experimentalists are no longer so self-assured about gaining knowledge for knowledge's sake, nor are they likely to be as wrong about the application of their work as Medawar was.

Santiago Ramón y Cajal first showed the feasibility of nervous system transplantation and its regenerative potential. Tessler provides evidence for optimism in regard to transplantation for Parkinson's disease and spinal cord injury.

The ultimate limits to transplant treatment of human disease may well prove to be not scientific but ethical, as the recent raging debate on fetal transplantation in the British House of Lords suggests.

VCH

Transplants of embryonic nervous system tissue have been used since the end of the nineteenth century as an experimental strategy for studying the mechanisms by which axons develop and regenerate.[19] Although transplants have been the subject of a steadily increasing number of publications by basic scientists for the past 25 years, their interest for clinicians increased dramatically in the mid-1980s with reports from Sweden and Mexico that autografts of adrenal medulla produced modest[1] or major[35] improvement in the motor performance of patients with Parkinson's disease. Over 100 patients in the United States and additional patients abroad have undergone this operation, and the benefits of the procedure, as well as the mechanisms by which transplants exert their effects, remain a subject of considerable controversy and ongoing in-

vestigation. Transplants hold additional interest for neurologists and neurosurgeons because they have been reported to produce improvement in experimental models of human diseases that include not only Parkinson's but also Huntington's disease,[3] Alzheimer's disease,[12] and spinal cord injury.[46] Their potential clinical application is therefore extremely broad.

The mechanisms by which transplants promote behavioral recovery are likely to be complex and may differ depending on the identity of the tissue that is transplanted, the condition for which the tissue is transplanted, and the site into which the graft is placed.[18] The goal of transplantation, however, is to promote behavioral recovery by restoring or replacing as much of the damaged neuronal circuitry as is necessary to be functionally effective. The extent to which the circuitry will have to be restored to normal depends on the system that has been damaged. In some cases specific connections between neurons may need to be replaced, and the transplanted neurons may have to be thoroughly integrated into surviving neuronal circuitry. Such a complete restoration of circuitry might be necessary, for example, to restore the fine motor functions mediated by corticospinal neurons or the discriminatory sensations mediated by primary afferent neurons. In other cases it might suffice for transplants to act as pumps of neurotransmitter that would ensure a constant supply of neurotransmitter within the cerebrospinal fluid or close to the targets of damaged neurons. Restoring the functions mediated by still other systems of neurons might require intermediate degrees of specificity of connections between host neurons afferent to transplants and transplant neurons efferent to host target neurons. The present brief review will consider one experimental model in which transplants have been used to correct deficits that do not require complete restoration of specific connections between donor and host tissues and one model in which the restoration of function is likely to require the establishment of specific circuits. As an example of the restoration of function primarily through the release of neurotransmitter, we will consider the experimental background that led to the use of transplants for the treatment of Parkinson's disease. As an example of restoration of function that is likely to require the replacement of specific connections, we will consider experiments that may lead to a similar treatment of spinal cord injury.

TRANSPLANTS FOR PARKINSON'S DISEASE

Appropriateness of Transplant Therapy

Features of Parkinson's Disease

Several features of Parkinson's disease make it a promising candidate for treatment by the transplantation of neural tissue. First, the disordered motor function is largely ac-counted for by the degeneration of a single system of dopaminergic neurons whose cell bodies are in the substantia nigra and whose axons terminate in the ipsilateral caudate and putamen.[25] Transplanted tissue would therefore have only to replace the spatially restricted projections of a discrete population of neurons. Second, levels of striatal dopamine must be reduced by at least 80% before the disease becomes symptomatic.[25] Transplanted tissue might therefore improve function even if levels of dopamine remained far below normal. Third, the dopaminergic neurons whose degeneration is responsible for the motor dysfunction of Parkinson's disease are thought to be "permissive" neurons that modulate the level of activity of neurons in the striatum by providing nonspecific information related to arousal.[10,54] This background level of activity is necessary for neuronal interactions within the striatum to occur, but it is set not by precise point-to-point connections with postsynaptic targets but by the release of transmitter in proximity to these targets.[10] Transplants would therefore not necessarily have to restore the synaptic connections found in the normal striatum but might function usefully as reservoirs for the release of neurotransmitter in the vicinity of their targets in the striatum. Fourth, treatment with levodopa or carbidopa often relieves, at least temporarily, the motor impairments of Parkinson's disease in spite of the continuing degeneration of substantia nigra neurons. Because the exogenous replacement of neurotransmitter is effective, transplants might function even in the absence of either a normal complement of connections between transplant and target neurons or an extensive network of afferent neurons from the host.

Availability of Experimental Model

Information available from studies performed in several laboratories encouraged attempts to use transplants in the treatment of experimental parkinsonism. It was known, for example, that transplants of embryonic substantia nigra survived grafting to the anterior chamber of the eye and that neurites would grow out from these transplants and establish projections within pieces of embryonic corpus striatum that has been cotransplanted along with the substantia nigra.[41] A quantifiable and particularly useful laboratory model for Parkinson's disease also existed in which one substantia nigra – corpus striatum projection was destroyed in rats by a unilateral sterotaxic injection of the neurotoxin 6-hydroxydopamine (6-OHDA).[10,41] Destruction of one projection produced supersensitivity of the denervated dopaminergic receptors and consequently a syndrome in which rats turned away from the lesion following the systemic injection of apomorphine. This is a dopamine receptor agonist that stimulates denervated receptors to a greater extent than those that are intact. The systemic administration of amphetamine, which causes the release of dopamine from intact terminals, caused the animal to rotate toward the side of the injection.[10,41] Because the circling behavior of these rats could be quantified, it was possible to transplant embryonic substantia nigra adjacent to the corpus striatum of rats that had received a unilateral 6-OHDA lesion and to expect (1) that the grafts would survive and establish projections into the corpus striatum and (2) that the behavioral consequences of the transplantation could be studied quantitatively.

Transplants in Experimental Parkinsonism

Fetal Substantia Nigra Transplants in 6-OHDA Rodent Model

In one of the early demonstrations that transplants could reverse experimental parkinsonism, fetal substantia nigra was placed into the lateral ventricle adjacent to the caudate nucleus, which had been denervated by an injection of 6-OHDA.[44] The grafted neurons survived and established a dense dopaminergic innervation within the transplant, but very little outgrowth into host parenchyma occurred. Nevertheless, rats that had received a transplant of fetal substantia nigra, but not those that had received a control transplant of sciatic nerve, demonstrated behavioral improvement on the apomorphine-induced rotation test. This result suggested that the test transplants had re-

duced the supersensitivity of denervated dopaminergic receptors and that the mechanism did not require reinnervation of the denervated receptor sites. Release of dopamine into the cerebrospinal fluid and elsewhere in the vicinity of the denervated striatum appeared to suffice. When, however, solid pieces of fetal substantia nigra are grafted onto the surface of the neostriatum denervated by 6-OHDA injections,[27] or nigral cell suspensions are injected into the striatum,[4] large numbers of dopaminergic axons grow for distances of up to 2 mm into the adjacent denervated host striatum. Dopamine is released from transplanted neurons,[48] and levels of dopamine[17] as well as the density of postsynaptic dopamine receptor binding sites[15] in the striatum denervated by 6-OHDA return toward normal. Both behavioral and morphologic observations support the idea that the recovery is mediated at least in part by reinnervation of host striatum as well as by local release of neurotransmitter. For example, dopaminergic axons originating in the transplants form synapses in host neuropil.[36] In addition, outgrowth appears to be correlated with behavioral improvement, since asymmetries in rotation induced by 6-OHDA injection are corrected by transplants that send projections into the dorsal striatum but not into the lateral neostriatum, whereas the sensorimotor "neglect" of the side contralateral to a unilateral injection of 6-OHDA is counteracted by transplants that send axons into the ventrolateral portions of the neostriatum.[41]

Fetal Substantia Nigra Transplants in MHTP Primate Model

The administration systemically of the meperidine analog MPTP produces in monkeys,[9] as well as in humans,[30] a selective degeneration of nigrostriatal dopamine neurons, which results in impairments in motor behavior similar to those of Parkinson's disease. This neurotoxin therefore provides an experimental model in monkeys in which the morphologic, biochemical, and behavioral consequences of transplants can be studied. When solid grafts of fetal substantia nigra are transplanted into the striatum of adult African green monkeys intoxicated with MPTP, large numbers of grafted tyrosine hydroxylase – containing, presumably dopaminergic neurons extend processes into the denervated striatum, and levels of the dopamine metabolite homovanillic acid in the cerebrospinal fluid, which are decreased by MPTP, return toward normal.[51] The impairments in motor performance also recover in the early days after transplantation, and improvement is found months later, although there may be an intervening period of relapse. This recovery is likely to be due to reinnervation, since a control monkey that received transplants of fetal substantia nigra into cingulate cortex, fetal hypothalamic dopaminergic neurons into one striatum, and noradrenergic neurons from locus ceruleus and subceruleus into the other striatum showed only transient improvement in spite of the survival of transplanted neurons.[51] Because the behavioral deficits are corrected by embryonic substantia nigra transplants that have been placed adjacent to the target rather than in the normal position of dopaminergic neurons in the midbrain, host afferent input to the transplant must differ from the pathways that modulate substantia nigra function in the normal brain. The restoration of motor function that is mediated by transplants in the 6-OHDA and MPTP models of Parkinson's disease therefore does not require the restoration of normal neuronal circuitry.

Adrenal Medulla Transplants in Rodent and Primate Models

To avoid the complicated practical and legal problems that would be raised by transplants of fetal tissue in humans, the behavioral effects of other sources of dopaminergic neurons have been investigated. When separated from the adrenal cortex and cultured in an environment that contains nerve growth factor (NGF), chromaffin cells of the adrenal medulla have been shown to extend neurites and synthesize catecholamines including dopamine.[42] Intraventricular transplants of adrenal chromaffin tissue reverse apomorphine-induced turning behavior to about the same extent as fetal substantia nigra transplants in rats whose striatum has been unilaterally denervated by 6-OHDA; very few neurites are produced by

these transplants.[16] Intrastriatal transplants of adrenal medulla also produce behavioral improvement in the 6-OHDA – treated rodent model, but, unlike transplants of embryonic substantia nigra, this is not due to reinnervation of the denervated striatum, since intraparenchymal transplants of adrenal medulla form very limited projections.[14,43] Diffusion of dopamine is also unlikely to account for recovery after adrenal medulla transplants, because neither cerebrospinal[2,55] nor striatal[2] levels of catecholamines are persistently elevated after intrastriatal transplantation.

An alternative explanation is that the transplant or the transplantation procedure itself induces dopaminergic neurons in the host striatum to regenerate, to form collateral axons, or to increase their synthesis of catecholamines[39] and that it is this compensatory response of dopaminergic host neurons that is crucial for the behavioral recovery. Transplantation of adrenal medullary cells into the striatum of mice intoxicated with MPTP, for example, is associated with increased density of host tyrosine hydroxylase – containing axons that occurs despite a very limited survival of grafted cells.[5] This result suggests that the transplant exerts a trophic effect on the host neurons that is independent of graft survival. Enhanced outgrowth of tyrosine hydroxylase – positive fibers is also observed near graft sites in the caudate of normal Cebus monkeys or of Cebus monkeys treated with MPTP,[21] although very few adrenal chromaffin cells survive transplantation.[11] However, tyrosine hydroxylase – immunoreactive fibers were also induced in a control monkey that had received an implant consisting only of a metal tissue carrier.[11] One implication of this experiment is, therefore, that the injury caused by the transplant procedure, rather than the tissue implanted, produces compensatory responses in the host that contribute to behavioral recovery.[11,29,38]

Transplants in Parkinson's Disease Patients

Whether or not transplants of adrenal medulla produce behavioral improvement in the primary model for Parkinson's disease has received surprisingly little attention. In human beings with Parkinson's disease the results have been mixed. As reported from Sweden, four patients received transplants of solid pieces of their own adrenal medulla into either the caudate[1] or the putamen.[33] At best the procedures produced transient improvement shown by brief reversal of motor deficits and temporary decrease in the need for medication. More dramatic and sustained improvement was reported by Madrazo and colleagues[35] in a series of patients that now totals over 40. The two patients described in their initial report showed a marked reduction in rigidity, akinesia, and tremor that persisted for the duration of the follow-up periods of 3 and 10 months. The operation as performed in Mexico differed technically from that performed in Sweden because the procedure was performed as an open craniotomy, and the solid graft implanted into the caudate remained in contact with the cerebrospinal fluid of the lateral ventricle. Differences in surgical technique alone, however, are unlikely to have accounted for the differing outcomes, because other groups that have employed the same surgical procedure as was used by the Mexican surgeons have been unable to reproduce their results. A study of 19 patients that combined the results of three medical centers in the United States, for example, found only an increase in the periods in which patients responded to medication ("on" time) and a decrease in the severity of impairment during the periods when the medication was ineffective ("off" time).[20] Postoperative medical and behavioral complications were also frequent. In general, the results of the more than 100 operations performed in the United States have shown that the procedure produces "modest to slight benefits in only a proportion of patients"[52] and have prompted considerable skepticism about the success reported by Madrazo and co-workers.[32] The operation has failed when the transplant has not survived,[45] and when chromaffin cells have survived in the transplant but not synthesized dopamine,[22] suggesting that in the human with Parkinson's disease, graft survival and dopamine synthesis are necessary to improve motor performance and that

compensatory changes in the host produced by the transplant or the transplantation procedure do not suffice.

If the capacity to reinnervate the striatum and to deliver dopamine close to the normal target neurons is a prerequisite for transplants to mediate locomotor recovery, then the available experimental evidence suggests that transplants of embryonic substantia nigra provide a more promising therapeutic possibility than adrenal medulla transplants. Two patients who received transplants of human fetal substantia nigra tissue have not, however, shown major functional improvement after a 6-month period of study.[34] Formidable technical problems need to be solved in the rodent and primate models of Parkinson's disease before the still more difficult technical challenges as well as complicated legal and ethical issues in humans are confronted.

TRANSPLANTS FOR SPINAL CORD INJURY

State of the Art

Transplantation is far from providing a practical approach to the treatment of patients with spinal cord disease or spinal cord injury. Areas of embryonic brain as well as whole pieces and cell suspensions prepared from embryonic spinal cord have been shown to survive transplantation into the spinal cord of newborn and adult host rats, and the possibility that connections form between neurons in the host and neurons in the transplant has begun to be evaluated using a variety of morphologic methods. The electrophysiologic and behavioral function of these transplants is at an earlier stage of study, and very little work has been done yet in the cat or primate.

Transplant Strategies

Transplants of Fetal Supraspinal Neurons

One implication of the transplant studies in the experimental models of Parkinson's disease is that some types of behavior can be improved by transplants that deliver neurotransmitters and/or neurotrophic substances to the vicinity of their targets, even if the transplants cannot reconstitute the damaged neuronal circuits in detail. One strategy for using transplants to correct experimental spinal cord injury has followed similar reasoning: that the appropriate neurons placed in proximity to their targets can restore some behaviors abolished by spinal cord injury even without the complete restoration of damaged circuits.[40] It is known, for example, that the intravenous administration of dopamine or the alpha$_2$-adrenergic agonist clonidine can elicit stepping movements in cats with spinal cord transection that allow them to walk on a treadmill.[13] This action is thought to be due to the activation of circuitry for locomotion that is intrinsic to the spinal cord. It is also known that serotonergic neurons are important in the supraspinal control of the spinal reflexes that mediate penile erection and ejaculation and that administration of a serotonin receptor agonist to rats with spinal cord transection can induce ejaculation.[37] Therefore, one approach has been to transplant supraspinal monoaminergic neurons into the distal portion of spinal cord isolated by a lesion. Both catecholaminergic neurons known to be important for locomotor behavior and serotonergic neurons that mediate autonomic function have been used. Embryonic noradrenergic neurons taken from locus ceruleus and serotonergic neurons taken from the rhombencephalic raphe region extend processes up to 2 cm in length into host spinal cord and restore levels of neurotransmitters that have been depleted experimentally by the use of neurotoxins[40] or by spinal cord section.[46] Axons of transplanted serotonergic neurons grow into the regions of spinal cord that receive 5-HT innervation normally and establish morphologically normal synaptic terminals with motoneurons in the ventral horn and with neurons in the intermediolateral column.[46] In addition, reflex ejaculation, which is abolished in rats with spinal cord transection, recovers in rats that receive transplants of embryonic raphe,[46] suggesting that behavioral recovery is related to the recovery of serotonergic innervation.

Transplanted noradrenergic neurons originating in the locus ceruleus also extend axons into the regions of spinal cord to which locus ceruleus axons project in normal spinal cord and appear to contribute to the recovery of reflex stepping activity.[57] The question of whether transplanted noradrenergic axons establish synapses with their target neurons has not been studied, and therefore the anatomic basis for the recovery mediated by noradrenergic neurons remains to be determined. Like transplants of embryonic substantia nigra in experimental Parkinson's disease, these embryonic transplants of brainstem nuclei appear to contribute to behavioral recovery by extending axons into host neuropil, where they function by releasing neurotransmitter or neurotrophic substances close to their normal targets. As in the parkinsonism models, the transplants are successful even though they have not been placed in their normal location and the neuronal circuits in which they participate normally have not been restored.

Transplants of Fetal Spinal Cord

Because the recovery of other behaviors abolished by spinal cord injury may require more faithful reconstruction of damaged circuits, a second strategy has been to use transplants of embryonic spinal cord in an effort to replace populations of damaged neurons and restore neuronal connections.[47] The transplant might then function as a bridge across injured tissue, either by permitting the direct growth of lesioned axons into intact spinal segments or by permitting the formation of relays within the graft. Embryonic spinal cord transplanted into a cavity in host spinal cord survives and becomes integrated with host neuropil.[47] Grafts lack the characteristic butterfly appearance of normal spinal cord but contain differentiated areas that resemble substantia gelatinosa.[24] This resemblance to normal spinal cord encourages the expectation that transplants might replace damaged populations of neurons and, with them, their normal connections. One additional way in which transplants of embryonic spinal cord may contribute to recovery of behavioral function has already been demonstrated in newborn hosts, where transplants have been shown to rescue injured host rubro-spinal neurons otherwise destined to die.[8] Whether transplants to spinal cord can also rescue axotomized neurons in adult hosts is currently being studied in several laboratories.

In newborn hosts, spinal cord transplants have the capacity to act as bridges that support the elongation of supraspinal axons into regions of intact spinal cord well below the level of injury. Both serotonergic axons originating in neurons in the brainstem raphe nuclei[6] and the axons of corticospinal neurons[7] traverse transplants placed into lesioned newborn thoracic spinal cord and establish projections within host spinal cord as far caudal as the lower lumbar levels. Animals with transplants perform better than littermates with lesions alone on several tests of locomotor function,[28] consistent with the idea that the axons that grow into host spinal cord caudal to the lesion contribute to the improved performance. If so, then transplants into newborn spinal cord have assisted in the recovery of complex behavior that requires not only the reconstitution of precise input by supraspinal neurons but also intact afferent control of these supraspinal neurons.

In adults, projections from host into transplant and from transplant into host are more modest, and damaged host axons do not traverse the full extent of the graft.[47] However, serotonergic axons from brainstem raphe nuclei,[47] axons from corticospinal neurons,[7] and primary afferent axons originating in dorsal root ganglion neurons[56] regenerate into transplants, whereas they are unable to elongate into spinal cord in the absence of a transplant (Fig. 14–1). Dorsal root ganglion axons not only establish synapses with neurons within transplants (Fig. 14–2), but these synapses resemble in several respects those formed by dorsal root ganglion axons within the dorsal horn of normal spinal cord.[23] The establishment of

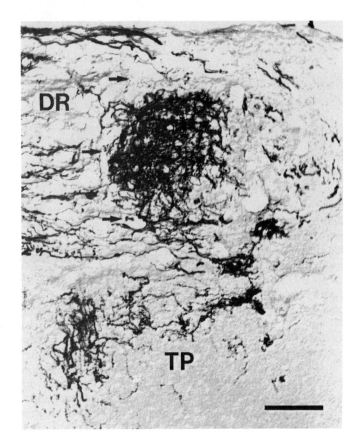

FIGURE 14–1. Sagittal section of the interface (*arrows*) between fetal spinal cord transplant (TP) and host dorsal root (DR) showing regenerated host dorsal root axons within the transplant. The dorsal axons have been labeled to demonstrate calcitonin gene-related peptide immunoreactivity, since this is a specific label for many of the primary different axons that terminate in the dorsal horn of normal spinal cord. (Bar = 100 μm.)

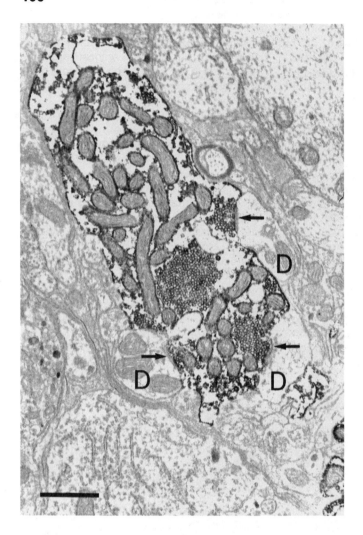

FIGURE 14-2. Electron micrograph showing synapses formed by host dorsal root axon which has regenerated into the fetal spinal cord transplant. A complex terminal makes asymmetric synaptic contacts (*arrows*) upon three different dendritic profiles (D). The dorsal root has been labeled by the direct application of wheat germ agglutinin-conjugated horseradish peroxidase. (Bar = 1 μm.)

morphologically normal synapses by an identified population of host neurons afferent to the transplant encourages the idea that relays of synaptically coupled neurons formed within transplants may allow the transplants to act as bridges across damaged spinal cord. Donor neurons in transplants have in fact been shown to send axons through the transplant into the peripheral nervous system of the host[56] (Fig. 14-3). Therefore it is at least possible that transplants of fetal spinal cord have the capacity to restore a damaged motor reflex arc as well as to stimulate or support the regeneration of axons otherwise unable to regrow. An important component of these transplants is

thought to be the contribution of the glia, especially the astrocytes.

Prostheses of Fetal Astrocytes

A third strategy for using transplants to mediate behavioral recovery after spinal cord injury is to use prostheses prepared from immature astrocytes as bridges that will promote the regeneration of damaged central nervous system (CNS) axons. In the developing CNS, the surfaces of astrocytes and astrocyte precursors provide an important substrate for neuron migration[31] and the outgrowth of neuronal processes.[49,50] Injured adult axons may retain or reacquire

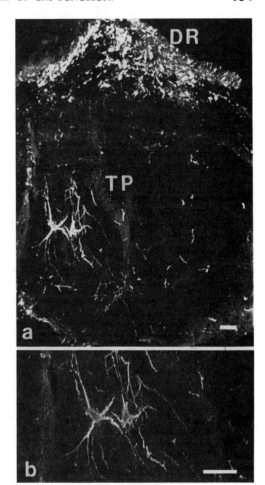

FIGURE 14-3. Dark-field photomicrographs of transverse sections through a fetal spinal cord transplant following injection of cholera toxin–conjugated horseradish peroxidase into the ipsilateral sciatic nerve A. Within the transplant (TP) are the cell bodies of neurons whose axons have grown out from the transplant and down the sciatic nerve of the host. Regenerated host dorsal root axons (DR) are also shown at the margin of the transplant. (Bar = 200 μm.) B, The labeled cell bodies are shown at higher magnification. (Bar = 100 μm.)

the capacity to growth along immature glia, since astrocytes isolated from newborn corpus callosum and trapped on a piece of Millipore filter can stimulate the regrowth of damaged corpus callosum axons and guide them across the site of injury to project into normal regions of termination.[53] In a first attempt to apply the same technique to the repair of the damaged spinal cord, the L-5 dorsal root was crushed approximately 2 to 3 mm from the dorsal root entry zone, and a prosthesis consisting of a pennant-shaped piece of Millipore filter was coated with astrocytes isolated from embryonic spinal cord and inserted into the spinal cord so as to direct the crushed dorsal root axons into the dorsal horn.[26] Control animals that received implants not coated with astrocytes showed an intense inflammatory reaction to the implant, along with hemorrhage and cavitation in the adjacent spinal cord and no ingrowth of regenerating axons into the dorsal horn. Animals that received implants coated with astrocytes showed a reduced inflammatory response and little hemorrhage or cavitation. In these animals, regenerated axons grew along the implant and terminated within the dorsal horn, some after first following an aberrant circumferential path around the dorsal horn. Although the experimental injury was mild compared with the massive tissue destruction seen in human spinal cord injury, and although the functional significance of the regeneration remains to be explored, the results of this experiment suggest that transplanted astrocytes can both reduce the necrosis that accompanies spinal cord injury and promote the regeneration of axons past the site of injury. Moreover, once past the site of crush, the elongating axons are able to recognize cues that enable them to return to their normal sites of termination within the dorsal horn.

SUMMARY

Transplants of embryonic CNS tissue have for many years contributed to the study of axon development and regeneration. Neurologists and neurosurgeons became interested when grafts were reported to provide a method of therapy for Parkinson's disease and potentially for other illnesses. Several features of Parkinson's disease made it a promising candidate for treatment by transplantation, and both fetal substantia nigra and adult adrenal medulla grafts have restored locomotor function in experimental models of parkinsonism. The mechanisms by which transplants improve function are debated, as is the role of transplantation in the treatment of patients with Parkinson's disease. Several strategies have also been proposed for using transplants to treat experimental spinal cord injury, including the use of transplants of brainstem monoaminergic neurons, transplants of embryonic spinal cord, and prostheses of embryonic astrocytes. The functional effects of transplants into spinal cord are in the early stages of investigation. However, transplants continue to provide insights into the mechanisms by which axons grow, and they represent a first step toward the development of a rational treatment of human spinal cord injury.

ACKNOWLEDGMENTS

I am grateful to B. T. Himes, C. Rogahn, and Dr. Y. Itoh for their help in all aspects of my laboratory's work and to K. Golden and C. Stewart for their help in preparation of this chapter. My laboratory's research is supported by the Research Service of the Veterans Administration, USAMRDC grant 51930002 and NIH grant NS 24707.

REFERENCES

1. Backlund, E-O, Granberg, P-O, Hamberger, B, Knutsson, E, Mårtensson, A, Sedvall, G, Seiger, Å, and Olson, L: Transplantation of adrenal medullary tissue to striatum in parkinsonism. J Neurosurg 62:169–173, 1985.
2. Becker, JB and Freed, WJ: Adrenal medulla grafts enhance functional activity of the striatal dopamine system following substantia nigra lesions. Brain Res 462:401–406, 1988.
3. Björklund, A, Lindvall, O, Isacson, O, Brundin, P, Wictorin, K, Strecker, RE, Clarke, DJ, and Dunnett, SB: Mechanisms of action of intracerebral neural implants: Studies on nigral and striatal grafts to the lesioned striatum. Trends Neurosci 10:509–516, 1987.
4. Björklund, A, Schmidt, RH, and Stenevi, U: Functional reinnervation of the neostriatum in the adult rat by use of intraparenchymal grafting of dissociated cell suspensions from the substantia nigra. Cell Tissue Res 212:39–45, 1980.
5. Bohn, MC, Cupit, L, Marciano, F, and Gash, DM: Adrenal medulla grafts enhance recovery of striatal dopaminergic fibers. Science 237:913–916, 1987.
6. Bregman, BS: Spinal cord transplants permit the growth of serotonergic axons across the site of neonatal spinal cord transection. Dev Brain Res 34:265–279, 1987.
7. Bregman, BS, Kunkel-Bagden, E, McAtee, M, and O'Neill, A: Extension of the critical period for developmental plasticity of the corticospinal pathway. J Comp Neurol 282:355–370, 1989.
8. Bregman, BS and Reier, PJ: Neural tissue transplants rescue axotomized rubrospinal cells from retrograde death. J Comp Neurol 244:86–95, 1986.
9. Burns, RS, Chiueh, CC, Markey, SP, Ebert, MH, Jacobowitz, DM, and Kopin, IJ: A primate model of parkinsonism: Selective destruction of dopaminergic neurons in the pars compacta of the substantia nigra by N-methyl-4-phenyl-1,2,3,6-tetrahydropyridine. Proc Natl Acad Sci U S A 80:4546–4550, 1983.
10. Dunnett, SB, Björklund, A, and Stenevi, U: Dopamine-rich transplants in experimental parkinsonism. Trends Neurosci 6:266–270, 1983.
11. Fiandaca, MS, Kordower, JH, Hansen, JT, Jiao, SS, and Gash, DM: Adrenal medullary autografts into the basal ganglia of cebus monkeys: Injury-induced regeneration. Exp Neurol 102:76–91, 1988.
12. Fine, A, Dunnett, SB, Björklund, A, and Iverson, SD: Cholinergic ventral forebrain grafts into the neocortex improve passive avoidance memory in a rat model of Alzheimer disease. Proc Natl Acad Sci U S A 82:5227–5230, 1985.
13. Forssberg, H and Grillner, S: The locomotion of the acute spinal cat injected with clonidine i.v. Brain Res 50:184–186, 1973.
14. Freed, WJ, Cannon-Spoor, HE, and Krauthamer, E: Intrastriatal adrenal medulla grafts in rats:

Long-term survival and behavioral effects. J Neurosurg 65:664–670, 1986.

15. Freed, WJ, Ko, GN, Niehoff, DL, Kuhar, MJ, Hoffer, BJ, Olson, L, Cannon-Spoor, HE, Morihisa, JM, and Wyatt, RJ: Normalization of spiroperidol binding in the denervated rat striatum by homologous grafts of substantia nigra. Science 222:937–939, 1983.

16. Freed, WJ, Morihisa, JM, Spoor, E, Hoffer, B, Olson, L, Seiger, Å, and Wyatt, RJ: Transplanted adrenal chromaffin cells in rat brain reduce lesion-induced rotational behaviour. Nature 292: 351–352, 1981.

17. Freed, WJ, Perlow, MJ, Karoum, F, Seiger, Å, Olson, L, Seiger, Å, and Wyatt, RJ: Restoration of dopaminergic function by grafting of fetal rat substantia nigra to the caudate nucleus: Long-term behavioral, biochemical, and histochemical studies. Ann Neurol 8:510–519, 1980.

18. Gage, FH, and Buzáki, G: CNS grafting: Potential mechanisms of action. In Seil, FJ (ed): Neural Regeneration and Transplantation. Frontiers of Clinical Neuroscience. Alan R Liss, New York, 1989, p 211.

19. Gash, DM: Neural transplants in mammals: A historical overview. In Sladek, JR Jr and Gash, DM (eds): Neural Transplants Development and Function. Plenum Press, New York, 1984, p 1.

20. Goetz, CG, Olanow, CW, Koller, WC, Penn, RD, Cahill, D, Morantz, R, Stebbings, G, Tanner, CM, Klawans, HL, Shannon, KM, Comella, CL, Witt, T, Cox, C, Waxman, M, and Gauger, L: Multicenter study of autologous adrenal medullary transplantation to the corpus striatum in patients with advanced Parkinson's disease. N Engl J Med 320:337–341, 1989.

21. Hansen, JT, Kordower, JH, Fiandaca, MS, Jiao, SS, Notter, MFD, and Gash, DM: Adrenal medullary autografts into the basal ganglia of cebus monkeys: Graft viability and fine structure. Exp Neurol 102:65–75, 1988.

22. Hurtig, H, Joyce, J, Sladek, JR Jr and Trojanowski, JQ: Postmortem analysis of adrenal-medulla-to-caudate autograft in a patient with Parkinson's disease. Ann Neurol 25:607–614, 1989.

23. Itoh, Y and Tessler, A: Ultrastructural organization of adult dorsal root ganglion neurons regenerated into transplants of fetal spinal cord. J Comp Neurol 292:369–411, 1990.

24. Jakeman, LB, Reier, PJ, Bregman, BS, Wade, EB, Dailey, M, Kastner, RJ, Himes, BT and Tessler, A: Differentiation of substantia gelatinosa–like regions in intraspinal and intracerebral transplants of embryonic spinal cord tissue in the rat. Exp Neurol 103:17–33, 1989.

25. Kish, SJ, Shannak, K, and Hornykiewicz, O: Uneven pattern of dopamine loss in the striatum of patients with idiopathic Parkinson's disease. N Engl J Med 318:876–880, 1988.

26. Kliot, M, Smith, GM, Siegal, J, Tyrrell, S, and Silver, J: Induced regeneration of dorsal root fibers into the adult mammalian spinal cord. Current Issues in Neural Regeneration Research. Alan R Liss, New York, pp 311–328, 1988.

27. Kromer, LE, Björklund, A, and Stenevi, U: Intracephalic implants: A technique for studying neuronal interactions. Science 204:1117–1119, 1979.

28. Kunkel-Bagden, E, and Bregman, BS: Transplants alter the development of sensorimotor function after neonatal spinal cord damage. Society for Neurosciences Abstracts 14:1003, 1988.

29. Landau, WM: Mucking around with Peter Pan. Ann Neurol 24:464, 1988.

30. Langston, JW, Ballard, P, Tetrud, JW and Irwine, I: Chronic parkinsonism in humans due to a product of meperidine-analog synthesis. Science 219:979–980, 1983.

31. Levitt, P, and Rakic, P: Immunoperoxidase localization of glial fibrillary acidic protein in radial glial cells and astrocytes of the developing Rhesus monkey brain. J Comp Neur 193: 817–848, 1980.

32. Lewin, R: Cloud over Parkinson's therapy. Science 240:390–392, 1988.

33. Lindvall, O, Backlund, EO, Farde, L, Sedvall, G, Freedman, R, Hoffer, B, Nobin, A, Seiger, Å and Olson, L: Transplantation in Parkinson's disease: Two cases of adrenal medullary grafts to the putamen. Ann Neurol 22:457–468, 1987.

34. Lindvall, O, Rehncrona, S, Brundin, P, Gustavii, B, Åstedt, B, Widner, H, Lindholm, T, Björklund, A, Leenders, KL, Rothwell, JC, Frackowiak, R, Marsden, CD, Johnels, B, Steg, G, Freedman, R, Hoffer, BJ, Seiger, Å, Bygdeman, M, Strömberg, I, and Olson, L: Human fetal dopamine neurons grafted into the striatum in two patients with severe Parkinson's disease: A detailed account of methodology and a 6-month follow-up. Arch Neurol 46:615–631, 1989.

35. Madrazo, I, Drucker-Colín, D, Diaz, V, Martínez-Mata, J, Torres, C, and Becerril, JJ: Open microsurgical autograft of adrenal medulla to the right caudate nucleus in two patients with intractable Parkinson's disease. N Engl J Med 316:831–834, 1987.

36. Mahalik, TJ, Finger, TE, Strömberg, I, and Olson, L: Substantia nigra transplants into denervated striatum of the rat: Ultrastructure of graft and host interconnections. J Comp Neurol 240: 60–70, 1985.

37. Mas, M, Zahradnik, MA, Martino, V, and Davidson, JM: Stimulation of spinal serotonergic receptors facilitates seminal emission and suppresses penile erectile reflexes. Brain Res 342:128–134, 1985.

38. Nieto-Sampedro, M, Manthrope, M, Barbin, G, Varon, S, and Cotman, CW: Injury-induced neuronotrophic activity in adult rat brain: Correlation with survival of delayed implants in the wound cavity. N Neurosci 2:2219–2229, 1983.

39. Norman, AB, Lehman, MN, and Sanberg, PR: Functional effects of fetal striatal transplants. Brain Res Bull 22:163–172, 1989.

40. Nornes, H, Björklund, A, and Stenevi, U: Transplantation strategies in spinal cord regeneration. In Sladek, JR Jr and Gash, DM (eds): Neural

Transplants: Development and Function. Plenum Press, New York, 1984, p 407.

41. Olson, L: On the use of transplants to counteract the symptoms of Parkinson's disease: Background, experimental models, and possible clinical applications. In Cotman, CW (eds): Synaptic Plasticity. Guilford Press, New York, 1985, p 485.

42. Olson, L, Hamberger, B, Hoffer, B, Miller, R and Seiger, Å: Nerve fiber formation by grafted adult adrenal medullary cells. In Stjärne, L, Lagercrantz, H, Hedqvist, P, and Wennmalm, Å (eds): Chemical neurotransmission: 75 years. Academic Press, London, 1982, p 35.

43. Patel-Vaidya, U, Wells, MR, and Freed, WJ: Survival of dissociated adrenal chromaffin cells of rat and monkey transplanted into rat brain. Cell Tissue Res 240:281–285, 1985.

44. Perlow, MJ, Freed, WJ, Hoffer, BJ, Seiger, Å, Olson, L, and Wyatt, RJ: Brain grafts reduce motor abnormalities produced by destruction of nigrostriatal dopamine system. Science 204:643–647, 1979.

45. Peterson, DI, Price, ML, and Small, CS: Autopsy findings in a patient that had an adrenal-to-brain transplant for Parkinson's disease. Neurology 39:235–238, 1989.

46. Privat, A, Mansour, H, Rajaofetra, N, and Geffard, M: Intraspinal transplants of serotonergic neurons in the adult rat. Brain Res Bull 22:123–129, 1989.

47. Reier, PJ, Bregman, BS and Wujek, JR: Intraspinal transplantation of embryonic spinal cord tissue in neonatal and adult rats. J Comp Neur 247:275–296, 1986.

48. Rose, G, Gerhardt, G, Strömberg, I, Olson, L, and Hoffer, B: Monoamine release from dopamine-depleted rat caudate nucleus reinnervated by substantia nigra transplants: An in vivo electrochemical study. Brain Res 341:92–100, 1985.

49. Silver, J, Lorenz, SE, Wahlsten, D and Coughlin, J: Axonal guidance during development of the great cerebral commissures: Descriptive and experimental studies, in vivo, on the role of preformed glial pathways. J Comp Neur 210:10–29, 1982.

50. Silver, J and Rutishauser, U: Guidance of axons in vivo by a preformed adhesive pathway on neuroepithelial endfeet. Dev Biol 106:485–499, 1984.

51. Sladek, JR Jr, Collier, TJ, Haber, SN, Deutch, AY, Elsworth, JD, Roth, RH, and Redmond, DE Jr: Reversal of parkinsonism by fetal nerve cell transplants in primate brain. In Azmitia, EC and Bjorklund, A (eds): Cell and Tissue Transplantation into the Adult Brain. Ann NY Acad Sci 495:641, 1987.

52. Sladek, JR Jr and Shoulson, I: Neural transplantation: A call for patience rather than patients. Science 240:1386–1388, 1988.

53. Smith, GM, Miller, RH, and Silver, J: Changing role of forebrain astocytes during development, regenerative failure, and induced regeneration upon transplantation. J Comp Neur 251:23–43, 1986.

54. Stricker, EM and Zigmond, MJ: Recovery of function after damage to central catecholamine-containing neurons: A neurochemical model for the lateral hypothalamic syndrome. In Sprague, JM and Epstein, AN (eds): Progress in Psychobiology and Physiological Psychology. Academic Press, New York, 1976, p 121.

55. Strömberg, I, Herrera-Marschitz, M, Hultgren, L, Ungerstedt, U, and Olson, L: Adrenal medullary implants in the domapine-denervated rat striatum. I. Acute catecholamine levels in grafts and host caudate as determined by HPLC-electrochemistry and fluorescence histochemical image analysis. Brain Res 297:41–51, 1984.

56. Tessler, A, Himes, BT, Houlé, and Reier, PJ: Regeneration of adult dorsal root axons into transplants of embryonic spinal cord. J Comp Neur 270:537–548, 1988.

57. Yakovleff, A, Roby-Brami, A, Guezard, B, Mansour, H, Bussell, B, and Privat, A: Locomotion in rats transplanted with noradrenergic neurons. Brain Res Bull 22:115–121, 1989.

CHAPTER 15

• •

Managing the Refractive Parkinsonian Patient

A. Jon Stoessl, M.D., F.R.C.P(C)

A refractive Parkinsonian patient is one referred by a colleague. Stoessl has had ample experience in this regard. As may be expected from an expert, his pathophysiologic discussion is substantial and his therapeutic enthusiasm is qualified by the realization of the complexity of the disease and the multiple effects of any drug.

His discussion of selective D_2 agonists and nondopaminergic neurotransmitters is particularly intriguing and makes us aware of the fundamental importance of the concept of homeostasis. Biological organisms are infinitely complex, and any attempt to alter this equilibrium, even in disease, leads to consequences that are not always predictable.

Although we have a long way to go in the treatment of Parkinson's disease, almost all patients can be offered an improvement in the quality of their lives, albeit temporarily.

VCH

THE EXTENT OF THE PROBLEM

Incidence of Parkinson's Disease and Complications

Parkinson's disease is one of the commonest neurologic disorders, affecting approximately 150 individuals per 100,000.[59,113] Whereas the early response to therapy is gratifying in the majority of cases, only one third of patients will have sustained (5 years or more) benefit from levodopa. The majority develop disabling complications of therapy that limit the maximum tolerated dose of medication or become largely refractory to available treatments.[71] Formulating an approach to this group of patients requires that the underlying pathogenesis of the disease and its complications be sufficiently understood.

Description of the Complication

The major therapeutic complications of levodopa therapy are fluctuations in response, dyskinesias, and loss of efficacy. These often go hand in hand, and the pathogenesis may be related. Certain fluctuations in disability were noted to occur prior to the introduction of levodopa and are therefore presumed to reflect the underlying disease process. These would include variations related to emotional state (including paradoxic kinesia), freezing, and sleep benefit. Nowadays, most fluctuations are seen in patients on drug therapy. The commonest of these is the phenomenon known as "wearing off," the more-or-less predictable decline in response seen toward the end of the dose interval. In the early stage of therapy, levodopa may be given on a thrice-daily schedule, with sustained benefit implying a duration of action of 4 to 6 hours. As the disease progresses, this duration may decline to 2 or 3 hours. The duration of benefit derived from a given dose of levodopa may vary throughout the course of the day, so that a first morning dose may last for 3 to 4 hours, whereas a late afternoon dose may only provide relief for 1 to 2 hours. Such variations will differ from patient to patient and must be determined individually. Predictable wearing off may respond well to simple modifications in dosing intervals.

Much attention is paid to the so-called "on-off" phenomenon. In my opinion, this term should be reserved for rapid, unpredictable oscillations in motor performance that bear no apparent relationship to drug administration. This is actually a relatively uncommon occurrence if the degree of disability is carefully plotted out over the course of the day. It may be necessary to admit the patient to hospital for direct observation to do this, rather than to rely on the history. It may also be necessary to plot charts of disability over several days before a pattern emerges. Furthermore, one must take into account freezing episodes (which may simply reflect progression of the underlying disease process) and the occurrence of drug-resistant "off" periods. Freezing episodes are brief and may affect a single motor function (e.g., gait) only, while other capacities are preserved. Potential explanations for drug-resistant "off" periods will be discussed below.

The occurrence of fluctuations in response to therapy is often accompanied by dyskinesias, or involuntary movements, which may take any form, including chorea (most common), dystonia, tics, and myoclonus. Although these can appear very dramatic and are most distressing to others, especially health care providers, most patients prefer to be mobile, even if this entails the presence of severe dyskinesias. Furthermore, both patients and inexperienced staff may misinterpret the dyskinesias as parkin-

sonian tremor and will request an increase in medication when the opposite may be required. For this reason, careful observation and charting are vitally important in the management of the resistant patient.

The commonest form of dyskinesia occurs when the patient is obtaining maximum therapeutic benefit in terms of reversing parkinsonian disability. Such "peak-dose" (or "I-D-I," for immobile-dyskinetic-immobile[81a]) dyskinesias may respond to a small reduction in dose or to a simple alteration in which the same total daily dose is given but with smaller doses on a more frequent basis. Unfortunately, as the disease progresses, more and more patients develop a "square-wave" pattern of dyskinesias, in which dyskinesias are present throughout the period of therapeutic benefit. Both the patient and the physician are then confronted with the unenviable choice of being free of dyskinesias but frozen or mobile but choreic. As noted above, a majority of patients will choose the latter. A less common form of dyskinesia occurs at the beginning and/or end of the period of benefit. The patient will take his or her medication and just before the improvement in parkinsonian disability occurs may suffer from involuntary movements, particularly affecting the legs and/or the side on which parkinsonian disability is greater. Unlike the peak-dose dyskinesias described above, such "diphasic" or "D-I-D" (dyskinetic-improved-dyskinetic[81a]) dyskinesias may respond better to an *increase* in medication. Once again, lack of familiarity with this phenomenon or inadequate attention to the details of the patient's disability may lead to inappropriate therapeutic decisions. A somewhat related phenomenon is "early-morning dystonia," which typically affects a single foot. Early-morning dystonia occurs only in patients on chronic levodopa therapy, and it abates when levodopa is withheld for several days. Although it may paradoxically appear to be precipitated by the first morning dose of levodopa, it is often relieved or forestalled by moving forward the time of the first dose, and it appears to reflect a period of critical dopamine deficiency.[76,98] Rarely, peak-dose akinesia may occur, and this probably represents a form of drug-induced dystonia.[19]

Other manifestations of chronic Parkinson's disease may not be attributable to the therapy but may nonetheless significantly complicate both the course of the disease and the tolerance of medication. It should be remembered that dopamine replacement therapy for Parkinson's disease is most effective for the rigidity and bradykinesia, and sometimes for the tremor. Postural disturbance is a cardinal manifestation of more advanced Parkinsonism, whose pathogenesis is only poorly understood. Certainly it has been recognized for many years that the basal ganglia play an important role in postural control, but dopaminergic therapy has little effect on instability. Finally, cognitive impairment affects approximately 20% of patients with Parkinson's disease.[8] The mechanisms are controversial, likely multifactorial, and are discussed below. Significant cognitive impairment is not only refractory to therapy in its own right but may substantially limit the tolerance to standard antiparkinson medications, which may result in unacceptable psychiatric side effects.

PATHOPHYSIOLOGY

Etiology

The etiology of Parkinson's disease is still unknown. However, a number of points can be made with relative certainty. First, evidence from twin studies indicates that in the majority of cases, genetic factors are probably not important.[133] Second, while encephalitis lethargica was the commonest cause of parkinsonism in the earlier half of this century, modern attempts to demonstrate a viral agent that is consistently associated with the development of Parkinson's disease have failed,[30] nor is there evidence of transmissibility, which might suggest a slow viral/prion process.[39] A number of features suggest that some environmental factor(s) may play a causal role. Individuals brought up in rural communities and exposed to well water during childhood are more likely to develop Parkinson's disease.[101,122] Other studies have shown an increased risk among people exposed to pesticide sprays.[101] Finally, the extraordinary occurrence of severe parkinsonism among individuals

exposed to the meperidine analogue N-methyl-4-phenyl-1,2,3,6-tetrahydropyridine (MPTP) and the induction of clinical, pathologic, and biochemical features of parkinsonism in subhuman primates treated with MPTP lend further credence to the hypothesis that some environmental toxin(s) may be responsible for the idiopathic disorder.[10,61] Indeed, it has been suggested that parkinsonism may result from early exposure to a subclinical environmental insult unmasked in later life by the continued, physiologic decline in nigral neurons and the consequent decrease in striatal dopamine production.[13] Ongoing nigral cell death may alternatively reflect an active process of mitochondrial dysfunction and generation of superoxide radicals.[54]

Pathology

The cardinal pathologic features of Parkinson's disease are well known and do not require extensive review here. The primary abnormality is the death of neuromelanin-containing dopamine neurons of the pars compacta of the substantia nigra. Other pigmented brainstem neurons, including those of the ventral tegmental area, locus ceruleus, and dorsal motor nucleus of the vagus are also affected.[33,53] The raphe nuclei also are affected. Degenerating neurons may contain characteristic eosinophilic intracytoplasmic inclusion (Lewy) bodies, and areas of neuronal degeneration are infiltrated by glial tissue. That the process of cell destruction is an active, ongoing one (and therefore potentially amenable to therapeutic intervention) is indicated by the presence of microglia that stain positively for HLA-DR2.[75]

Neurochemistry

The predictable result of the degeneration of affected neurons is the progressive loss of the monoamine neurotransmitters they produce. Thus the major biochemical abnormality of the disease is a decrease in dopamine and its metabolites affecting the substantia nigra, the ventral tegmental area, and their projections: the striatum, nucleus accumbens, and limbic cortex.[28,112] Striatal dopamine loss seems to affect the putamen more than the caudate, particularly in the earlier stages of the disease.[60] This is of interest, because on the basis of their connections to cortical regions, the putamen is thought to be more directly involved in motor function, whereas the caudate may have a more integrative function.[23] In a similar fashion, degeneration of the locus ceruleus leads to widespread decreases in noradrenaline, whereas raphe cell loss is associated with diminished levels of 5-hydroxytryptamine.[1,16,28,104,112]

In addition to the predicted changes in classic transmitter systems, levels of numerous other putative transmitters, chiefly neuropeptides, are affected. These include substance P,[73] cholecystokinin,[121] Leu- and Met-enkephalin,[124] neurotensin, and bombesin.[3] Since similar changes are not seen following MPTP administration to subhuman primates or in individuals dying of progressive supranuclear palsy (also characterized by degeneration of midbrain dopamine systems), it is still not entirely clear whether changes in peptide systems reflect primary degeneration of peptide-containing neurons or whether these are secondary to longstanding changes in dopamine content.

Numerous alterations in receptors also have been reported. Destruction of midbrain dopamine neurons results in denervation supersensitivity of D2 receptors experimentally.[22] An analogous increase in D2 binding density in parkinsonian striatum has been observed by some investigators,[63] while others have found no change or decreases in some patients.[102,108] Guttman and co-workers[45] confirmed the early increase in striatal D2 binding, but found that treatment with levodopa resulted in a return to normal of D2 receptor density. They found no correlation between D2 binding, disease duration, or response to therapy. The effects of disease on D1 binding density are equally controversial. Both increased and unchanged levels have been reported in the striatum,[95,100,106] whereas binding is decreased in the substantia nigra pars compacta.[17]

Receptors for other transmitters are also affected in Parkinson's disease. These include 5-hydroxytryptamine (decreased

5-HT$_1$ binding in cortex of demented individuals[93]); mu- (decreased in striatum and substantia nigra[103,129]); and kappa-opiate receptors (decreased in nigra[129]), neurotensin, and somatostatin (decreased in nigra[129,130]). Not all investigators can reproduce the abnormalities in opiate binding.[24]

Dopamine Systems: Anatomy and Pharmacology

There are three major dopamine systems in the brain: the nigrostriatal, mesolimbic/mesocortical, and tuberohypophyseal. Fibers from the pars compacta of the substantia nigra project to both the caudate and putamen. Striatal inhomogeneities (cholinesterase-deficient "patches" and cholinesterase-positive matrix) occur,[44] but dopaminergic terminals are found in both sites.[37] Although dopamine is traditionally regarded as an "inhibitory" transmitter (striatal turnover of acetylcholine is decreased in response to dopaminergic stimulation), this is an oversimplification. Electrophysiologically, dopamine may have excitatory effects, and it furthermore appears that dopamine behaves differently depending on the precise site within the striatum and its ultimate area of projection.[91] Classical pharmacologic studies have suggested the existence of two major subtypes of dopamine receptor: D1, which is linked in a stimulatory fashion to adenylate cyclase, and D2, which is cyclase-independent.[55] Actually, D2 stimulation has an inhibitory effect on D1-mediated formation of cyclic adenosine monophosphate (cAMP).[120] The potency of neuroleptic drugs in terms of antipsychotic efficacy, their capacity to induce parkinsonian features, and stimulation of prolactin release all seem to correlate with their ability to displace D2 binding, and until recently it was therefore thought that all of the important functional effects of dopamine in the nervous system are D2-mediated. Behaviorally, dopaminergic stimulation results in increased locomotion and stereotypic (repetitive and nonpurposive) behavior. Lesion studies in rodents suggest that increased locomotion actually results from stimulation of mesolimbic dopamine systems, whereas stereotypy is striatally mediated.[56] Unilateral stimulation of ascending dopamine projections in experimental animals results in contraversive turning. All of these responses may be seen after treatment with mixed D1/D2 or selective D2 dopamine agonists, thus lending further support to clinical impressions that D2 stimulation is of primary importance. However, recent work indicates that D2-mediated responses can be attenuated by the administration of selective D1 antagonists[6,69,78,99] and that the effects of selective D2 agonists are potentiated by D1 agonists.[132,134] Furthermore, contrary to initial impressions, selective D1 stimulation does have behavioral correlates, although these are somewhat controversial. These include grooming[79] and the induction of vacuous chewing movements.[109] For certain behaviors (locomotion, rearing, sniffing, and grooming), there appears to be synergism between D1 and D2 systems, whereas D1 and D2 stimulation may have antagonistic effects in the regulation of chewing movements.[82] The implications of such observations for the treatment of Parkinson's disease are not known at this time, but they may be substantial.

In the last few months, molecular biologic techniques have led to the identification of D3, D4, and D5 receptors.[114a,121a,131a] The function of these receptors is as yet undetermined, but they may be of importance for neuroleptic effects (D3 and D4[114a,131a]) and as dopamine autoreceptors (D3[114a]).

Pathophysiology of Motor Fluctuations and Postural Disorders

Alterations in dopamine function undoubtedly play a role in many of the motoric complications of long-term therapy, but the precise relationship is far from clear. Explanations for these complications can be considered to fall into three categories: pharmacokinetic variations in dopamine availability, pharmacodynamic alterations in the response to available dopamine, and mechanisms independent of dopamine (Table 15–1). The first category has received the most attention. While there is some correlation between plasma levels of levodopa and the clinical state, this is

TABLE 15–1. **POSSIBLE MECHANISMS UNDERLYING FLUCTUATIONS IN PARKINSONIAN DISABILITY**

Failure to absorb medication from GI tract
Competition for transport of levodopa across the blood-brain barrier
Inadequate central decarboxylation of levodopa
Inadequate "storage capacity" for dopamine due to loss of synaptic vesicles
Altered affinity of dopamine receptors
Inappropriate balance of D1 vs. D2 stimulation (Do dyskinesias reflect excessive D1 stimulation?)
Dysregulation of dopaminergic activity due to abnormalities in other neurotransmitter systems

imperfect, particularly in patients with unpredictable "on-off" reactions.[80,114] Drug-resistant off periods may in some circumstances reflect failed absorption of levodopa, perhaps secondary to impaired gastric emptying or competition with other amino acids for transport across the gut mucosal membrane.[77,85] The importance of such mechanisms is supported by the beneficial response to continuous administration of levodopa by intravenous or nasoduodenal routes.[47,88,111] Also, even though levodopa may be present in adequate concentrations in plasma, it may fail to cross the blood-brain barrier. Contenders for competitive inhibition of transport include 3-0-methyldopa, formed by the ubiquitous action of catechol O-methyltransferase (COMT) and other large neutral amino acids.[85]

In rats with unilateral lesions of the substantia nigra, the duration and amplitude of levodopa-induced elevations in striatal dopamine are lower ipsilateral to the lesion.[115] This has led to the suggestion that fluctuations in advanced disease reflect decreased storage capacity in degenerating nigrostriatal terminals and consequent impairment of buffering capacity. Shorter duration of benefit in fluctuating patients has been noted in some clinical trials[32] but not others.[36,58] There can be little question that peripheral kinetic factors play an important role in fluctuating responses to levodopa, but the precise degree remains controversial. Even in patients treated with continuous intravenous infusions of levodopa, some fluctuations persist, suggesting that other factors are at play.[47,88]

Other investigators have postulated that alterations in dopamine receptors underlie the variation in function. They suggest that dyskinesias reflect stimulation of receptors rendered supersensitive by denervation. Indeed, D2 receptors are upregulated in Parkinson's disease,[63] and normal individuals treated with levodopa do not develop dyskinesias, suggesting that these reflect a pathologic response to the drug. However, postmortem studies indicate that upregulation only occurs in untreated Parkinson patients and that treatment with levodopa results in a return of D2 binding density to normal levels. Furthermore, there is no correlation between disease state, response to therapy, and D2 binding.[45] In vivo studies using positron emission tomography have failed to reveal consistent changes in dopamine receptor binding in Parkinson's disease,[118] and there is no experimental support for the hypothesis that sudden fluctuations in clinical state reflect rapid swings in dopamine receptor affinity. If anything, clinical studies would suggest the opposite, since patients who are off maintain the ability to respond to dopamine receptor agonist therapy.[35,47]

As indicated above, there is evidence for both synergistic and antagonistic relationships between D1 and D2 receptor stimulation. A number of authorities feel that the incidence of dyskinesias is lower in individuals treated with D2 agonists such as bromocriptine than in those treated with levodopa alone,[107] and consequently, a contribution of D1 stimulation to dyskinesias has been postulated. At present, there is far too little clinical experience with selective D1 agents to test this hypothesis, and the relationship, if any, between putative D1-mediated behaviors in rodents (grooming and chewing movements) to clinical effects in humans is unknown.

Finally, it is obvious that despite careful attempts to maintain an even delivery of dopamine to the striatum, fluctuations in disability still occur, and it is therefore prudent to consider the possible contribution of abnormalities in other transmitters to parkinsonian disability. As previously noted, a wide variety of transmitters and their receptors may be affected by the disease, and in general the effects of these alterations are unknown. Particularly striking candidates for a role here are the numerous peptides in the basal ganglia, many of which are affected in Parkinson's disease and which also appear to exert some of their actions by modulating activity in mesostriatal and/or mesolimbic dopamine systems.[117]

It has long been recognized that the basal ganglia play a role in postural control. Subhuman primates with lesions of the basal ganglia lose postural reflexes, and postural instability is one of the cardinal features of Parkinson's disease. The neurochemical basis for postural control is unknown, and treatments aimed at ameliorating dopamine deficiency often have little effect on the postural disturbance in Parkinson patients.

Pathophysiology of Dementia and Other Mental Changes

Dementia occurs in approximately 20% of patients with Parkinson's disease, and lesser degrees of cognitive impairment may be even more common. Considerable controversy surrounds the question of whether the dementia associated with basal ganglia disease (i.e., subcortical dementia) is qualitatively different from that seen in Alzheimer's disease (i.e., cortical dementia). Studies attempting to address this issue have been hampered by numerous methodologic problems, including the difficulties arising when one attempts to equate disability from dementia with disability from motor dysfunction and the whole question of whether the tests employed truly assess cognition or whether they are only dependent on intact motor function. From a histologic point of view, at least three pathologic processes may underlie cognitive impairment in Parkinson's disease: (1) concurrent Alzheimer's disease — that is, cortical plaques and neurofibrillary tangles[46]; (2) the subcortical component of Alzheimer's disease — that is, degeneration of the nucleus basalis of Meynert, but in the absence of cortical plaques and tangles[135]; and (3) diffuse cortical degeneration associated with Lewy bodies (Lewy body disease).[9,11,38] Undoubtedly, this pathologic heterogeneity may explain some of the difficulties encountered when trying to define a characteristic clinical expression of dementia in Parkinson's disease. Furthermore, the cognitive impairment of Parkinson's disease may in part reflect underlying basal ganglia dysfunction. The neurochemical substrates of dementia in Parkinson's disease are not fully determined, but again some overlap with Alzheimer's disease appears likely. Thus, demented Parkinson patients demonstrate a loss of cortical cholinergic markers, regardless of the presence of cortical plaques and tangles, and this change is either not seen or is less profound in cognitively intact patients with Parkinson's disease.[26,92] Hippocampal somatostatin is also depressed in demented Parkinson patients, as it is in Alzheimer's disease.[31]

Mental changes other than dementia are seen in Parkinson 's disease. Depression is common and is associated with decreased levels of the 5-HT metabolite 5-HIAA in the cerebrospinal fluid.[74] Psychosis may also occur independently of dementia, and it is then usually attributable to drug therapy. This represents one of the most difficult therapeutic problems in Parkinson's disease and will be discussed further in the following section.

TREATMENT

Levodopa

Regardless of changes in other systems, the primary abnormality in Parkinson's disease is deficiency of nigrostriatal dopamine, and therefore the backbone of therapy rests on dopamine replacement. This is primarily achieved by the administration of levodopa, which with very few exceptions should be given in combination with a peripheral decarboxylase inhibitor, such as carbidopa or benserazide. Use of a decarboxylase inhibitor allows the use of approximately 25% of the dose of levodopa that would otherwise be required and results in substantial attenuation of peripherally mediated side effects, including nausea and other gastrointestinal upset, postural dizziness, and cardiac arrhythmias. Levodopa given in this fashion produces benefit within 30 minutes, with a duration of action of approxi-

mately 3 hours. Sustained-release forms of levodopa/carbidopa and levodopa/benserazide are available and have demonstrated modest benefit in patients suffering from predictable end-of-dose deterioration ("wearing off").[18,41,97] The latency to benefit is prolonged, and maximum efficacy is diminished compared with the standard preparations, however, and a combination of standard and sustained-release forms may be required. In patients with marked response fluctuations, substantial benefit may be derived from the controlled and continuous administration of levodopa, either by duodenal[111] or intravenous[47,87] routes (Table 15–2). These routes allow one to attain relatively constant plasma levels of levodopa but are cumbersome and still do not entirely overcome the problems of sudden freezing and the difficult choice between dyskinesias and bradykinesia. Finally, a simple but frequently effective means of stabilizing levodopa levels and response is the avoidance of high protein intake, which interferes with levodopa transport by competing for sites on the large neutral amino acid transport carrier system. Many patients will note a profound deterioration in association

TABLE 15–2. **THERAPEUTIC STRATEGIES FOR FLUCTUATIONS IN RESPONSE TO THERAPY**

Optimize dosage schedule to avoid excessive peaks and troughs
Ensure adequate and even delivery of levodopa to striatum
Avoid taking medication with large meals that:
Delay gastric emptying
Allow competition for transport across blood-brain barrier
Alternate forms of administering levodopa:
Controlled release
Duodenal or intravenous infusion
Delay breakdown of dopamine
Deprenyl (prolongs and enhances action of levodopa)
Dopamine agonists
Longer duration of action than levodopa
Allow the use of a lower dose of levodopa
Fewer dyskinesias than the equivalent dose of levodopa
May be able to administer by alternate routes:
Subcutaneous (apomorphine*, lisuride*)
Intravenous (lisuride*)
Transdermal (PHNO*)

* Not available in the United States.

with a heavy protein meal, and they benefit from taking small snacks during the daytime, with the major protein intake redistributed toward the evening.[96,105]

Dopamine Agonists

When the benefits derived from levodopa become increasingly limited, the second strategy employed is frequently the addition of a dopamine agonist (Table 15–3). These agents have the advantage of directly stimulating dopamine receptors, thereby bypassing the requirement for native decarboxylase. One can achieve a certain degree of selective stimulation of D2 (or D1) receptors, and this may confer some advantage, although this is as yet not entirely clear. The dopamine agonists currently available are ergot derivatives, and the prototype of these is bromocriptine, whose use in Parkinson's disease was first reported in 1974 by Calne and colleagues.[15] Bromocriptine has a longer duration of action than levodopa (4 to 6 hours) and is highly selective for D2 receptors. The addition of bromocriptine to levodopa tends to smooth out fluctuations, with longer on periods between doses and probably fewer dyskinesias than when levodopa is used alone. This tendency for fewer dyskinesias has been attributed to D2 selectivity, but the synergistic relationship between D1 and D2 stimulation described above has also been cited as an explanation for the improved efficacy of bromocriptine when given in addition to levodopa rather than as the sole agent, at least in patients with more advanced disease.[49,108] Currently, most experts add an agonist such as bromocriptine once a modest dose of levodopa (300 to 600 mg/d) is ineffective as sole therapy.[14,107]

Other ergot derivatives include pergolide,[25,51,66] lisuride,[*43,90] and mesulergine.[11,52,126*] In general, all of the agonists are comparable if one assesses the effects in a group of patients. For any individual patient, however, one agent may be better than

another. Certain potential advantages accrue to each. Pergolide is more potent and has a longer duration of action than bromocriptine (approximately 8 hours). Earlier concerns about cardiotoxicity have not withstood more rigorous analysis.[123] Lisuride is highly water soluble, and this allows its administration by continuous intravenous[89] or subcutaneous[89a] infusion. Its disadvantage is a high incidence of adverse psychiatric effects. The closely related compound transdihydrolisuride (TDHL)* is a partial D2 agonist. This means that it should preferentially stimulate supersensitive receptors. Although limited benefit has been reported, partial agonists also have antagonistic properties on the basis of receptor occupancy, and this may lead to exacerbation of Parkinsonian deficits. Mesulergine is another agent whose effect was found to be comparable to that of bromocriptine,[11,52,126] but which was withdrawn from further development because of possible carcinogenicity when very high doses were given for long periods to experimental rats.

The other major category of dopamine agonists is the group derived from apomorphine.* Apomorphine itself is a mixed D1/D2 agonist that was used for Parkinson's disease in the 1960s and 1970s but was abandoned because of unacceptable toxicity, including not only nausea and emesis but also azotemia.[21] At that time the drug was being administered orally, and very high doses were required. Recently apomorphine has been reintroduced but given by either intermittent or continuous subcutaneous injection.[116] In patients with severe fluctuations in disability, this seems to be an extremely promising therapeutic modality. Patients who suddenly and unpredictably go off can be trained to self-administer a "booster" dose of apomorphine, which will take effect within 10 minutes and last for approximately 1 hour. To date, no major adverse effects have been noted in patients undergoing subcutaneous administration, provided that peripheral D2 receptors are blocked with domperidone.

Some novel D2 dopamine agonists are being developed that are chemically distinct from ergot or apomorphine derivatives. (+)-4-propyl-9-hydroxynaphthoxa-

---

*Not available in the United States.

TABLE 15–3. DRUGS FOR THE TREATMENT OF PARKINSON'S DISEASE*

	Drug	Availability	Initial Dose	Maintenance Dose	Comments
EARLY DISEASE	Levodopa/carbidopa	100/10 100/25 250/25 scored tabs	50/12.5 mg tid	Increase by 50 mg q 5–7 d to 100/25 mg tid–qid	Further increases in dose possible, but frequently preferable to add a second drug at this point (see below). Side effects minimized by taking with food, but this may decrease efficacy.
	or				
	Levodopa/benserazide	50/12.5 100/25 200/50 capsules			
	Amantadine	100-mg caps	100 mg daily–bid	100 mg bid	Helpful for tremor. Long-term usefulness limited.
FLUCTUATORS	Controlled-release Levodopa/carbidopa (Sinemet CR)†	200/50-mg tabs	Switch to same total daily dose as standard preparation, but decrease dose frequency by 30%–50%. May require approximately 25% higher total daily dose than with standard preparation.		May need to supplement first A.M. dose with a low dose of standard levodopa/carbidopa. To prevent loss of sustained-release properties, do not break into doses smaller than ½ tab.
	Deprenyl (Selegiline)	5-mg tabs	2.5 mg bid	Increase by 2.5 mg q 5–7 d to 5 mg bid	Avoid exceeding 5 mg bid. Loses selectivity for MAO-B and no further advantage conferred.
	Bromocriptine	2.5-mg scored tabs 5-mg caps	1.25 mg test dose, then 1.25 mg tid	Increase by 1.25 mg q 5–7 d to 15–20 mg/d in 3–4 doses	Confusion and sleep disturbance may be minimized by taking second dose no later than lunch. Peripheral side effects may be attenuated by taking with food and adding domperidone 10 mg qid (½ h ac meal + h).
	Pergolide	0.05-mg, 0.25-mg, 1.0-mg scored tabs	0.05 mg bid	Increase to 1–3 mg/d in three divided doses over approximately 4 wk	As above. Mixed D1/D2 agonist.

* These are suggested guidelines only. The treatment is highly individualized, and adjustments may be necessary.
† A comparable preparation of sustained-release levodopa/benserazide (Madopar HBS) is available in Europe.

zine (PHNO)[*] is a highly selective D2 agonist[72] that is effective in reversing cardinal parkinsonian features.[81,119] This drug is particularly interesting in that it is rapidly absorbed through skin. Preliminary studies in MPTP-treated monkeys[110] and humans[20] suggest that it may be feasible to use a patch impregnated with PHNO to continuously deliver a relatively constant amount of drug. At the end of the day, or in case of adverse reactions, the patch could be removed. Another novel agent is ciladopa,[*] which like TDHL is also a partial agonist.[67] Its development has been held back because of potential toxicity.

As noted above, the potential role for D1 stimulation in Parkinson's disease is not clear at this time. On the one hand, indirect evidence accruing from the use of selective D2 agonists suggests that it might be preferable to minimize D1 stimulation to decrease the incidence of dyskinesias. On the other hand, a growing body of evidence based on work with experimental animals (mostly rats, which may not be strictly comparable) suggests a synergistic relationship between D1 and D2 receptors. Trials with SKF 38393,[*] a selective D1 agonist, have failed to demonstrate benefit in Parkinson's disease, even when the drug is given in combination with levodopa[7] or bromocriptine.[65] Another agonist with somewhat less D1 selectivity is CY 208-243,[*] which may be modestly useful.[125,128]

Amantadine and Anticholinergics

Many neurologists prefer to delay the use of levodopa and have traditionally started therapy with amantadine and/or anticholinergics. In my opinion, the evidence condemning early use is not strong, and it has therefore been my practice to initiate therapy with levodopa and avoid these alternate agents in most cases. In some situations, however, they may be beneficial. Amantadine is thought to enhance dopamine release from surviving neurons. The profile of side effects suggests that it may also possess some anticholinergic properties. As a rule, it

may buy a few months' time if one is trying to delay the use of levodopa. It is not very effective for the treatment of bradykinesia. It is frequently helpful in the treatment of tremor, and in a patient with minimal disability apart from tremor, it is a very reasonable alternative. The same can be said for the anticholinergics, the use of which is diminishing largely because of the high incidence of confusion in elderly patients and concerns that these drugs may exacerbate dementia.

MAO Inhibition

Another potential approach to prolonging and potentiating the effect of levodopa is to prevent the breakdown of dopamine. Like other monoamines, dopamine is catabolized by oxidative deamination to dihydroxyphenylacetic acid (DOPAC). This reaction can be inhibited by the selective monoamine oxidase (MAO)-B inhibitor deprenyl, which because it fails to inhibit MAO-A is devoid of the "cheese" effect. After deprenyl was introduced in the 1970s, some investigators were cautiously optimistic that it might smooth out fluctuations and enhance the benefit derived from levodopa.[64] Others found no objective evidence of benefit, even though patients reported subjective improvement.[29] Currently deprenyl is finding use as adjunctive therapy in Parkinson's disease, but unfortunately somewhat less than 50% of patients ever derive substantial benefit, and in these individuals the effects are not sustained.[42] Limiting factors include exacerbation of dyskinesias and confusion. Recently there has been a great deal of excitement over another potentially beneficial effect of deprenyl: the possibility that it may retard progression of the underlying disease process. This will be discussed further in the final section.

Adverse Effects of Dopaminergic Stimulation

Peripherally Mediated Effects

Dopaminergic therapy is frequently limited by medication-induced side effects. Those that are peripherally mediated, in-

---

[*]Not available in the United States.

cluding nausea, postural dizziness, and cardiac arrhythmias, may respond to treatment with a peripherally selective dopamine D2 antagonist, such as domperidone. The usual dose is 10 mg tid given 30 minutes prior to meals, but this can be doubled if necessary. It is often possible to wean individuals off domperidone as tolerance to the toxic effects of dopaminergic stimulation develops. Another approach in the case of levodopa is optimization of the levodopa/decarboxylase inhibitor (DCI) ratio. The typical daily requirement for DCI (carbidopa or benserazide) is 75 to 100 mg. Thus, if one administers a modest dose (300 to 500 mg) of a preparation with a high levodopa/DCI ratio of 10 : 1, the total daily intake of DCI will be inadequate. Switching to a preparation with a ratio of 4 : 1 will often be sufficient not only to suppress side effects but also to enhance the benefit, because more active drug is transported across the blood-brain barrier.

Central Effects

Central side effects from dopaminergic stimulation are much more difficult to manage. Dyskinesias may respond to lowering the individual dose, and this may require shortening the interval between doses. Replacing some of the levodopa with a dopamine agonist may help. However, even with optimum regulation of dosage, dyskinesias are likely to appear, particularly in patients with more advanced disease. Even more problematic is the emergence of drug-induced psychoses. These may develop relatively insidiously, with just a "funny feeling in the head," which over the next few days progresses to florid paranoia, hallucinations, and violent behavior. All drugs used to treat Parkinson's disease have the potential to provoke this reaction. In dealing with this situation, the first step is to search for and correct any other contributing factors, such as intercurrent illness, toxic or metabolic upsets, sleep deprivation (particularly in hospitalized patients), and, especially, other medications (Table 15 – 4). Any medications not clearly necessary for the patient's management should be discontinued. Should these measures fail, the next step is cautious reduction of dopaminergic therapy. Abrupt discontinuation of all anti-

TABLE 15–4. MANAGEMENT OF DRUG-INDUCED PSYCHOSIS

Rule out other contributory factors
    Intercurrent illness
    Metabolic upset
    Other psychotropic medications
    Sleep deprivation
Decrease anti-Parkinson medication in order of
    toxicity vs. efficacy
    Anticholinergics
    Dopamine agonists, levodopa
Benzodiazepines if necessary for agitation
Avoid typical neuroleptics
Atypical neuroleptics under observation
    Thioridazine
    Clozapine
Electroconvulsive therapy

Parkinson therapy is to be avoided if possible, since it may result in life-threatening akinesia and its attendant complications of hypostatic pneumonia and pulmonary embolus or even in the neuroleptic malignant syndrome. If possible, neuroleptics should be avoided, for obvious reasons, and if medication is necessary for agitation, it is worth attempting the use of benzodiazepines. Where one is caught between the options of immobility and psychosis, a cautious trial of dopaminergic therapy in combination with atypical neuroleptics may be warranted. Thioridazine is a weak antipsychotic agent with sedating and anticholinergic properties, but which also acts preferentially on the A10 (mesolimbic/mesocortical) dopamine neurons. Therefore, of antipsychotic agents readily available, it is the least likely to exacerbate parkinsonian features. Another choice is clozapine, which is a preferential D1 antagonist and also A10 selective. Recent trials suggest that clozapine may be helpful in this situation.[34,94] Finally, desperate situations may justify the use of electroconvulsive therapy (ECT). A pilot trial suggests that suppression of psychosis with ECT may allow continuation of life-saving anti-Parkinson therapy.[50]

Surgical Therapies
Symptomatic Therapy

Surgical treatment for Parkinson's disease is not new but has become largely unnecessary with the advent of levodopa and other pharmacologic innovations. As is the case with amantadine and anticholinergics, surgery may be quite effective for the management of tremor and/or rigidity, but it has little effect on akinesia, which is probably the most disabling feature of the disease. Nevertheless, in patients with tremor, one can demonstrate rhythmic bursting activity in the ventral intermediate nucleus of the thalamus, and surgical lesions in this location or in the ventral lateral nucleus may be beneficial.[57,83]

Transplantation

The role of grafting using autologus adrenal medullary tissue or fetal substantia nigra is uncertain, controversial, and dealt with by others in this monograph (see Chapter 14). At this stage, transplantation should be considered an experimental therapy, and the position regarding clinical use of these procedures can be fairly summarized by the following observations. (1) The efficacy of grafting for parkinsonism is undetermined. Most observers have been unable to reproduce the dramatic results described by Madrazo and colleagues.[40,68,70] (2) The mechanism of benefit from grafting is undetermined. Explanations include increased dopamine release and enhanced sprouting of surviving host dopamine fibres,[4,5] but some more cynical observers have even suggested that improvement is related to coincidental lesions of the caudate nucleus, in effect representing the resurrection of an old surgical technique for treating Parkinson's disease.[131] (3) The incidence of significant morbidity and mortality is relatively high.

THE FUTURE

The ideal approach to the refractive state in Parkinson's disease would be its prevention. Although the etiology and mechanism of disease progression in Parkinson's disease are unknown, growing evidence suggests environmental factors and the formation of oxidative metabolites. The discovery and further elucidation of the mechanisms of MPTP-induced parkinsonism may provide

clues to treatment of the idiopathic disorder. Thus, MPTP itself is nontoxic, but damage is mediated by the oxidative radical MPP^+, and the formation of this latter compound, as well as the induction of Parkinsonism in subhuman primates, can be blocked by co-administration of MAO-B inhibitors.[48,62]

At around the same time that this was becoming apparent, Birkmayer and his colleagues[2] in Vienna reported that Parkinson patients treated with levodopa/benserazide plus deprenyl had a longer life expectancy than those treated with levodopa/benserazide alone. This study was flawed, however, by its retrospective nature and by a number of baseline differences in the two treatment groups. A recent study by Tetrud and Langston[127] indicated that treatment with deprenyl may delay the requirement for symptomatic treatment of disease using levodopa. This pilot observation has been confirmed by a similar, larger, multicenter (DATATOP) trial.[90a] The latter study was designed to assess the effects of deprenyl, alpha-tocopherol, or a combination of the two, on the progression of early Parkinson's disease. Safety monitoring prompted a preliminary analysis of the data, as it was found that deprenyl either alone or in combination with vitamin E significantly delayed the requirement for levodopa. An interaction between tocopherol and deprenyl, or an independent effect of tocopherol has not yet been assessed, as the trial is ongoing. Neither the Tetrud and Langston[127] nor the DATATOP[90a] study found significant "washout" effects. In the latter study, there was a statistically significant "wash-in" effect of deprenyl, but this was felt to be of no biologic significance. Although these results from carefully performed studies are extremely exciting, it should be noted that a protective effect on disease progression has not yet been adequately demonstrated in patients whose disease has advanced to the point that symptomatic therapy is required.

The discussion of pathophysiology earlier in this chapter indicates the importance of steady rates of delivery of medication to the striatum. Although the infusion of levodopa is somewhat cumbersome, improved technology may lead to more widespread use of infusion pumps for the continuous subcutaneous administration of dopamine agonists.[89a,116] At least one dopamine agonist is readily absorbed transdermally,[20,110] and this raises hopes for a simple and efficacious means of assuring steady rates of drug administration. Finally, implantable matrix "pumps" allowing the sustained administration of dopamine over long periods of time are being developed but are still relatively far from clinical trials.[27]

Research concerning the widespread abnormalities found in Parkinson's disease in transmitter systems other than dopamine is also ongoing. Noradrenaline is depleted, and it has been suggested that freezing attacks may respond to the noradrenaline precursor L-threo-dihydroxyphenylserine.[84] Other investigators have had difficulty substantiating this claim. Depression in Parkinson's disease may respond well to tricyclics, presumed to act by preventing the reuptake of noradrenaline and/or 5-HT, but these agents have little effect on the motor manifestations of the disease. To date, manipulation of GABA (e.g., with valproate[87]) and opiate (e.g., administration of the opiate antagonist naloxone[86]) systems have not found widespread use in the treatment of Parkinson's disease. Many other nonopioid peptides are affected, and their manipulation offers another approach to the management of complications.[117] Finally, improved understanding of the efficacy, mechanisms, and best techniques for grafting may ultimately offer tremendous hope for a devastating illness.

SUMMARY

This chapter has dealt with the drug therapy of Parkinson's disease only, and the importance of other approaches, particularly physical, occupational, and speech therapy, has not been touched on. From a pharmacologic point of view, the first approach to treatment is the use of precursor therapy with levodopa. This is initially effective in most patients, but a high incidence of complications emerges by 5 years of therapy. Failure to respond to levodopa may be approached by ensuring better delivery to the striatum, delaying the breakdown of dopamine, or the use of agonists that directly stimulate dopamine receptors. Dyskinesias and psychiatric complications reflect dopaminergic toxicity and may respond to reduction and/or redistribution of medication, but the price in terms of akinesia may be unacceptably high. Improved therapy will depend on a better understanding of the basic mechanisms underlying parkinsonian disability, and directions for further development will include treatment to slow disease progression, novel systems for drug delivery, and manipulation of nondopaminergic transmitters.

ACKNOWLEDGMENT

AJS is supported by a Career Scientist Award from the Ontario Ministry of Health.

REFERENCES

1. Bernheimer, H, Birkmayer, W, and Hornykiewicz, O: Verteilung des 5-Hydroxytriptamins (Serotonin) im Gehirn des Menschen und sein Verhälten, bei Patienten mit Parkinson Syndrom. Klin Wochenschr 39: 1056–1059, 1961.
2. Birkmayer, W, Knoll, J, Riederer, P, Youdim, MBH, Hars, C, and Marton, J: Increased life expectancy resulting from addition of L-deprenyl to Madopar treatment in Parkinson's disease: A longterm study. J Neural Transm 64:113–127, 1985.
3. Bissette, G, Nemeroff, CB, Decker, MW, Kizer, JS, Agid, Y and Javoy-Agid, F: Alterations in regional brain concentrations of neurotensin and bombesin in Parkinson's disease. Ann Neurol 17:324–328, 1985.
4. Björklund, A, Lindvall, O, Isacson, O, Brundin, P, Wictorin, K, Strecker, RE, Clarke, DJ, and Dunnett, SB: Mechanisms of action of intracerebral neural implants: Studies on nigral and striatal grafts to the lesioned striatum. Trends Neurosci 10:509–516, 1987.
5. Bohn, MC, Cupit, L, Marciano, F, and Gash, DM: Adrenal medulla grafts enhance recovery of striatal dopaminergic fibers. Science 237: 913–916, 1987.
6. Boyce, S, Kelly, E, Davis, A, Fleminger, S, Jenner, P, and Marsden, CD: SCH 23390 may alter dopamine-mediated motor behaviour via striatal D-1 receptors. Biochem Pharmacol 34:1665–1669, 1985.
7. Braun, AR, Fabbrini, G, Mouradian, MM, Serrati, C, Barone, P, and Chase, TN: Selective D-1 dopamine receptor agonist treatment of Parkinson's disease. J Neural Transm 68:41–50, 1987.

8. Brown, RG and Marsden, CD: How common is dementia in Parkinson's disease? Lancet 2: 1262–1265, 1984.

9. Burkhardt, CR, Filley, CM, Kleinschmidt-deMasters, BK, de la Monte, S, Norenberg, MD, and Schneck, SA: Diffuse Lewy body disease and progressive dementia. Neurology 38: 1520–1528, 1988.

10. Burns, RS, Chiueh, CC, Markey, SP, Ebert, MH, Jacobowitz, DM, and Kopin, IJ: A primate model of parkinsonism: Selective destruction of dopaminergic neurons in the pars compacta of the substantia nigra by N-methyl -4-phenyl -1,2,3,6- tetrahydropyridine. Proc Natl Acad Sci U S A 80:4546–4550, 1983.

11. Burton, K, Larsen, TA, Robinson, RG, Bratty, PJ, Martin, WRW, Schulzer, M, and Calne, DB: Parkinson's disease: A comparison of mesulergine and bromocriptine. Neurology 35: 1205–1208, 1985.

12. Byrne, EJ, Lennox, G, Lowe, J, and Godwin-Austen, RB: Diffuse Lewy body disease: Clinical features in 15 cases. J Neurol Neurosurg Psychiatry 52:709–717, 1989.

13. Calne, DB and Langston, JW: Aetiology of Parkinson's disease. Lancet 2:1457–1459, 1983.

14. Calne, DB and Stoessl, AJ: Approaches to the use of bromocriptine in Parkinson's disease. In Fahn, S, Marsden, CD, Jenner, P, and Teychenne, P (eds): Recent Developments in Parkinson's Disease. Raven Press, New York, 1986, pp 255–258.

15. Calne, DB, Teychenne, PF, Claveria, LE, Greenacre, JK, and Petrie, A: Bromocriptine in parkinsonism. BMJ 4:442–444, 1974.

16. Cash, R, Dennis, T, L'Heureux, R, Raisman, R, Javoy-Agid, F, and Scatton, B: Parkinson's disease and dementia: Norepinephrine and dopamine in locus ceruleus. Neurology 37: 42–46, 1987.

17. Cash, R, Raisman, R, Ploska, A, and Agid, Y: Dopamine D-1 receptor and cyclic AMP-dependent phosphorylation in Parkinson's disease. J Neurochem 49:1075–1083, 1987.

18. Cedarbaum, JM, Breck, L, Kutt, H, and McDowell, FH: Controlled-release levodopa/carbidopa. II. Sinemet CR4 treatment of response fluctuations in Parkinson's disease. Neurology 37:1607–1612, 1987.

19. Claveria, LE, Calne, DB, and Allen, JG: 'On-off' phenomena related to high plasma levodopa. BMJ 2:641–643, 1973.

20. Coleman, RJ, Lange, KW, Quinn, NP, Loper, AE, Bondi, JV, Hichens, M, Stahl, SM, and Marsden, CD: The antiparkinsonian actions and pharmacokinetics of transdermal (+)-4-propyl-9-hydroxynaphthoxazine (+PHNO): Preliminary results. Mov Disord 4:129–138, 1989.

21. Cotzias, GC, Papavasiliou, PS, Tolosa, ES, Mendez, JS, and Bell-Midura, M: Treatment of Parkinson's disease with apomorphines: Possible role of growth hormone. N Engl J Med 294:567–572, 1976.

22. Creese, I, Burt, DR, and Snyder, SH: Dopamine receptor binding enhancement accompanies lesion-induced behavioural supersensitivity. Science 197:596–598, 1977.

23. De Long, MR, Georgopoulos, AP, and Crutcher, MD: Cortico-basal ganglia relations and coding of motor performance. Exp Brain Res (Suppl.)7:30–40, 1983.

24. Delay-Goyet, P, Zajac, J-M, Javoy-Agid, F, Agid, Y, and Roques, BP: Regional distribution of mu, delta and kappa opioid receptors in human brains from controls and parkinsonian subjects. Brain Res 414:8–14, 1987.

25. Diamond, SG, Markham, CH, and Treciokas, IJ: Double-blind trial of pergolide for Parkinson's disease. Neurology 35:291–295, 1985.

26. Dubois, B, Rubert, M, Javoy-Agid, F, Ploska, A, and Agid, Y: A subcortico-cortical cholinergic system is affected in Parkinson's disease. Brain Res 288:213–218, 1983.

27. During, MJ, Freese, A, Sabel, BA, Saltzman, WM, Deutch, A, Roth, RH, and Langer, R: Controlled release of dopamine from a polymeric brain implant: In vivo characterization. Ann Neurol 25:351–356, 1989.

28. Ehringer, H and Hornykiewicz, O: Verteilung von Noradrenalin und Dopamin (3-Hydroxytyramin) im Gehirn des Menschen und ihr Verhälten bei Erkrankungen des extrapyramidalen Systems. Klin Wochenschr 38: 1236–1238, 1960.

29. Eisler, T, Teravainen, H, Nelson, R, Krebs, H, Weise, V, Lake, CR, Ebert, MH, Whetzel, N, Murphy, DL, Kopin IJ, and Calne, DB: Deprenyl in Parkinson disease. Neurology 31:19–23, 1981.

30. Elizan, TS and Casals, J: The viral hypothesis in Parkinsonism. J Neural Trans Park Dis Dement Sect (Suppl)19:75–88, 1983.

31. Epelbaum, J, Ruberg, M, Moyse, E, Javoy-Agid, F, Dubois, B, and Agid, Y: Somatostatin and dementia in Parkinson's disease. Brain Res 278:376–379, 1983.

32. Fabbrini, G, Juncos, J, Mouradian, MM, Serrati, C, and Chase, TN: Levodopa pharmacokinetic mechanisms and motor fluctuations in Parkinson's disease. Ann Neurol 21:370–376, 1987.

33. Forno, LS: Pathology of Parkinson's disease. In Marsden, CD and Fahn, S (eds): Movement Disorders. Butterworth Scientific, London, 1982, pp 25–40.

34. Friedman, JH and Lannon, MC: Clozapine in the treatment of psychosis in Parkinson's disease. Neurology 39:1219–1221, 1989.

35. Gancher, ST and Nutt, JG: Diurnal responsiveness to apomorphine. Neurology 37: 1250–1253, 1987.

36. Gancher, ST, Nutt, JG, and Woodward, W: Response to brief levodopa infusions in parkinsonian patients with and without motor fluctuations. Neurology 38:712–716, 1988.

37. Gerfen, CR, Herkenham, M, and Thibault, J: The neostriatal mosaic: II. Patch- and matrix-

directed mesostriatal and non-dopaminergic systems. J Neurosci 7:3915–3934, 1987.

38. Gibb, WRG, Esiri, MM, and Lees, AJ: Clinical and pathological features of diffuse cortical Lewy body disease (Lewy body dementia). Brain 110:1131–1153, 1985.

39. Gibbs, CJ and Gajdusek, DC: An update on long-term in vivo and in vitro studies designed to identify a virus as the cause of amyotrophic lateral sclerosis, parkinsonism dementia, and Parkinson's disease. Adv Neurol 36:343–351, 1982.

40. Goetz, CG, Olanow, CW, Koller, WC, Penn, RD, Cahill, D, Morantz, R, Stebbins, G, Tanner, CM, Klausaus, HL, Shannon, KM, Comella, CL, Witt, T, Cot, C, Waxman, M and Ganger, L: Multicenter study of autologous adrenal medullary transplantation to the corpus striatum in patients with advanced Parkinson's disease. N Engl J Med 320:337–341, 1989.

41. Goetz, CG, Tanner, CM, Klawans, HL, Shannon, KM, and Carroll, VS: Parkinson's disease and motor fluctuations: Long-acting carbidopa/levodopa (CR-4-Sinemet). Neurology 37:875–878, 1987.

42. Golbe, LI: Long-term efficacy and safety of deprenyl (selegiline) in advanced Parkinson's disease. Neurology 39:1109–1111, 1989.

43. Gopinathan, G, Teravainen, H, Dambrosia, JM, Ward, CD, Sanes, JN, Stuart, WK, Evarts, EV, and Calne, DB: Lisuride in parkinsonism. Neurology 31:371–376, 1981.

44. Graybiel, AM and Ragsdale, CW Jr: Histochemically distinct compartments in the striatum of human, monkey and cat demonstrated by acetylcholinesterase staining. Proc Natl Acad Sci U S A 75:5723–5726, 1978.

45. Guttman, M, Seeman, P, Reynolds, GP, Riederer, P, Jellinger, K, and Tourtellotte, WW: Dopamine D2 receptor density remains constant in treated Parkinson's disease. Ann Neurol 19:487–492, 1986.

46. Hakim, A and Mathieson, G: Dementia in Parkinson disease: A neuropathologic study. Neurology 29:1209–1214, 1979.

47. Hardie, RJ, Lees, AJ, and Stern, GM: On-off fluctuations in Parkinson's disease: A clinical and neuropharmacological study. Brain 107:487–506, 1984.

48. Heikkila, RE, Manzino, L, Cabbat, FS, and Duvoisin, RC: Protection against the dopaminergic neurotoxicity of 1-methyl-4-phenyl-1,2,5,6-tetrahydropyridine by monoamine oxidase inhibitors. Nature 311:467–469, 1984.

49. Hoehn, MMM and Elton, RL: Low dosages of bromocriptine added to levodopa in Parkinson's disease. Neurology 35:199–206, 1985.

50. Hurwitz, TA, Calne, DB, and Waterman, K: Treatment of dopaminomimetic psychosis in Parkinson's disease with electroconvul-

sive therapy. Can J Neurol Sci 15:32–34, 1988.

51. Jankovic, J: Long-term study of pergolide in Parkinson's disease. Neurology 35:296–299, 1985.

52. Jankovic, J, Orman, J, and Jansson, B: Placebo-controlled study of mesulergine in Parkinson's disease. Neurology 35:161–165, 1985.

53. Jellinger, K: The pathology of parkinsonism. In Marsden, CD and Fahn, S (eds): Movement Disorders, ed 2. Butterworth Scientific, London, 1987, pp 124–165.

54. Jenner, P: Clues to the mechanism underlying dopamine cell death in Parkinson's disease. J Neurol Neurosurg Psychiatry (Suppl):22–28, 1989.

55. Kebabian, JW and Calne, DB: Multiple receptors for dopamine. Nature 277:93–96, 1979.

56. Kelly, PH, Seviour, PW, and Iversen, SD: Amphetamine and apomorphine responses in the rat following 6-OHDA lesions of the nucleus accumbens septi and corpus striatum. Brain Res 94:507–522, 1975.

57. Kelly, PJ, Ahlskog, JE, Goerss, SJ, Daube, JR, Duffy, JR, and Kall, BA: Computer-assisted stereotactic ventralis lateralis thalamotomy with microelectrode recording control in patients with Parkinson's disease. Mayo Clin Proc 62:655–664, 1987.

58. Kempster, PA, Frankel, JP, Bovingdon, M, Webster, R, Lees, AJ, and Stern, GM: Levodopa peripheral pharamcokinetics and duration of motor response in Parkinson's disease. J Neurol Neurosurg Psychiatry 52:718–723, 1989.

59. Kessler, II: Parkinson's disease in epidemiologic perspective. Adv Neurol 19:355–383, 1978.

60. Kish, SJ, Shannak, K, and Hornykiewicz, O: Uneven pattern of dopamine loss in the striatum of patients with idiopathic Parkinson's disease: Pathophysiologic and clinical implications. N Engl J Med 318:876–880, 1988.

61. Langston, JW, Ballard, P, Tetrud, JW, and Irwin, I: Chronic parkinsonism in humans due to a product of meperidine-analog synthesis. Science 219:979–980, 1983.

62. Langston, JW, Irwin, I, Langston, EB, and Forno, LS: Pargyline prevents MPTP-induced parkinsonism in primates. Science 225:1480–1482, 1984.

63. Lee, T, Seeman, P, Rajput, A, Farley, I, and Hornykiewicz, O: Receptor basis for dopaminergic supersensitivity in Parkinson's disease. Nature 273:59–61, 1978.

64. Lees, AJ, Shaw, KM, Kohout, LJ, Stern, GM, Elsworth, JD, Sandler, M, and Youdim, MBH: Deprenyl in Parkinson's disease. Lancet 2:791–795, 1977.

65. LeWitt, P, Schlick, P, Hussain, M, Kesaree, N, Kareti, D, and Berchou, R: Selective D-1 agonist (SK&F 38393) in parkinsonism. Neurology (Suppl 1)38:258, 1988.

66. Lieberman, AN, Goldstein, M, Leibowitz, M, Go-

pinathan, G, Neophytides, A, Hiesiger, E, Nelson, J, and Walker, R: Long-term treatment with pergolide: Decreased efficacy with time. Neurology 34:223–226, 1984.

67. Lieberman, A, Gopinathan, G, Neophytides, A, Pasternack, P, and Goldstein, M: Advanced Parkinson's disease: Use of a partial dopamine agonist, ciladopa. Neurology 37:863–865, 1987.

68. Lindvall, O, Backlund, E-O, Farde, L, Sedvall, G, Freedman, R, Hoffer, B, Nobin, A, Seiger, A, and Olson, L: Transplantation in Parkinson's disease: Two cases of adrenal medullary grafts to the putamen. Ann Neurol 22:457–468, 1987.

69. Longoni, R, Spina, L, and Di Chiara, G: Permissive role of D-1 receptor stimulation for the expression of D-2 mediated behavioral responses: A quantitative phenomenological study in rats. Life Sci 41:2135–2145, 1987.

70. Madrazo, I, Drucker-Colín, R, Díaz, V, Martínez-Mata, J, Torres, C, and Becerril, JJ: Open microsurgical autograft of adrenal medulla to the right caudate nucleus in two patients with intractable Parkinson's disease. N Engl J Med 346:831–834, 1987.

71. Marsden, CD, Parkes, JD, and Quinn, N: Fluctuations of disability in Parkinson's disease: Clinical aspects. In Marsden, CD and Fahn, S (eds). Movement Disorders. London: Butterworth Scientific, 1982, pp 96–122.

72. Martin, GE, Williams, M, Pettibone, DJ, Yarbrough, GG, Jones, JH, and Clineschmidt, BV: Pharmacological profile of a novel potent direct-acting dopamine agonist, (+) - 4 - propyl - 9 - hydroxynaphthoxazine [(+)-PHNO]. J Pharmacol Exp Therap 230:569–576, 1984.

73. Mauborgne, A, Javoy-Agid, F, Legrand, JC, Agid, Y, and Cesselin, F: Decrease of substance P–like immunoreactivity in the substantia nigra and pallidum of parkinsonian brains. Brain Res 268:167–170, 1983.

74. Mayeux, R, Stern, Y, Cote, L, and Williams, JBW: Altered serotonin metabolism in depressed patients with Parkinson's disease. Neurology 34:642–646, 1984.

75. McGeer, PL, Itagaki, S, Boyes, B, and McGeer, EG: Reactive microglia are positive for HLA-DR in the substantia nigra of Parkinson's and Alzheimer's disease brains. Neurology 38: 1285–1291, 1988.

76. Melamed, E: Early-morning dystonia: A late side effect of long term levodopa therapy in Parkinson's disease. Arch Neurol 36:308–310, 1979.

77. Melamed, E, Bitton, V, and Zelig, O: Episodic unresponsiveness to single doses of L-dopa in parkinsonian fluctuators. Neurology 36:100–103, 1986.

78. Molloy, AG, O'Boyle, KM, Pugh, MT, and Waddington, JL: Locomotor behaviors in response to new selective D-1 and D-2 dopamine receptor agonists, and the influence of selectifve antagonists. Pharmacol Biochem Behav 25:249–253, 1986.

79. Molloy, AG and Waddington, JL: Assessment of grooming and other behavioural responses to the D-1 dopamine receptor agonist SK&F 38393 and its R- and S-enantiomers in the intact adult rat. Psychopharmacology (Berl) 92:164–168, 1987.

80. Mouradian, MM, Juncos, JL, Fabbrini, G, and Chase, TN: Motor fluctuations in Parkinson's disease: Pathogenetic and therapeutic strategies. Ann Neurol 22:475–479, 1987.

81. Muenter, MD, Ahlskog, JE, Bell, G, and McManis, P: PHNO [(+)-4-propyl-9-hydroxynaphthoxazine]: A new and effective anti–Parkinson's disease agent. Neurology 38:1541–1545, 1988.

81a. Muenter, MD, Sharpless, NS, Tyce, GM, and Darley, FL: Patterns of dystonia ('I-D-I' and 'D-I-D') in response to L-dopa therapy for Parkinson's disease. Mayo Clin Proc 52:163–174, 1977.

82. Murray, AM and Waddington, JL: The induction of grooming and vacuous chewing by a series of selective D-1 dopamine receptor agonists: Two directions of D-1:D-2 interaction. Eur J Pharmacol 160:377–384, 1989.

83. Narabayashi, H: Surgical approach to tremor. In Marsden, CD and Fahn, S (eds): Movement Disorders. Butterworth Scientific, London, 1982, pp 292–299.

84. Narabayashi, H, Kondo, T, Hayashi, A, Suzuki, T, and Nagatsu, T: L-threo-3,4-dihydroxyphenylserine treatment for akinesia and freezing of parkinsonism. Proc Japan Acad (Ser B) 57:351–354, 1981.

85. Nutt, JG: On-off phenomenon: Relation to levodopa pharmacokinetics and pharmacodynamics. Ann Neurol 22:535–540, 1987.

86. Nutt, JG, Rosin, AJ, Eisler, T, Calne, DB, and Chase, TN: Effect of an opiate antagonist on movement disorders. Arch Neurol 35:810–811, 1978.

87. Nutt, J, Williams, A, Plotkin, C, Eng, N, Ziegler, M, and Calne, DB: Treatment of Parkinson's disease with sodium valproate: Clinical, pharmacological, and biochemical observations. Can J Neurol Sci 6:337–343, 1979.

88. Nutt, JG, Woodward, WR, Hammerstad, JP, Carter, JH, and Anderson, JL: The "on-off" phenomenon in Parkinson's disease: Relation to levodopa absorption and transport. New Engl J Med 310:483–488, 1984.

89. Obeso, JA, Luquín, MR, and Martínez-Lage, JM. Intravenous lisuride corrects oscillations of motor performance in Parkinson's disease. Ann Neurol 19:31–35, 1986.

89a. Obeso, JA, Luquín, MR, and Martínez-Lage, JM: Lisuride infusion pump: A device for the treatment of motor fluctuations in Parkinson's disease. Lancet 1:467–470, 1986.

90. Parkes, JD, Schachter, M, Marsden, CD, Smith, B, and Wilson, A: Lisuride in parkinsonism. Ann Neurol 9:48–52, 1981.

90a. Parkinson Study Group: Effect of deprenyl on the progression of disability in early Parkinson's disease. New Engl J Med 321:1364–1371, 1989.

91. Penney, JB and Young, AB: Striatal inhomogeneities and basal ganglia function. Mov Disord 1:3–15, 1986.

92. Perry, EK, Curtis, M, Dick, DJ, Candy, JM, Atack, JR, Bloxham, CA, Blessed, G, Fairbairn, A, Tomlinson, BE, and Perry, RH: Cholinergic correlates of cognitive impairment in Parkinson's disease: Comparisons with Alzheimer's disease. J Neurol Neurosurg Psychiatry 48:413–421, 1985.

93. Perry, EK, Perry, RH, Candy, JM, Fairbairn, AF, Blessed, G, Dick, DJ, and Tomlinson, BE: Cortical serotonin S-2 receptor binding abnormalities in patients with Alzheimer's disease: Comparisons with Parkinson's disease. Neurosci Lett 51:353–357, 1984.

94. Pfeiffer, RF, Kang, J, Graber, B, and Wilson, J: Clozapine for psychosis in Parkinson's disease. Neurology (Suppl 1)39:231, 1989.

95. Pimoule, C, Schoemaker, H, Reynolds, GP, and Langer, SZ: [3H]SCH 23390 labelled D1 dopamine receptors are unchanged in schizophrenia and Parkinson's disease. Eur J Pharmacol 114:235–237, 1985.

96. Pincus, JH and Barry, K: Protein redistribution diet restores motor function in patients with dopa-resistant "off" periods. Neurology 38:481–483, 1988.

97. Poewe, WH, Lees, AJ, and Stern, GM: Treatment of motor fluctuations in Parkinson's disease with an oral sustained-release preparation of L-dopa. Clinical and pharmacokinetic observations. Clin Neuropharmacol 9:430–439, 1986.

98. Poewe, WH, Lees, AJ, and Stern, GM: Dystonia in Parkinson's disease: Clinical and pharmacological features. Ann Neurol 23:73–78, 1988.

99. Pugh, MT, O'Boyle, KM, Molloy, AG, and Waddington, JL: Effects of the putative D-1 antagonist SCH 23390 on stereotyped behaviour induced by the D-2 agonist RU24213. Psychopharmacology (Berl) 87:308–312, 1985.

100. Raisman, R, Cash, R, Ruberg, M, Javoy-Agid, F and Agid, Y: Binding of [3H]SCH 23390 to D-1 receptors in the putamen of control and parkinsonian subjects. Eur J Pharmacol 113:467–468, 1985.

101. Rajput, AH, Uitti, RJ, Stern, W, Laverty, W, O'Donnell, K, Yuen, WK, O'Donnell, D, and Dua, A: Geography, drinking water chemistry, pesticides and herbicides and the etiology of Parkinson's disease. Can J Neurol Sci 14:414–418, 1987.

102. Reisine, TD, Fields, JZ, Yamamura, HI, Bird, ED, Spokes, E, Schreiner, PS, and Enna, SJ: Neurotransmitter receptor alterations in Parkinson's disease. Life Sci 21:335–344, 1977.

103. Reisine, TD, Rossor, M, Spokes, E, Iversen, LL, and Yamamura, HI: Alterations in brain opiate receptors in Parkinson's disease. Brain Res 173:378–382, 1979.

104. Riederer, P and Wuketich, ST: Time course of nigrostriatal degeneration in Parkinson's disease. J Neural Transm Park Dis Dement Sect 38:277–301, 1976.

105. Riley, D and Lang, AE: Practical application of a low-protein diet for Parkinson's disease. Neurology 38:1026–1031, 1988.

106. Rinne, JO, Rinne, JK, Laakso, K, Lonnberg, P, and Rinne, UK: Dopamine D-1 receptors in the parkinsonian brain. Brain Res 359:306–310, 1985.

107. Rinne, UK: Combined bromocriptine-levodopa therapy early in Parkinson's disease. Neurology 35:1196–1198, 1985.

108. Rinne, UK, Lonnberg, P, and Koskinen, V: Dopamine receptors in the parkinsonian brain. J Neural Transm Park Dis Dement Sect 51:97–106, 1981.

109. Rosengarten, H, Schweftzer, JW, and Friedhoff, AJ: Selective dopamine D2 receptor reduction enhances a D1 mediated oral dyskinesia in rats. Life Sci 39:29–35, 1986.

110. Rupniak, NMJ, Tye, SJ, Jennings, CA, Loper, AE, Bondi, JV, Hichens, M, Hand, E, Iversen, SD, and Stahl, SM: Antiparkinsonian efficacy of a novel transdermal delivery system for (+)-PHNO in MPTP-treated squirrel monkeys. Neurology 39:329–335, 1989.

111. Sage, JI, McHale, DM, Sonsalla, P, Vitagliano, D, and Heikkila, RE: Continuous levodopa infusions to treat complex dystonia in Parkinson's disease. Neurology 39:888–891, 1989.

112. Scatton, B, Javoy-Agid, F, Rouquier, L, Dubois, B, and Agid, Y: Reduction of cortical dopamine, noradrenaline, serotonin and their metabolites in Parkinson's disease. Brain Res 275:321–328, 1983.

113. Schoenberg, BS, Anderson, DW, and Haerer, AF: Prevalence of Parkinson's disease in the biracial population of Copiah County, Mississippi. Neurology 35:841–845, 1985.

114. Shoulson, I, Glaubiger, GA, and Chase, TN: On-off response: Clinical and biochemical correlations during oral and intravenous levodopa administration in Parkinsonian patients. Neurology 25:1144–1148, 1975.

114a. Sokoluff, P, Giros, B, Martres, M-P, Bouthenet, M-L, and Schwartz, JC: Molecular cloning and characterization of a novel dopamine receptor (D3) as a target for neuroleptics. Nature 347:146–151, 1990.

115. Spencer, SE and Wooten, GF: Altered pharmacokinetics of L-dopa metabolism in rat striatum deprived of dopaminergic innervation. Neurology 34:1105–1108, 1984.

116. Stibe, CMH, Lees, AJ, Kempster, PA, and Stern, GM: Subcutaneous apomorphine in parkinsonian on-off oscillations. Lancet 1:403–406, 1988.

117. Stoessl, AJ: Peptide-dopamine interactions in the central nervous system: Implications for

neuropsychiatric disorders. J Psychopharmacol 3:99–120, 1989.

118. Stoessl, AJ and Calne, DB: The dopaminergic system in Parkinsonism: In-vivo studies. In Rose, FC (ed): Parkinson's Disease: Clinical and Experimental Advances. Libbey, London, 1987, pp 33–45.

119. Stoessl, AJ, Mak, E, and Calne, DB: (+)-4-propyl-9-hydroxynaphthoxazine (PHNO), a new dopaminomimetic, in treatment of parkinsonism. Lancet 2:1330–1331, 1985.

120. Stoof, JC and Kebabian, JW: Opposing roles for D-1 and D-2 dopamine receptors in efflux of cyclic AMP from rat neostriatum. Nature 294:366–368, 1981.

121. Studler, JM, Javoy-Agid, F, Cesselin, F, Legrand, JC, and Agid, Y: CCK-8-immunoreactivity distribution in human brain: Selective decrease in the substantia nigra from parkinsonian patients. Brain Res 243:176–179, 1982.

121a. Sunahara, RK, Guan, H-C, O'Dowd, BF, Seeman, P, Laurier, LG, NgG, G Sr, Torchia, J, van Tol, HHM, and Niznik, HB: Cloning of the gene for a human dopamine D5 receptor with higher affinity for dopamine than D1. Nature 350:614–619, 1991.

122. Tanner, CM: The role of environmental toxins in the etiology of Parkinson's disease. Trends Neurosci 12:49–54, 1989.

123. Tanner, CM, Chablani, R, Goetz, CG, and Klawans, HL: Pergolide mesylate: Lack of cardiac toxicity in patients with cardiac disease. Neurology 35:918–921, 1985.

124. Taquet, H, Javoy-Agid, F, Hamon, M, Legrand, JC, Agid, Y, and Cesselin, F: Parkinson's disease affects differently Met5- and Leu5-enkephalin in the human brain. Brain Res 280:379–382, 1983.

125. Temlett, JA, Quinn, NP, Jenner, PG, Marsden, CD, Pourcher, E, Bonnet, A-M, Agid, Y, Markstein, R, and Lataste, X: Antiparkinsonian activity of CY 208-243, a partial D-1 dopamine receptor agonist, in MPTP-treated marmosets and patients with Parkinson's disease. Mov Disord 4:261–265, 1989.

126. Teravainen, H, Huttunen, J, and Hietanen, M: Initial treatment of parkinsonism with 8-alpha-amino-ergoline. Neurology 35:83–87, 1985.

127. Tetrud, JW and Langston, JW: The effect of deprenyl (selegiline) on the natural history of Parkinson's disease. Science 245:519–522, 1989.

128. Tsui, JKC, Wolters, ECH, Peppard, RF, and Calne, DB: A double-blind, placebo-controlled, dose-ranging study to investigate the safety and efficacy of CY 208-243 in patients with Parkinson's disease. Neurology 39:856–858, 1989.

129. Uhl, GR, Hackney, GO, Torchia, M, Stranov, V, Tourtellotte, WW, Whitehouse, PJ, Tran, V, and Strittmatter, S: Parkinson's disease: Nigral receptor changes support peptidergic role in nigrostriatal modulation. Ann Neurol 20:194–203, 1986.

130. Uhl, GR, Whitehouse, PJ, Price, DL, Tourtellotte, WW, and Kuhar, MJ: Parkinson's disease: Depletion of substantia nigra neurotensin receptors. Brain Res 308:186–190, 1984.

131. van Manen, J and Speelman, JD: Caudate lesions as surgical treatment in Parkinson's disease. Lancet 1:175, 1988.

131a. Van Tol, HHM, Bunzow, JR, Guan, H-C, Sunahara, RK, Seeman, P, Niznik, HB, and Civelli, O: Cloning of the gene for a human dopamine D4 receptor with high affinity for the antipsychotic clozapine. Nature 350:610–614, 1991.

132. Walters, JR, Bergstrom, DA, Carlson, JH, Chase, TN, and Braun, AR: D1 dopamine receptor activation required for postsynaptic expression of D2 agonist effects. Science 236:719–722, 1987.

133. Ward, CD, Duvoisin, RC, Ince, SE, Nutt, JD, Eldridge, R, and Calne, DB: Parkinson's disease in 65 pairs of twins and in a set of quadruplets. Neurology 33:815–824, 1983.

134. White, FJ: D-1 dopamine receptor stimulation enables the inhibition of nucleus accumbens neurons by a D-2 receptor agonist. Eur J Pharmacol 135:101–105, 1987.

135. Whitehouse, PJ, Hedreen, JC, White, CL, and Price, DL: Basal forebrain neurons in the dementia of Parkinson's disease. Ann Neurol 13:243–248, 1983.

SECTION SIX

• • • • • • • • • • •

TUMORS

EDITOR'S COMMENTARY

Tumors anywhere intimidate. This is particularly true if they occur within the skull, wherein there is little space and much that can go wrong. McDermott and Wilson detail how far we have come since the days of Harvey Cushing. We understand much more about the biology of tumors and the complexities of immune reactions. We also have available increasingly more sophisticated means of imaging and studying brain tumors. Most exciting of all are the steady steps taken by radiosurgery and the new approaches with polyamine inhibitors, monoclonal antibodies, and adoptive immunotherapy.

While primary brain tumors have always carried a varying prognosis, the presence of cerebral metastasis has been viewed with gloom. And yet, DeAngelis makes a persuasive case for the aggressive management of single metastasis with growing evidence that this approach results in improved quality and length of life.

A case is even made by Dropcho for the treatment of patients with multiple brain metastases, although questions must always arise as to when a possible improvement in the patient's life quality or longevity is negated by side effects of the treatment and by psychologic, economic, and emotional costs. Progress does not deny choices; it only makes them more difficult.

VCH

CHAPTER 16

• •

MANAGEMENT OF PRIMARY BRAIN TUMORS

Michael W. McDermott, M.D., F.R.C.S(C) and Charles B. Wilson, M.D.

Brain tumors are becoming more common. As the genetics of primary gliomas of the brain are unravelled, we may discover that they are also more familial than we realized. This has both negative and positive aspects — negative in the sense that relatives may harbor a higher risk and positive in that with modern imaging techniques it may be possible to detect brain tumors earlier, particularly in a prone population.

McDermott and Wilson provide a comprehensive and data-buttressed overview of primary brain tumors, ranging from the biology of tumors to the latest (albeit unproven) therapy. It is of interest that some techniques, such as sterotaxic brain surgery, which had declined after the introduction of levodopa for the treatment of Parkinson's disease, have made a successful comeback in brain tumor management.

Brain tumor diagnosis has become easier, treatment broader, and prognosis less abysmal.

VCH

Tumors of the central nervous system (CNS) account for less than 1.5% of all malignant disease and 2.1% of all cancer-related deaths.[7,47] Of the 1654 malignant tumors initially diagnosed and/or treated at the University of California, San Francisco (UCSF), 201 (12.2%) arose in the brain and nervous system.[232] In several population-based studies, the incidence of primary intracranial neoplasms ranges from 4 to 16 per 100,000; it was estimated that, in 1987, there would be 14,700 new cases of brain and other CNS tumors diagnosed in the United States.[7,32,92,117,194,224,235,236]

Malignant gliomas, the most common primary brain tumor in adults, have a peak incidence in people who are between the sixth and eighth decades of life, the portion of the population that is increasing most rapidly (Fig. 16 – 1). Coupled with an increased detection rate of intracranial pathology as a result of the increasing sensitivity and availability of radiologic imaging methods, this pattern makes it likely that we will be confronted with an increasing number of patients with brain tumor in the years ahead. The field of neuro-oncology is thus presented with a challenge to improve on past results by developing new technologies or by combining existing ones in more efficacious ways.

The past 15 years have produced impressive developments in imaging modalities, assisting in diagnoses, and in intraoperative techniques with the operating microscope, microsurgical instrumentation, ultrasound

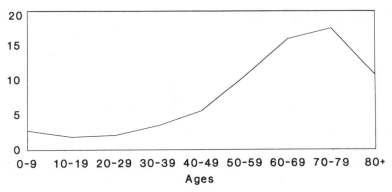

FIGURE 16–1. Age-related incidence of brain tumors per 100,000 population. (Adapted from Horm, et al,[92] p. 53.)

and stereotaxic biopsy, computer-surgeon interfacing systems, and neuroanesthesia, all of which have helped reduce the morbidity and mortality of surgery for brain tumors.[8] Whereas the aims of surgery are to establish a diagnosis, to reduce tumor burden so that other forms of therapy may be more effective, and to do so without creating new neurologic deficit, surgery is only one phase of the diagnosis and treatment sequence.

Some tumors begin to produce symptoms when they reach a size of 10 g, approximately 10^8 cells or 2.72 cm on computed tomography (CT) scan.[205] Most tumors of 100 g, 10^{11} cells or 5.85 cm on CT, cause significant increase in the intracranial pressure (ICP) and may be life-threatening. Even if 99% of the tumor mass is removed at this point, about 10^8 cells still remain, and the most malignant tumors, if nothing more is done, theoretically can regain their original size in 2 to 3 weeks.[205] Radiation therapy and adjuvant chemotherapy are directed at the residual tumor mass and at present complete the customary care for patients with malignant tumors. Newer forms of treatment include interstitial brachytherapy, intra-arterial chemotherapy, the use of biological response modifiers, and adoptive immunotherapy. However, these developments have yet to make a significant impact on the survival of patients with malignant brain tumors. The immunobiology and molecular genetics of brain tumors are two areas of active research that are rapidly increasing our knowledge base and may provide the means to improve on past therapeutic results.

In this chapter, we discuss neuro-oncogenesis and pathophysiology and the current neurosurgical management of selected primary brain tumors, emphasizing new therapies, results, and future directions. The medical management of patients with such tumors and the chemotherapy of malignant tumors are discussed elsewhere in this book.

PATHOGENESIS OF CENTRAL NERVOUS SYSTEM TUMORS

Almost certainly, the mechanism of neoplastic transformation in neuroepithelial cells is a multistep process. Cells may become neoplastic either through spontaneous mutation or after exposure to environmental agents such as chemicals, viruses, and radiation.[19,144,191,194,208] In experimental models of brain tumors, neoplastic change can be brought about by a number of agents.

The N-nitrosoureas methylnitrosourea (MNU) and ethylnitrosourea (ENU) display remarkable neurotropism and produce gliomas when given prenatally or postnatally to rats by way of several different routes.[194,225] The carcinogenicity of these agents relates to the brain's inability to repair alkylation of guanine bases at the 0^6 position.[194] Viruses of both the RNA and DNA type have been shown to produce neuroepithelial tumors in rats following intracerebral inoculation.[18] The avian sarcoma virus, an RNA virus, produces a spectrum of astrocytic neoplasms.[45] The human adenovirus type 12, a DNA virus, produces tumors resembling neuroblastoma.[156]

Observations from clinical series confirm an association between radiation therapy and neuro-oncogenesis. Sarcomas and meningiomas are the most common tumors seen following radiation therapy, but an increasing number of gliomas are similarly being reported.[260] In most instances radiation has been administered in childhood with a latency of 1 to 26 years between treatment and the appearance of tumor. Radiation doses have ranged between 400 and 6000 rad (4 and 60 Gy), and most of the tumors produced are malignant astrocytomas.

Recent experimental work on the initiation of neoplastic changes in the brain has focused on the role of oncogenes; the subject has recently been reviewed by Schmidek[208] and McDonald and Dohrmann.[144] Oncogenes are found in the DNA of all eukaryotic cells and are though to be involved normally in the control of cell division.[74] Activation of these oncogenes may occur at a chromosomal level by translocations or rearrangements and at the gene level by the loss of regulator sequences, point mutations, or gene amplification.[74,144,207] Irrespective of how activation of these oncogenes occurs, their de-repression is regarded as pivotal to the molecular basis of neoplastic change. Products of these oncogenes act as powerful mitogens, causing the affected cell to produce growth factors or increase the number of cell surface growth factor receptors.

The oncogene erb-B, the most common oncogene found in human brain tumors, codes for epidermal growth factor receptor (EGFR).[74,191,207] C-sis, an oncogene associated with the simian sarcoma virus, encodes for platelet-derived growth factor (PDGF).[191,207] Secretion of PDGF-like proteins and amplification of the sis oncogene have been observed in glioma cell cultures.[168] Both EGFR and PDGF can stimulate cell division of normal glial cells in culture.

The clinical correlate of oncogene expression and amplification has been demonstrated with the oncogene n-myc and neuroblastoma.[188,209,231] Higher levels of n-myc are associated with a more advanced stage of the disease at diagnosis and with a worse prognosis. Seeger and associates[210] found that n-myc amplification occurred in 38% of

89 patients with neuroblastoma. Gene amplification was present in 12.5%, 65%, and 47.5% of patients with tumors in clinical stages II, III, and IV, respectively. The 18-month progression-free period of survival was 70% for those with only one copy of n-myc and only 5% in those with more than 10 copies of the gene ($P < 0.0001$). Similarly, Tsuda and colleagues,[231] in analyzing 52 cases of neuroblastoma, found that 14% of patients with stage II and 67% with stage IV disease had n-myc amplification. The 24-month survival rate was 81% for patients without, and 12% for those with, n-myc amplification ($P < 0.001$).

Recently another oncogene, the gli oncogene, localized to chromosome 12, has been found amplified more than 50-fold and highly expressed in a human malignant glioma.[111] Although its exact role is still unknown, it was not found to be related to other known oncogenes, suggesting that a select group of genes may be altered and play a role in the development of human malignant gliomas. Although the molecular biology of malignant brain tumors is in its infancy, further work in this area should improve our understanding of biology and pathophysiology and may have implications for the treatment of brain tumors.

Following the initiation of neoplastic change, tumor growth depends on a number of factors and represents the net result between the processes of cell proliferation and cell loss.[94,191] In malignant gliomas the growth fraction, or proportion of cells in the proliferating pool, is 0.31 on the average, and the cell cycle time is 2 to 3 days.[94,96] The cell loss fraction may be as high as 0.85 in glioblastoma. Cell proliferation depends on an adequate blood supply, oxygenation, and continued mitogenic stimulation. Recently, the extracellular matrix (ECM) has been recognized as having an important role in tumor growth by its ability to bind growth factors and present them to the cell surface.[195] Components of the ECM may also be important in mediating cell-cell contact inhibition and have direct antiproliferative effects on tumor cells. Rutka and co-workers[196] have observed inhibition and differentiation of a glioma cell line exposed to the ECM proteins of leptomeningeal cells. Further work in this area will improve our understanding of the mechanisms of tumor cell infiltration, growth, and distant spread.

PATHOPHYSIOLOGY OF TUMOR GROWTH

Primary brain tumors in an intra-axial location produce symptoms based on their location, growth rate, and growth pattern. Their effects may be either local — related to tumor infiltration and invasion of the surrounding brain, mechanical pressure effects, or vascular compression — or distant, primarily due to increased ICP. The clinical syndromes related to tumor location are well known. Slow-growing, infiltrating neoplasms may produce few symptoms early on, as tumor cells interdigitate with functioning normal glial and neuronal cells. In contrast, rapidly growing tumors may produce symptoms early, displacing normal tissue to the periphery as centrally placed clonogenic tumor cells grow exponentially. These different growth rates and patterns have implications for surgical treatment: removal of slow-growing, infiltrating neoplasms may include functioning neural tissue, whereas the bulk of malignant, rapidly growing tumors consists of solid tumor tissue and necrosis, the normal brain having been largely displaced to the periphery.

Locally, tumors compress surrounding brain, interfering with interstitial bulk flow of extracellular fluid and with venous and arterial blood flow. As a result, metabolic and toxic tumor metabolites and products are not cleared as readily as normal. A relative ischemia of the surrounding brain, resulting from vascular compression, may be increased by arteriovenous shunting through abnormal tumor vessels.[81,119] Local cell destruction by invading tumor or deefferentation of overlying neurons may produce focal neurologic signs, while deafferentation may cause irritative disturbances and seizures.[249]

The distant effects of tumors relate largely to their effects on ICP. Taking into consideration the volume-pressure relationship between the rigid cranial vault and its contents, an elevation in ICP may be caused by a tumor, surrounding edema, hemorrhage into tumor, obstruction of cerebrospinal fluid (CSF) pathways, or venous occlusion. In all such cases, surgical removal of tumor can have a dramatic and immediate effect in improving the patient's condition.

DIAGNOSTIC MODALITIES

Imaging

For patients with brain tumors, CT has been the standard of radiologic imaging for diagnosing and assessing the response to treatment. A CT scan may not define the margins of, or even identify, low-grade tumors that do not show contrast enhancement, and there is a 3% to 5% rate of false-negative findings.[114] Magnetic resonance imaging (MRI) resolves some of these problems, and now, with the availability of paramagnetic contrast agents that increase the sensitivity of the technique, MRI has become the standard of imaging (Fig. 16–2).[83,226] The absence of bone artifact and the ability to image in the coronal as well as sagittal planes makes MRI the procedure of choice for evaluating brainstem, posterior fossa, midline hemispheric, and nonenhancing lesions. However, the correlation between the information obtained from imaging and the actual pathology is not exact, and neither CT nor MRI can differentiate radiation necrosis from active tumor. Tumor biopsy is the definitive diagnostic test.

MRI phosphorus 31 (^{31}P) spectroscopy is a technique being developed for use with available MRI machines that permits an in vivo assessment of high-energy phosphorus-containing compounds in tumors and normal brain. With this technique, up to seven different ^{31}P peaks can be resolved, reflecting information about the make-up and metabolic state of a region of interest.[98,228] Experimental and clinical studies using this technique have demonstrated changes in ^{31}P spectroscopy before and after treatment and before any change is observed with standard proton-based MRI.[84,211,228] MR spectroscopy using a head coil can define small volumes of interest from a proton-based MR image, and the same volume of interest can be studied using ^{31}P spectroscopy (Fig. 16–3).[98,210] This method eliminates the back-

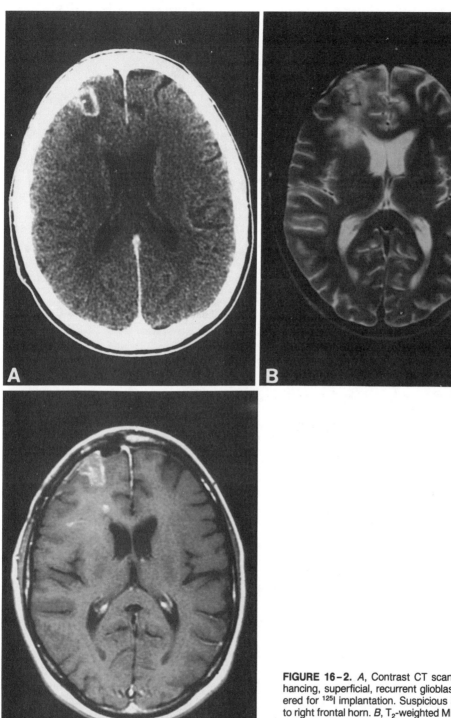

FIGURE 16–2. *A*, Contrast CT scan showing enhancing, superficial, recurrent glioblastoma considered for ^{125}I implantation. Suspicious area adjacent to right frontal horn. *B*, T_2-weighted MR image demonstrating increased signal intensity in the area of concern. *C*, Gadolinium-DTPA-enhanced scan confirms deeper recurrence, making the patient ineligible for implant.

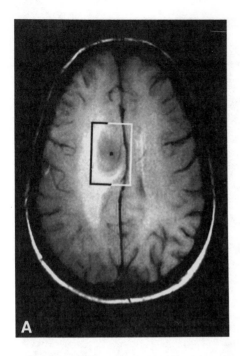

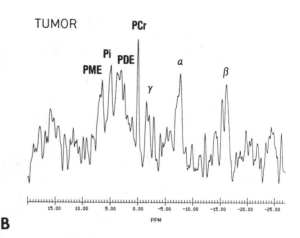

FIGURE 16-3. *A*, T$_1$-weighted MR image of right parasagittal astrocytoma. Volume of interest (VOI) for spectroscopy outlined with cursor. *B*, ^{31}P spectrum demonstrating reduced metabolite concentrations as compared to surrounding normal brain. (From Hubesch, et al,[98] pp. 406–407, with permission.)

ground information and surface tissue information obtained with surface coils. Using this technique, Hubesch and colleagues[98] have observed reductions in phosphate metabolites of between 20% and 70% in brain tumors as compared with normal brain. Phosphocreatine, phosphate monoesters, and phosphate diesters showed the largest decrease, whereas inorganic phosphate showed the least. In the future this technique may be useful in assessing response to various forms of treatment and for potentially differentiating areas of active tumor from those of radiation necrosis.

Positron emission tomography (PET) is an imaging technique that, although not widely available, allows for an assessment of local brain metabolism using fluorine 18-fluorodeoxyglucose (^{18}F-FDG). Malignant gliomas demonstrate hypermetabolism as compared to surrounding brain, and in one study PET was used as a predictor of degeneration in low-grade gliomas.[66] PET also differentiates radiation necrosis from tumor with a high degree of accuracy. This distinction is clinically important, considering the 30% to 50% incidence of radiation necrosis following interstitial brachytherapy (Fig. 16–4). Valk and associates[234] studied 34 patients who had undergone brachytherapy who presented with clinical or radiologic evidence suggesting a recurrence of tumor. Areas of high activity on both the rubidium 82 (^{82}Rb) and ^{18}F-FDG studies indicated tumor recurrence, whereas high activity with ^{82}Rb and low activity following ^{18}F-FDG predicted radiation necrosis. The findings with PET correlated with the follow-up diagnosis in 15 of the 17 cases of recurrent tumor and in 17 of the 21 cases of radiation necrosis, for an overall accuracy of 84%. Other authors[51] have confirmed the utility of PET for differentiating recurrent tumor from radiation necrosis.

Tumor Biopsy

Despite the improvements in radiologic imaging techniques, there is still no exact correlation between tumor characteristics observed on either CT or MR images at presentation and the actual pathology. To direct therapy accurately and appropriately, an exact knowledge of the tumor type is necessary. In obtaining biopsy specimens a sampling error, whether large or small, is always possible, but this should not be a reason to

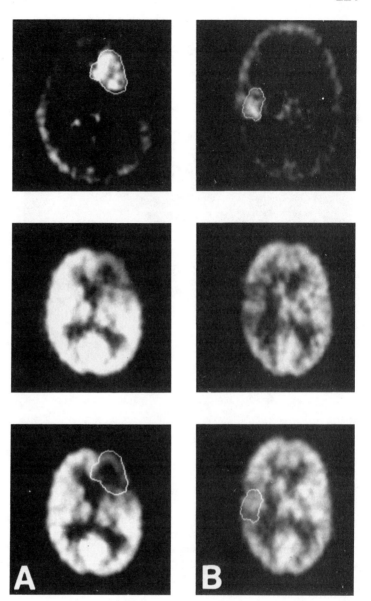

FIGURE 16-4. *A*, Top: ^{82}Rb PET scan demonstrating area of blood-brain barrier (BBB) breakdown after interstitial implant therapy. Area outlined by cursor. Middle: ^{18}F-FDG study showing lower metabolic rate of left frontal lobe. Bottom: Images superimposed confirming lesion as radiation necrosis. *B*, Top: ^{82}Rb image revealing BBB breakdown in right fronto-parietal region. Middle: ^{18}F-FDG study showing central area of increased metabolism. Bottom: Superimposition of images reveals increased metabolism in same area as BBB breakdown, highly suspicious for recurrence. (From Valk et al,[234] pp. 833-834, with permission.)

defer the chance of a definitive diagnosis. No longer is it acceptable simply to follow a patient who has a low-density lesion observed on CT scanning, because the biologic behavior and pathology of these lesions are not predictable.

Tumor tissue can be obtained through either open or closed surgical techniques. Open techniques for biopsy are applicable to those tumors extending to the surface of the brain or located just subcortically.

Closed techniques include stereotaxic CT-directed or MRI-directed biopsy, CT-directed nonstereotaxic biopsy, and ultrasound-directed biopsy. Present-day stereotaxic systems permit a microscopic diagnosis to be obtained in 81% to 95.6% of cases.[9,25,44,105,165] The procedure can be done using local anesthesia in adults and is most suitable for those tumors that are ill-defined or in a deep location. The mortality and morbidity associated with sterotaxic

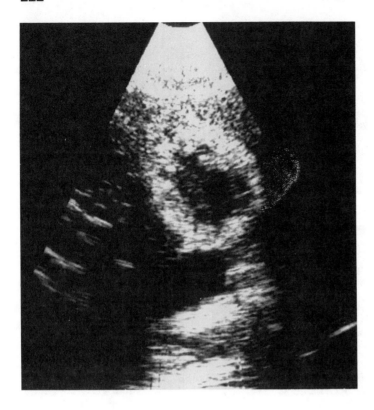

FIGURE 16–5. Intraoperative ultrasound of subcortical tumor. (Courtesy of Dr. M. L. Rosenblum.)

biopsies range from 0% to 4.3% and 0.2% to 8%, respectively.

Ultrasound-directed biopsy can be done either through a burr hole or at open craniotomy. Different ultrasound heads allow for satisfactory resolution of superficial as well as deep lesions (Fig. 16–5). During open craniotomy for subcortical, low-grade, and/or cystic lesions, ultrasound has become an indispensable tool in correctly and safely placing the cortical incision. Low-density tumors that do not show contrast enhancement on CT are hyperechogenic and well defined by ultrasound.[112,145] Repeat ultrasound imaging during the course of surgery permits an intraoperative assessment of the completeness of resection. Ultrasound can also differentiate cystic from necrotic tumor centers, and with real-time imaging, it allows for the quick and safe drainage of tumor cysts.[34]

GLIOMAS

Astrocytomas

Pathology

The pathologic classification of gliomas in current use is based on the system of Bailey and Cushing.[11] Since that system was devised, new systems of classification have emerged, creating confusion in published clinical series.[30,46,109,162,186,194,261]

The system of Kernohan[109] divides astrocytic neoplasms by their degree of histologic malignancy into one of four grades. In this system, glioblastoma multiforme is equivalent to astrocytomas grades III and IV. Subsequent studies have shown no difference in rates of patients' survival between these grades of malignancy.[46,162,207]

Burger and co-workers[31] reviewed 1440 astrocytic gliomas from three phase III trials of the Brain Tumor Study Group to assess the usefulness of a three-tiered histologic grading scheme (astrocytoma, anaplastic astrocytoma, glioblastoma multiforme). In each study there was a significant difference in the 1-year survival rate for those patients with anaplastic astrocytoma (60% to 73%) as compared to those with glioblastoma multiforme (35% to 44%). Earlier, Ringertz[186] had published similar results of his three-tiered system of classifying astrocytic neoplasms as astrocytoma, an intermediate type of astrocytoma, and glioblastoma multiforme.

At UCSF, astrocytic neoplasms are divided into a four-tiered system based on cytoplasmic and nuclear pleomorphism, degree of cellularity, vascular proliferation, and number of mitoses. Histologic features define four levels of astrocytic neoplasms as mildly anaplastic, moderately anaplastic, highly anaplastic, and glioblastoma multiforme; however, more than 99% of the tumors that are examined belong to one of the latter three categories.[48] The median survival for patients with moderately anaplastic astrocytoma is 220 weeks, for those with highly anaplastic astrocytoma, 116 weeks, and for those with glioblastoma, 66 weeks.[134]

A recent report by Daumas-Duport and colleagues[46] documents a new method of grading astrocytic neoplasms based on the presence or absence of four criteria: (1) nuclear atypia, (2) mitoses, (3) endothelial proliferation, and (4) necrosis. Grade I neoplasms have none of the criteria, grade II have one, grade III have two, and grade IV have three or four criteria present. Using this system, the authors reviewed 338 cases previously classified under the Kernohan system and treated at the Mayo Clinic between 1960 and 1969. A 15-year period of followup review was available for all surviving patients. Among the 287 patients with "ordinary" astrocytomas, 0.7% were grade I, 17% were grade II, 18% were grade III, and 63% were grade IV. The median survival rates for grades II through IV were significantly different at 4 years, 1.6 years, and 0.7 years, respectively ($P < 0.0001$). The presence of only two patients who had a grade I astrocytoma raises questions again about the value of a four-tiered system. Analysis of the same group of patients using the Kernohan system failed to identify any significant difference in survival between Kernohan grades I and II or between Kernohan grades III and IV.

Whereas most major studies at present use a three-tiered system, any interpretation of results published in clinical series must take into account the pathologic classification or grading system used. Unfortunately, the confusion between series will persist until a single pathologic grading system is adopted universally for reporting major phase II and phase III clinical trials.

Tumor Labeling Index

As with the measurement of n-myc amplification in neuroblastoma, other measures of the proliferative potential of tumors may provide further information with regard to prognosis. Hoshino[93] has shown that the percentage of cells labeled with bromodeoxyuridine (BUdR), a thymidine analogue, reflects the proliferative potential of the tumor, which in turn determines the patient's prognosis. The labeling index (LI), defined as the proportion of cells labeled with BUdR on the histologic preparation of tumor obtained at the time of surgery, is indicative of the percentage of cells in DNA synthesis and correlates well with the histology of astrocytic neoplasms. The mean LI was 9.3% for glioblastoma multiforme, 4% for anaplastic astrocytoma, and 1% or less for astrocytomas. Irrespective of the pathologic diagnosis, those patients with LIs greater than 5% had a significantly poorer survival rate than those with indices less than 5%. Even within the group of low-grade astrocytomas, the LI is predictive of clinical behavior. In a recent report by Hoshino and associates,[95] 29 of 47 (60%) of patients with low-grade astrocytomas had an LI less than 1%, and in 18 (40%) the LI was greater than 1%. The 3-year survival rate was 85% for LI less than 1% and 10% for LI greater than 1% ($P < 0.01$). Other techniques using the monoclonal antibody Ki-67 directed against a nuclear antigen present only in proliferating cells, as well as flow cytometry to demonstrate DNA content and aneuploidy, may assist in a more objective assessment of the proliferative potential of tumors.[38,167,258,259]

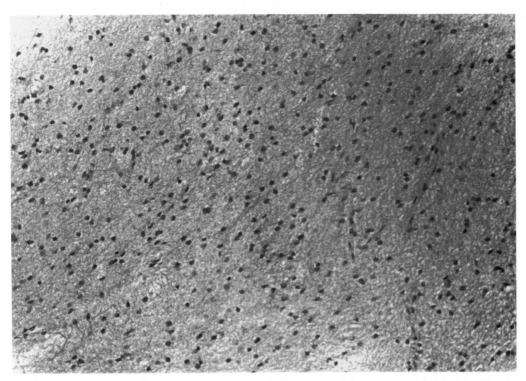

FIGURE 16-6. Low-grade astrocytoma demonstrating mild increase in cellularity, little cytoplasmic or nuclear pleomorphism, and no mitotic activity (H & E ×40). (Courtesy of Dr. R. L. Davis.)

This information may assist in more clearly defining the prognosis and predicting a response to treatment.

Low-Grade Astrocytomas

Low-grade astrocytomas account for between 5% and 8% of all primary brain tumors and for 18% of all astrocytomas.[81,120,121,194] In surgical series, these tumors represent 15% to 32% of the case material.[121,178,246] They occur most commonly in the temporal (42%) and frontal (41%) lobes, followed by the parietal (15%) and occipital (2%) lobes of adults, and they most often become symptomatic during the third to fifth decades of life.[121] In children, CNS tumors are the most common type of solid tumor, and astrocytomas represent 26% to 28% of all gliomas.[85,194] Dohrmann and colleagues,[57] in reporting on 174 astrocytomas in children, found that 55% of these tumors occurred in the cerebellum, 18% in the cerebral hemispheres, 17% in the brainstem, and 2% in the optic chiasm.

The microscopic pathology of low-grade astrocytomas reveals a regular, uniform population of cells with a mild-to-moderate increase in cellularity and little in the way of cytoplasmic pleomorphism (Fig. 16-6).[30,194] Despite this benign appearance, however, tumors may have variable clinical behavior as predicted by BUdR LIs. Their infiltrative growth pattern and lack of a clear border with the surrounding brain give them "malignant" characteristics that prove fatal without treatment.[95]

The clinical manifestations of slow-growing tumors are well known to all clinicians: 66% to 90% of patients present with a history of seizures, approximately half of them with a history of headaches, and a third present with a history of increased ICP or focal motor deficits.[81,178,219] With these tumors the interval between onset of symptoms and diagnosis has been as long as 10 years, in part owing to the inability of previous imaging studies to identify small, low-grade tumors.[121] Characteristically, on CT scans these tumors have a lower density than

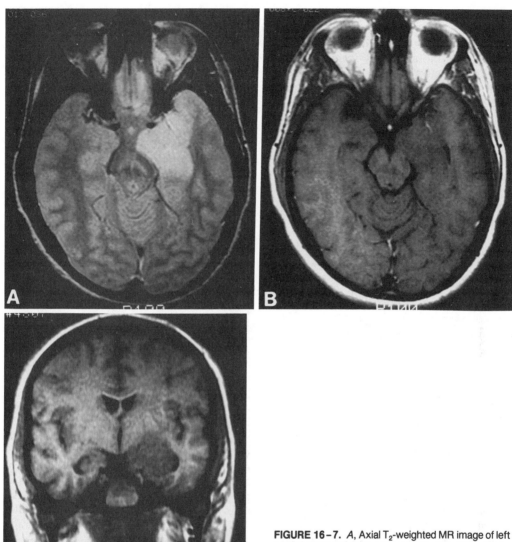

FIGURE 16–7. *A*, Axial T_2-weighted MR image of left medial temporal lobe astrocytoma showing well-defined area of increased signal intensity. *B*, Gadolinium-DTPA-enhanced T_1-weighted study in the same plane and coronal plane. *C*, Revealing no enhancement.

surrounding normal brain and are not contrast-enhancing. Piepmeier,[178] in reporting on 60 low-grade tumors of the cerebral hemispheres, found that the presence of contrast enhancement adversely affected survival. The mean survival for 13 patients *with evidence of enhancement* was 4.79 years, as compared with 7.92 years in the 45 patients *without enhancement* ($P =$ 0.012). Cysts are most common with a cerebellar location and occur in 20% to 30% of hemispheric tumors. With MRI, these low-

grade tumors appear as areas of increased signal intensity on T_2-weighted images and are nonenhancing with the paramagnetic contrast-enhancing agent gadolinium-DTPA (Fig. 16–7). Kelly and colleagues[108] have demonstrated by sterotaxic biopsy specimens that the area of increased signal intensity of T_2 images, as well as the area of low density on CT scans, consists of infiltrating tumor cells with intact parenchyma.

All patients with low-grade astrocytomas should be treated in standard medical fashion with anticonvulsants to control seizures. Corticosteroid medication should be reserved for those patients who show clinical or radiologic indications of increased ICP. Patients suspected of harboring a low-grade tumor who have a negative CT scan should be studied with MRI. If an abnormality is identified, the diagnosis should be confirmed by either stereotaxic biopsy, open biopsy, or surgical debulking, depending on the tumor's location. For superficial lesions and for those involving subcortical or polar areas of noneloquent cortex, consideration should be given to an open procedure for an attempt at gross total resection. In areas of eloquent cortex, intraoperative functional localization with somatosensory evoked potentials, direct cortical stimulation, and cortical mapping can assist in determining the extent of surgical resection that is possible without producing neurologic deficits.[16,20,252]

The extent of surgery necessary in the management of low-grade astrocytomas is a controversial issue.* As early as 1960 there was evidence that the extent of surgical resection of low-grade astrocytomas correlated with survival. Gol,[73] in reporting on the management of 194 cases, found that those patients diagnosed through biopsy and treated with or without radiation therapy had a median survival of 8 months, whereas those who underwent resection, with or without radiation therapy, survived a median of 34 months. The mortality rate was 16% for surgical resection and 37% for biopsy only. Later reports also supported increasing survival rates for increasing degrees of resection.[65,126,220,246] Laws and co-workers[120,121] noted a progressive increase in the 5-year survival for patients with low-grade supratentorial astrocytomas undergoing biopsy/subtotal removal, radical subtotal removal, and total removal. In this study, and contrary to a widely held opinion, lobectomy did not produce a significant increase in survival over that achieved with gross total resection.

In their review of low-grade astrocytomas, Scanlon and Taylor[207] found that patients undergoing simple biopsy combined with

radiation therapy did as well as those who had surgical resection. However, during the interval of study the surgical mortality for patients with low-grade astrocytomas was nearly 20%. Two more recent series[178,214] have failed to show any benefit of an increased extent of surgical resection for those patients undergoing irradiation postoperatively.

The results of radiation therapy for low-grade astrocytomas have not been studied in a prospective randomized trial, although such studies are underway. Weir and Grace[246] reported an improved survival rate for all surgical groups who received radiation therapy up to a period of 3 years after diagnosis and treatment. Leibel and associates,[126] in reviewing 122 patients with low-grade astrocytomas, reported 5-year and 10-year survival rates of 46% and 35% in patients with incomplete resection and postoperative radiation therapy and of 19% and 11% in a group of patients with incompletely resected tumors who did not undergo irradiation. Fazekas[65] found that the 5-year survival rate for patients with low-grade astrocytomas was improved from 32% to 54% with postoperative radiation therapy, but irradiation added nothing to the 5-year survival in patients whose tumor was completely resected, and it had little effect on 10-year survival. From his experience Fazekas concluded that radiation therapy played a palliative rather than a curative role. Laws and colleagues[121] in reviewing 461 patients, found that radiation therapy was of benefit to those patients more than 40 years of age with subtotal resection and that a dose of greater than 4000 cGy was necessary to improve survival. A recent report by Shaw and associates,[214] where the authors distinguished between pilocytic and "ordinary" astrocytomas and mixed oligoastrocytomas, found that patients who received more than 53 cGy had significantly better survival times than those who received less than the amount or surgery alone. The 5-year survival rate for patients receiving higher-dose radiation therapy was 68%, 47% for low-dose irradiation, and 32% for surgery only. At present, the overall survival rate for adults with low-grade astrocytomas treated with surgery and irradiation is approximately 50%, while chil-

---

*References 121, 125,148, 178, 207, 214, 246, 251.

TABLE 16-1. **SURVIVAL OF
LOW-GRADE ASTROCYTOMAS
AFTER SURGERY AND
RADIATION THERAPY**

Series	n	5-Year Survival
Rutten, et al[197] (1981)	27	44%
Silverman and Marks[219] (1981)	22	58%–65%*
Laws, et al[121] (1984)	74	49%
Medberry, et al[148] (1988)	50	45%
Soffietti, et al[220] (1989)	11 (>40 Gy)	9.1%
	21 (<40 Gy)	25.2%
Shaw, et al[214,†] (1989)	35 (>53 Gy)	68%
	67 (<53 Gy)	47%

* 4-year survival.
†Includes mixed oligoastrocytoma.

dren have a more favorable course (Table 16-1).[121,153,197,214,219,220]

In the management of patients who have low-grade astrocytomas (Fig. 16-8), the diagnosis is first confirmed by obtaining tissue for histopathologic examination. For superficial lesions of the cerebral hemispheres, an open operation is undertaken, and gross total resection is attempted in noneloquent areas of cortex. For those patients who by radiologic criteria have achieved gross total resection, an initial period of observation with follow-up radiologic studies at 3-month intervals for the first year, 4-month intervals for the second year, and 6-month intervals thereafter is warranted. With evidence of clinical or radiologic recurrence, a decision regarding reoperation or irradiation can be made. A high percentage of recurrent tumors show evidence of malignant change (49% to 76%).[121,158] Patients with recurrence are then treated with focal external-beam irradiation to a dose of at least 5400 cGy and subsequently observed as just described. If there is recurrence, consideration is again given to reoperation, and treatment with nitrosourea-based multiagent chemotherapy is begun. Patients with further recurrence are entered on experimental protocols.

Those patients who by radiologic criteria initially have subtotal tumor resection are treated with focal external-beam radiation therapy and are then observed and treated for recurrence, as just described.

Following gross total or subtotal resection, patients with juvenile pilocytic astrocytomas initially are followed with interval imaging studies; reoperation and radiation therapy are reserved for patients with recurrence. Wallner and co-workers,[242] and Shaw and co-workers[216] have both reported 93% and 79% 10-year survival rates for this group of patients. Microcystic cerebellar astrocytomas can be cured by gross total resection. Radiation therapy should be reserved for recurrence or for when reoperation is not possible. Children with hemispheric astrocytomas have a better prognosis than do adults; moreover, children are susceptible to the long-term adverse effects of radiation therapy on a developing brain.[85,251] The recent report by Hirsch and associates[85] documents the favorable response of these childhood tumors to operation alone. Of 42 patients (22 astrocytoma, 12 oligoastrocytoma, 8 oligodendroglioma) observed for 6 months to 17 years, there were no recurrences in 82% of patients after surgery. Therefore, after gross or subtotal resection, children with astrocytomas are observed initially, reserving radiation therapy for tumor recurrence.

Malignant Astrocytomas

Malignant astrocytomas are the most common form of primary brain tumor, with glioblastomas accounting for approximately 50% and anaplastic astrocytomas for 30% of all neuroepithelial tumors.[81] At diagnosis, 3% to 7% of tumors are found to be multicentric. The anaplastic astrocytoma is characterized by a marked increase in cellularity, moderate nuclear and cytoplasmic pleomorphism, mitotic figures, and vascular endothelial proliferation (Fig. 16-9A). Necrosis has been identified as an important feature differentiating anaplastic astrocytoma from glioblastoma multiforme.[31,162] Other histologic features of glioblastoma include pseudopalisading around areas of necrosis, vascular endothelial proliferation, and moderate-to-marked hypercellularity

MANAGEMENT OF LOW GRADE ASTROCYTOMAS

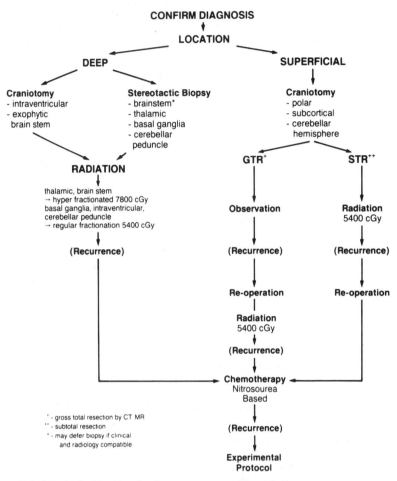

FIGURE 16–8. Algorithm for the management of low-grade astrocytomas.

and pleomorphism (Fig. 16–9B).[30,194] A variant of glioblastoma, the giant-cell type, is reported to have a slightly better prognosis.[143,175] Three of seven patients with this diagnosis reported by Margetts and colleagues[143] had a survival of more than 36 months, although our experience does not support this distinction.

The most common symptoms in patients with malignant gliomas are headache, focal motor deficit, mental change, and seizures.[40,81,201] Seizures that occur for the first time in adulthood should suggest the diagnosis of brain tumor until proven otherwise.

The appearance of these tumors on CT scan is variable. Anaplastic astrocytomas may be nonenhancing or homogeneously enhancing, whereas, with few exceptions, glioblastoma multiforme is a heterogeneously enhancing or ring-enhancing lesion. MRI typically demonstrates a much larger area of abnormality on T_2-weighted images as compared to the region of low density seen on CT. On MR images with gadolinium-DTPA, enhancement is similar to that seen on CT, although MRI is more sensitive for multifocal enhancing lesions. Kelly and associates[108] have shown that the area of contrast

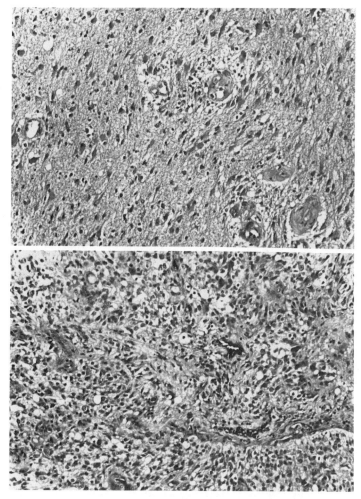

FIGURE 16-9. *A,* Anaplastic astrocytoma with marked cellular and nuclear pleomorphism, endothelial proliferation infiltrating white matter (H & E ×40). *B,* Glioblastoma multiforme showing hypercellularity, pleomorphism, and endothelial proliferation. No necrosis is in this section (H & E ×40). (Courtesy of Dr. R. L. Davis.)

enhancement on the CT scan represents solid tumor tissue, whereas the outer limit of increased signal intensity on T_2 indicates the limit for outside perimeter of isolated tumor cells that can be seen on histologic preparations after stereotaxic biopsy in these areas. In a postmortem study correlating the CT scan appearance of glioblastomas with histologic analysis, Burger[29] confirmed that the central area of low density on CT scan is necrosis, the enhancing rim is a hypercellular tumor, and the perimeter of low density includes infiltrating tumor cells. The maximum thickness of that area of infil-

trating cells constituted only 25% of the total tumor volume in most cases, and at the maximum thickness the infiltrating cell area varied between 4 and 33 mm. Both of these sets of data have implications for sterotaxic biopsy and radiation therapy.

The surgical approach to presumed malignant gliomas begins with a decision regarding the surgical suitability of the tumor, based on the patient's general and neurologic condition and the tumor's location.[202] Numerous studies have shown that age, Karnofsky performance status, and tumor type are the important prognostic variables.[6,35,50,81,203,213,238] These are also the factors to consider in evaluating the results of different treatment modalities.

The benefits of tumor resection include immediate mechanical cytoreduction, removal of resistant cells, and the possibility of bringing noncycling cells into the proliferating pool — in theory, rendering them more susceptible to radiation and chemotherapy. The likelihood of cells being resistant to treatment is directly proportional to cell number, and the literature indicates the benefits of tumor removal by showing that an increasing extent of tumor removal is associated with an improved rate of survival.[6,81,142,201,244] The immediate reduction in tumor mass achieved by surgery also provides relief from symptoms of increased ICP and allows for an improvement in neurologic function. Moreover, Ammirati and associates[6] have shown that the postoperative functional status of patients is significantly improved by gross total resection as opposed to subtotal resection. Up to 86% of extraganglionic hemispheric malignant gliomas can be grossly totally resected with minimal operative morbidity and a morbidity rate of nearly zero.[40] Figures for operative mortality range from 0% to 3%, and those for morbidity, from 8% to 14%.[6,81,201] Whereas Yasargil[253] has reported impressive results with the excision of thalamic and basal ganglionic tumors using open techniques, and while the Mayo Clinic[106] has reported removal of ganglionic tumors with computer-assisted techniques, in most centers tumors in these lesions are diagnosed through stereotaxic biopsy and treated with irradiation and chemotherapy. Coffey and associates[42] have confirmed the poorer prognosis in patients with malignant gliomas situated in a nonlobar location.

Radiation therapy is the single most effective form of treatment for malignant gliomas.[243,244] Walker and co-workers[238] in reporting a controlled, prospective, randomized study evaluating the use of 1,3-bis-(2-chloroethyl)-1-nitrosourea (BCNU) and/or radiation therapy in patients with anaplastic gliomas, reported a median survival of 14 weeks for patients having the best conventional care, 18.5 weeks for those receiving BCNU alone, 35 weeks for those undergoing irradiation, and 34.5 weeks for those

receiving BCNU plus radiation therapy. The Brain Tumor Study Group[239] analyzed 621 patients entered into randomized trials and divided these patients into groups receiving median doses of 50, 55, and 60 Gy. A significant dose-response effect was observed, with a median survival time of 28 weeks for the group receiving 50 Gy and 42 weeks for the group receiving 60 Gy ($P = 0.004$). No increase in toxicity occurred at the higher dose.

The issues related to radiation treatment volume, fractionation, and the use of radiation sensitizers deserve comment. In a study comparing CT scans made up to 2 months before death to the pathology observed at autopsy, Hochberg and Pruitt[87] found that, in 80% of patients, the perimeter of tumor observed on the CT scan plus a 2-cm margin defined the perimeter of microscopic tumor extension. In those patients treated and observed to recurrence, 90% of tumors recurred within a 2-cm margin of the primary tumor site. Wallner and co-workers[240] have reported similar results, 78% of tumors recurring within 2 cm and 56% within 1 cm of the initial tumor margin observed on CT scan. A recent report by the Brain Tumor Cooperative Group[213] concluded that giving part of the radiation as a focal boost was as effective as whole brain irradiation. This information, confirmed by the reports of Burger[29] and Kelly and associates[108] provides no justification for the use of whole brain radiation therapy, with its predictable radiation toxicity.

There are theoretical reasons to explain why hyperfractionated radiation therapy might be more effective than conventional radiation schedules. Increasing the number of fractions increases the proportion of cells treated during the most sensitive phase of the cell cycle. Reducing the fraction size has two effects that exploit the differences between normal and malignant cells: First, it reduces the degree of sublethal damage that normal cells are better able to repair; second, it reduces the dependence of radiation effect on the presence of oxygen, so that hypoxic cells are the more susceptible to multiple rather than single daily fractions.[161] Despite these theoretical advantages, however, several recent trials have failed to show any advantage of hyperfractionation.[50,137,161,213] In the Edmonton hyperfractionation trial,[233] higher total doses (to 80 Gy) produced some improvement in survival times. The median survival for patients receiving 80 Gy in three daily fractions was 60.5 weeks, as compared with 45.8 and 37.2 weeks for those receiving 61.41 and 71.20 Gy, respectively ($P = 0.003$).

Radiosensitizing agents are designed to enhance tumoricidal radiation effects without increasing radiotoxicity to normal tissues. Hypoxic cells, which are common in the center of a rapidly growing tumor, are relatively insensitive to the effects of radiation therapy. One class of radiosensitizers enhance tumor cell killing by delivering oxygen to the hypoxic region. Levin and associates[132] studied the radiation-sensitizing effects of hydroxyurea in the treatment of primary malignant tumors and found that the median time to tumor progression was significantly longer in the glioblastoma patients who received hydroxyurea (41 weeks) as compared with those who did not (31 weeks; $P = 0.03$). Since that study, we have incorporated hydroxyurea into the radiation therapy of all patients with malignant gliomas. The nitroimidazoles misonidazole and metronidazole can increase the sensitivity of an hypoxic cell mass to the effects of radiation therapy, but when the drugs have been studied in the CNS, clinical trials[50,125,160] have not shown a significant improvement in survival. Recent laboratory investigations with a combination of newer radiosensitizers indicate tumor concentrations that could have a significant advantage over former agents.[164] BUdR, a halogenated pyrimidine analogue that competes with thymidine, has also been studied as a radiation sensitizer administered through intra-arterial and intravenous routes of administration.[75] A summary of the radiation sensitizers used since 1981 has been provided by Kornblith and Walker.[113]

The chemotherapy of malignant gliomas has been subjected to intensive research and clinical investigation over the past 10 years, and these efforts are reviewed by McDonald elsewhere in this book.[60,113] Since 1978, BCNU has remained the standard of adjuvant therapy against which all other treatments are compared. The Brain Tumor Study Group,[237] reporting on the results of a controlled, prospective, randomized study of malignant gliomas (90% GBM), noted median survivals of 35 weeks for patients receiving postoperative radiation therapy of 50 Gy or more and of 34.5 weeks for those receiving BCNU plus radiation therapy. Although there was no significant difference between the median survival rate for the groups receiving radiation therapy only and those receiving radiation therapy plus BCNU, a significantly greater number of patients who had received combination therapy were alive at 18 months. In a subsequent study by Chang and associates[35] evaluating 535 patients randomized to postoperative radiation therapy and postoperative radiation therapy plus chemotherapy groups, BCNU was found to significantly increase the survival in the 40- to 60-year-old age group as compared with the control group ($P = 0.01$). The previous experience with single and combined chemotherapeutic regimens has been reviewed by Edwards and associates[60] and by Kornblith and Walker,[113] and no combination has proved superior to BCNU alone. Recent efforts combining high-dose BCNU with an autologous bone marrow transplant after surgery and conventional radiation therapy have not demonstrated any significant increase in survival over that obtained with the conventional treatment, but rather have shown a high incidence of fatal pulmonary toxicity.[250]

Despite the theoretical advantages of intra-arterial chemotherapy, it remains a controversial and largely experimental form of therapy, and studies have demonstrated that it is not without significant morbidity rates.[136] The potential advantages of intra-arterial chemotherapy are that a higher dose of drug may be delivered to the tumor and that the total dose may be reduced, thereby reducing systemic toxicity. The disadvantages of this modality include the associated risks of any endovascular technique, the requirements of a dedicated angiography suite and an in-hospital stay, and the potential of local toxicity in the infused region. Levin and co-workers[130] demonstrated a 190% to 280% increase in brain concentrations of BCNU following intra-arterial, as compared to intravenous, infusion in squirrel monkeys. Others have used hyperosmolar agents to open the blood-brain barrier prior to the administration of chemotherapeutic agents in the hope of further increasing drug delivery to the tumor.[163] However, the blood-tumor barrier is affected less than is the BBB by the hyperosmolar infusion, with the result that the concentration of a drug increases disproportionately in the normal brain.[136]

The focus of the largest clinical experience with intra-arterial chemotherapy has been BCNU. For BCNU used adjuvantly and at recurrence, response rates of 40% to 70% have been recorded, but there is also significant neurotoxicity, with a 10% to 25% incidence of leukoencephalopathy and 16% to 25% incidence of blindness.[14,76,88,103] The reported leukoencephalopathy was attributed partly to the drug and partly to the carrier, ethyl alcohol. Ocular toxicity was attributed to the catheter's being positioned below the ophthalmic artery. Although a supraophthalmic positioning of catheters reduced the incidence of ophthalmic toxicity, it appeared to increase the risk of leukoencephalopathy.[88]

The Brain Tumor Cooperative Group[212] has reported the only prospective randomized trial comparing intra-arterial versus intravenous BCNU with concurrent radiation therapy, and in this study there was no difference in survival.

Other nitrosourea compounds, like 3-(4-amino - 2 - methyl - 5 - pyrimidinyl)methyl -1- (2-chloroethyl)-3-nitrosourea (ACNU) and 1 - (2 - chloroethyl) - 3 - (2,6 - dioxo - 3 - piperidyl)-1-nitrosourea (PCNU), have demonstrated some activity but have not yet been subjected to a phase III study.[136] In a recent study by Mahaley and associates,[140] 35 patients with recurrent malignant gliomas received intra-arterial cisplatin, resulting in a partial response or stabilization in 74%. The median survival from recurrence was 35 weeks for those who responded and 27.5 weeks for those who did not. Cisplatin has also been studied in several phase I-II trials, in all of which the drug was associated with otologic, ophthalmic, and renal toxicity.[136,140,170]

Reoperation has not been proved an effective method of initial treatment for recurrent malignant gliomas (Table 16–2).[200,203,255] Ammirati and co-workers[5] reported a median survival of 36 weeks after reoperation for 55 patients with recurrent

TABLE 16–2. RESULTS OF REOPERATION FOR RECURRENT MALIGNANT GLIOMA

Series	n	Median Survival after Reoperation (wk)
Young, et al[255]	24	14
Salcman, et al[200]	40	37
Ammirati, et al[5]	20 (AA)	61
	35 (GM)	29
Harsh, et al[80]	31 (AA)	88
	39 (GM)	36

Abbreviations: AA = anaplastic astrocytoma; GBM = glioblastoma multiforme.

malignant glioma (35 glioblastoma multiforme [GBM], 20 with atypical or anaplastic features [AA]). They found that patients with a Karnofsky performance status of greater than 70, with anaplastic astrocytoma as opposed to glioblastoma, and with gross total resection at reoperation, had the longest survival period. In the series by Harsh and colleagues,[80] the median postoperative survival after reoperation for patients with glioblastoma was 36 weeks, and for those with anaplastic astrocytoma, 88 weeks. Age and functional status were not found to affect significantly the duration of survival after reoperation, but these factors did have a significant effect on the patient's quality of life after reoperation.

In patients with recurrent malignant gliomas, with or without reoperation, chemotherapeutic agents used alone or in combinations have demonstrated significant activity. In 1970, Wilson and associates[247] reported a 47% response rate to BCNU in the treatment of 36 recurrent primary brain tumors. Since then, numerous trials have demonstrated the activity of single and multiple drug regimens with response rates between 20% and 50%.[113]

Interstitial brachytherapy is a promising technique for the treatment of recurrent malignant gliomas. Theoretically, continuous low-dose-rate irradiation maximizes the differential cell killing effectiveness between neoplastic and normal tissue, enhancing the therapeutic ratio.[17] Gutin and co-workers[79] reported a median survival of 52 weeks for recurrent glioblastomas and 153 weeks for anaplastic astrocytoma after iodine[125] implantation. These results were superior to those in a group of historical controls treated with chemotherapy (GBM 28 weeks, AA 51 weeks; $P < 0.01$). A recent update of this report to cover patients treated between January 1980 and January 1988 included 45 patients with recurrent glioblastoma and 50 patients with anaplastic astrocytoma.[78] The median survival period after ^{125}I implantation for recurrence in these patients was 54 weeks and 87 weeks, respectively. Forty-six patients (48%) underwent reoperation after implantation for clinical deterioration and an increasing mass of radionecrosis observed on CT scan; these patients had a significantly improved survival as compared to survival in those not undergoing reopera-

tion. The quality of life in the long-term survivors appeared to be acceptable, with an average Karnofsky performance status of 79 in 29 survivors at 18 months and of 76 in 17 survivors at 36 months.

The current management of patients with malignant gliomas at UCSF is outlined in Figure 16–10. Within 3 days of operation, contrast-enhanced CT scans are used to determine the amount of residual tumor. Tumors of less than 5 cm in diameter that are not crossing the midline and are not in the parasagittal or basal ganglionic location are now being entered on an experimental protocol with the Northern California Oncology Group. This protocol combines focal external-beam radiation therapy with hydroxyurea administered orally, followed by ^{125}I implantation and adjuvant systemic

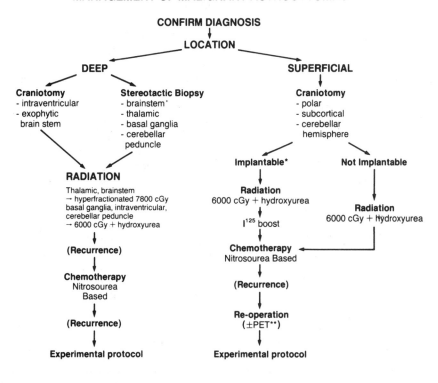

FIGURE 16–10. Algorithm for the management of malignant astrocytomas.

chemotherapy combining procarbazine, 1 - (2 - chloroethyl) - 3 - cyclohexyl - 1 - nitrosourea (CCNU), and vincristine (PCV-3). A tumor dose of between 4600 and 12,000 cGy is delivered with the implants at a maximum distance of 0.5 cm from the contrast-enhancing mass observed on the CT scan. The patients are observed with interval CT scans at 6- to 8-week intervals until the completion of chemotherapy and then at 3-month intervals thereafter for the following year. Those patients with evidence of an increased contrast-enhancing mass on CT scan are considered either for repeat operation, depending on clinical symptoms, or for evaluation with PET to assess the likelihood of radiation necrosis. Those patients not considered candidates for interstitial brachytherapy are treated with standard wide-field external-beam radiation therapy to a dose of 6000 cGy, again with adjuvant hydroxyurea chemotherapy, using conventional fractionation with a 2- to 3-cm margin on the enhancing tumor. After the radiation therapy, they are treated with adjuvant systemic chemotherapy on an experimental protocol including BCNU. For those patients with deep or basal ganglionic lesions, the diagnosis is confirmed with sterotaxic biopsy using either CT or MRI systems followed by radiation therapy, hydroxyurea, and nitrosourea-based chemotherapy.

Brainstem Gliomas

Brainstem gliomas account for 10% to 20% of childhood brain tumors and 2% of all tumors in adults.[81] The tumor most frequently affects children between the ages of 3 and 9 years. Brainstem gliomas are the third most common tumor in the posterior fossa, coming after cerebellar astrocytoma and medulloblastoma.[69,81,169]

Characteristically, patients with brainstem gliomas present with multiple cranial nerve palsies and cerebellar and long-tract signs. The sixth and seventh cranial nerves are most commonly involved followed, by the ninth, tenth, and fifth nerves.[169] Albright and colleagues[2] have found that multiple cranial nerve palsies are associated with a poor prognosis. Ataxia, strabismus, and personality change are often seen in children,

and symptoms of increased ICP occur in approximately one third. Ataxia and hydrocephalus may develop earlier in the clinical course of patients with dorsally exophytic tumors of the lower brainstem. In adults, gait disturbance, diplopia, and focal weakness are common, and these symptoms are often of slower onset in adults than in children.[61] The pons is the most frequent location for brainstem gliomas, and up to 60% to 70% of all brainstem tumors may show malignant features on postmortem examination.[169] Focal, cystic, and cervicomedullary tumors are usually low-grade, slow-growing lesions. Epstein and Wisoff,[64] Hoffman and associates,[89] and Stroink and associates[221] have described the successful surgical management of these low-grade, slow-growing cervicomedullary tumors, which account for 20% to 30% of all brainstem tumors.

CT scanning reveals that the majority of these lesions appear as diffuse, hypodense, and nonenhancing tumors. Albright and colleagues[2] have shown that patients with diffuse and hypodense lesions, as seen on CT, have a poor prognosis as compared with those with focal lesions. Tumors may be exophytic into the anterior or parapontine cisterns and cerebellopontine angle or dorsally into the fourth ventricle. Focal and homogeneously enhancing tumors are usually consistent with a low-grade pathology (juvenile pilocytic astrocytoma).[61]

MRI has replaced CT as the neurodiagnostic procedure of choice. The MR image frequently demonstrates a much more extensive abnormality than is seen on CT, and the tumors can be imaged on both the axial and sagittal planes.[174] Patients with hydrocephalus and a diagnosis of aqueductal stenosis should undergo MRI to rule out a periaqueductal brainstem glioma.

The differential diagnosis of brainstem glioma includes arteriovenous malformation, encephalitis, demyelinating disease, abscess, and neurofibromatosis. In children with neurofibromatosis, areas of increased signal intensity of T_2-weighted images frequently resolve spontaneously and are thought to represent areas of white matter not yet fully myelinated. The necessity of biopsy of brainstem tumors is controversial because sterotaxic biopsies may not be representative of the entire tumor, and there is the fear of significant morbidity.[1,3,61,62,204] For those tumors that are exophytic into the basal cisterns or fourth ventricle, an open operation allows for both pathologic diagnosis and the possibility of reestablishing CSF pathways with minimal morbidity. Intrinsic, diffuse lesions of the brainstem are most often malignant, and Epstein and McCleary[63] have shown that patients with these lesions do not benefit from operation. For cystic lesions where there is radiographic evidence of increasing cyst size that correlates with a deteriorating clinical course, cyst drainage by sterotaxic or open methods may provide significant improvement. If the clinical picture and imaging studies are consistent with typical brainstem gliomas, we have not recommended operation. When the diagnosis is in doubt, recent reports indicate, sterotaxic biopsy may be performed with high yield, low morbidity, and low mortality.[1,10,67,68,72,77,91] Using CT sterotaxic equipment and either a transfrontal or transcerebellar approach, diagnostic tissue is obtained in 92% to 100% of cases with morbidity-mortality figures of 0% to 3% and 0% to 8%. Coffey and Lunsford[41] reported on 13 sterotaxic biopsies in 12 patients with lesions of the pons and midbrain. A definitive diagnosis was obtained in all patients, and in none did postoperative CT demonstrate a hemorrhage at the biopsy site. The recent series of Abernathey and colleagues[1] included 26 patients who were studied with CT, MRI, and angiography. This information was used collectively for a stereotaxic suboccipital transcerebellar biopsy of pontine mass lesions and was not associated with any morbidity or mortality. The authors stated they could find no consistent correlation between the radiologic charac-

teristics of lesions and the histology as proven by biopsy. One patient proved to have a cryptococcal abscess, which responded to antibiotic therapy.

The 5-year survival rate for patients with brainstem tumors that are treated with conventionally fractionated radiation therapies is about 20% to 30%.[61] Adjuvant chemotherapy for brainstem tumors has not proved to be more effective than conventional radiation therapy alone.[102,129]

In an effort to improve the preceding results with conventional irradiation, several trials using hyperfractionated radiation therapy to a higher dose were initiated (Table 16–3). Packer and associates[172] reported the results of a pilot study in which 16 patients were treated with a dose of 6480 cGy using 120-cGy fractions. Patients with suspected low-grade tumors were excluded from the study. The median survival for the entire group was 9.8 months. In 1988, Freeman and co-workers[69] achieved a median survival of 11 months in 34 children using 110-cGy fractions to a total dose of 6600 cGy. Their study included three patients with juvenile pilocytic astrocytomas. Edwards and associates[62] recently reported the results of a phase I-II trial using 100-cGy fractions twice a day, 4 to 8 hours apart, to a total dose of 7200 cGy. There were 53 patients: 19 adults and 34 children. All patients were evaluated with MRI. No patients with low-grade tumors were presumed to have been included in this study, and all patients with biopsy-proved low-grade neoplasms were either observed or else treated with conventional radiation therapy. Pathologic confirmation of tumor was obtained in 23 of 53 patients: 72% were astrocytomas, 14% were anaplastic astrocytomas, and 14%

TABLE 16–3. **SURVIVAL AFTER HYPERFRACTIONATED RADIATION THERAPY FOR BRAINSTEM GLIOMAS**

Series	n	Dose	Median Survival
Packer, et al[172]	16	64.8 Gy	9.8 mo
Freeman, et al[69]	34	66.0 Gy	11 mo
	34 (children)		64 wk
Edwards, et al[61]	19 (adults)	72.0 Gy	92 wk

were glioblastomas. For the entire group, the median time to tumor progression (MTTP) was 59 weeks; median survival was 72 weeks. In regard to both median time to tumor progression and median survival, adults (MTTP 66 weeks, median survival 92 weeks) fared better than children (MTTP 44 weeks, median survival 64 weeks). There was no clinical evidence of increased toxicity with this dose, and two patients showed no evidence of radiation necrosis at autopsy. Patients with a poor prognosis included children, patients with diffuse tumors, and those with symptoms of less than 2 months' duration.

Based on this information, patients with tumors exophytic into the perimesencephalic, parapontine, or cerebellopontine angle cisterns and those exophytic into the fourth ventricle undergo open operation for biopsy and/or partial removal. At present, those patients with diffuse intrinsic brainstem gliomas with a typical clinical history and radiologic features are not subjected to either open operation or stereotactic biopsy. Enlarging tumor cysts are drained as clinical symptoms warrant. At UCSF we have begun a study of hyperfractionated radiation therapy to a dose of 7800 cGy based on the experience with 7200 cGy, and so far we have observed no adverse effects.[181]

Oligodendrogliomas

Oligodendrogliomas account for approximately 5% of all gliomas and most often occur between the third and fifth decades of life. In children, oligodendrogliomas account for 6% of tumors; the peak incidence is between the ages of 6 and 12 years.[37,154] Eighty percent of the tumors occur within the hemispheres. They are most common in the frontal lobe, followed by the parietal, temporal, and occipital lobes.[81] Three percent to 22.8% of these tumors occur within the ventricle.[81,154,223,241] Recent reports[166,194] indicate that tumors previously described by light microscopy as intraventricular oligodendrogliomas may have synapses and clear and dense core vesicles on electron microscopy and in fact may be of neuronal origin (intraventricular neurocytoma).

Clinically, the majority of patients with these tumors present with a history of seizures, headache, and personality change. Calcification is seen on plain skull x-rays in 28% to 56% of cases and tumor cysts in 20% to 34%.[81,154,194,245] CT scans commonly reveal a low-density, calcified, nonenhancing, infiltrative lesion of the subcortical white matter, whereas MRI reveals a lesion of increased signal intensity of T_2 images and of a slightly larger volume than appears on CT scans.

Pathologically, oligodendrogliomas appear as sheets of small, dark, uniform cells with a perinuclear halo, which represents an artifact of preservation.[194] Microcysts and endothelial proliferation may be seen, and calcospherites occur in an incidence exceeding that of astrocytoma or ependymoma.[30] Often these tumors contain a significant astrocytic component, and small areas of hemorrhage and infiltration of the leptomeninges are not unusual. The incidence of leptomeningeal spread detectable clinically ranges between 1% and 5.6%.[28,154,241]

The goal of surgery is gross total resection of tumor, when this is possible with a good neurologic outcome. Although the margins of oligodendrogliomas may be more distinct than astrocytomas, their infiltrative nature makes them difficult to remove completely. Cortical mapping and deep brain stimulation, with which there is recent experience, may improve on previous results.[16] In the early series of Earnest and colleagues,[58] gross total resection resulted in a larger number of patients alive beyond 5 years as compared to those who had subtotal resection, but there was no difference in mean postoperative survival (44.5 months versus 51.0 months). Mork and associates[154] reported that the median survival of patients in whom gross total resection was achieved was 14 months longer than that of other patients, while Lindegaard and co-workers[133] found that in the group treated without radiation therapy, the median survival for patients having gross total resection was 83.5 months versus 26 months for those having subtotal resection. Sun and associates,[223] reporting 57 cases undergoing combinations of therapy, found that the extent of removal did not significantly influence survival;

however, only two patients underwent gross total resection, with a median survival time of 108 months.

There is no prospective study that defines the role of radiation therapy in the postoperative management of these tumors (Table 16–4).[28,133,223,241] Mork and associates[154] found that the median survival of those patients receiving radiation therapy was 11 months longer than that for patients not treated. The recent report of Wallner and co-workers[241] documented the UCSF experience with oligodendrogliomas between 1940 and 1983. The 10-year survival rate for 14 patients who received greater than 45 Gy was 56%, as compared with 18% for 11 patients who did not have postoperative irradiation ($P = 0.09$).

Based on this information, adult patients with oligodendroglioma in noneloquent areas of brain should undergo operation for attempted surgical removal. Patients with subtotally resected tumors, as identified by postoperative imaging studies, are treated with focal external-beam radiation therapy to a dose of about 60 Gy. Chemotherapy is reserved for recurrent or malignant tumors.[33]

Ependymoma

Ependymomas account for 1.2% to 9% of all brain tumors and for 10% to 12% of all childhood tumors.[55,115,155,187,194] In the cerebral hemispheres they arise from the ventricular wall or trapped ependymal cell rests. Sixty percent of ependymomas occur in the posterior fossa; of all tumors in this location, 75% occur in children.[194] One third of the lesions are cystic, 25% show calcification, and 1% to 8% have anaplastic features.

Clinical symptomatology relates to the tumor's location. Patients with supratentorial tumors present with the symptom complex of headache, hemiparesis and seizures, whereas for patients with ependymomas in the posterior fossa, nausea, vomiting, and headache are the most common symptoms.[55,185] Because of the tumors' intraventricular location, metastasis through the CSF is possible, and reportedly its incidence is higher with malignant ependymomas and those located in the posterior fossa. The incidence of clinical CSF spread is 3% to 30%.[81,115,185,217] Most ependymomas are subtotally resected because of their ependymal origin and large size; this is so especially for tumors of the fourth ventricle, where intraoperative disturbance of cardiorespiratory centers can have grave consequences. With intraventricular tumors causing hydrocephalus, tumor removal is attempted first in an effort to avoid the need for a permanent shunt. Those patients presenting with increased ICP caused by hydrocephalus are managed with either a ventriculostomy preoperatively or a CSF shunting procedure, as the clinical situation dictates. Whereas previous operative mortality figures ranged between 22% and 32%, at present acceptable figures are 5% to 10%.[55,155]

Although no controversy exists regarding the radiosensitivity of these tumors and the need for postoperative radiation therapy, unresolved issues include the volume of ra-

TABLE 16–4. **RECENT RESULTS IN THE TREATMENT OF OLIGODENDROGLIOMAS WITH AND WITHOUT RADIATION**

Series	n	+RT	−RT	P
Bullard, et al (1978)	71	5.2 yr (37)	4.5 yr (34)	NS
Lindegaard, et al[133] (1987)	170	38 mo (108)	26.5 mo (62)	$P = 0.039$
Sun, et al[223] (1988)	56	47.5 mo (30)	54.0 mo (16)	NS
Wallner, et al[241] (1988)	25	56%* (14)	18%* (11)	$P = 0.09$

* 10-year survival rate.

diation necessary for low-grade tumors and the correlation between histologic grade and survival.[54,71,199]

There seems to be good information suggesting improved survival in those patients with malignant ependymomas treated with craniospinal axis irradiation (CSI). In 1983, Salazar and associates[199] reported a 5-year survival rate of 47% in patients with high-grade ependymomas treated with CSI, as compared with 8% in those undergoing only cranial irradiation ($P < 0.05$). All patients with malignant ependymoma should undergo craniospinal axis staging with focal irradiation of demonstrable masses distal to the primary tumor, in conjunction with CSI. However, in patients with low-grade tumors, leptomeningeal spread is rare, and in a review of four series by Leibel and Sheline,[125] the incidence was 3.1%. Shaw and colleagues[215] reported that for patients with low-grade tumors, the incidence of metastatic leptomeningeal spread was 14% in those who received CSI and 8% in those who did not and that CSI was not a significant factor in survival. Coupled with the fact that nearly all patients who died did so because of failure at the primary site, the authors concluded that CSI was not necessary for low-grade ependymoma and that localized irradiation was adequate.

The issue regarding the lack of correlation between tumor grade and survival was recently reported by Ross and Rubinstein.[193] In 15 patients with malignant ependymomas who were observed 15 months to 14 years postoperatively, the median survival was 8.8 years. Following surgery, 8 of 15 patients were treated with radiation therapy, 1 with chemotherapy, and 4 with the combination of radiation and chemotherapy. Among the one third who died with recurrence, the median survival was 2.5 years. The authors could make no correlation between the characteristics of cellular anaplasia and the clinical course. Mork and Loken[155] reported a 21% 7-year survival for typical ependymoma and 0% for the anaplastic form, whereas Shaw and colleagues[215] reported that the failure rate with high-grade tumors (67%) was twice that with the low-grade form (32%). Nagashima and co-workers[159] reported that 3 of 8 patients with ependymomas had a BUdR LI

greater than 1% (3.2%, 3.4%, and 4.8%). All 3 recurred within 2 years after gross or subtotal resection, while only 1 showed malignant histologic features. Currently we consider both the histologic features and BUdR LI in deciding on the most appropriate form of therapy for patients with ependymomas.

All patients with ependymomas should undergo operative removal of tumor and, following surgery, staging of the craniospinal axis to rule out dissemination. Our present practice is to perform a gadolinium-enhanced MRI of the entire spine and/or a complete myelogram and CSF cytology 2 weeks after operation. Localized, benign ependymomas are treated with focal external-beam radiation therapy to a dose of 54 Gy, while those tumors with dissemination are treated with CSI (30 Gy, whole brain and spinal axis; 54 Gy, primary site). Bulky intracranial or intraspinal disease should be treated with a focal boost. At UCSF, malignant ependymomas are now treated on an experimental protocol combining one cycle of neoadjuvant chemotherapy, followed by CSI at a reduced dose of 25 Gy with a dose of 60 Gy to the primary site, followed by 6 cycles of chemotherapy.

Subependymomas

Subependymomas are slow-growing neoplasms that occur most commonly in the ventricular system of adults. Composed of a mixture of astrocytes and ependymal cells, they are found in the region of the fourth ventricle and lateral recesses, in the wall of the lateral ventricle in the region of the foramen of Monro, in the septum pellucidum, and in the cerebral aqueduct.[194] The production of symptoms arises from obstruction of CSF pathways. The treatment of these tumors involves resection to reestablish CSF flow. Tumors of the lateral ventricle and septum pellucidum can be totally resected, but those in the floor or lateral recesses of the fourth ventricle cannot. In either situation, the patient is not treated further with adjuvant therapy and is simply observed at regular intervals with radiologic imaging studies.

Choroid Plexus Papilloma

Choroid plexus papillomas are rare tumors, accounting for 0.4% to 1% of all brain tumors.[23,82,101] Typically, it is a tumor of neonates and infants. In the series of Tomita and associates,[230] 82% occurred in children at an age of less than 24 months. Between 10% and 18% of choroid plexus papillomas are malignant, and calcification occurs in less than 20% of cases.[23,82,184] In children, tumors are located most often in the lateral ventricles. In adults, they most often arise in the fourth ventricle. The third ventricle is an unusual site for these tumors in both age groups. Blood is supplied from the appropriate choroidal artery (anterior, posterior, posterior medial, and/or posterior lateral), and during surgery an attempt is made to isolate these vessels before resection begins.

Commonly these patients present with symptoms of increased ICP related to hydrocephalus. Younger children have an enlarged head and papilledema. Hydrocephalus is thought to be related to one or a combination of factors: CSF overproduction, blockage of CSF pathways by intraventricular tumor, blockage of CSF absorption by recurrent small hemorrhages, or high CSF protein concentrations.[101] Tomita and colleagues[230] documented CSF production of greater than 700 mL/d in four out of five monitored patients. The differential diagnosis includes papillary ependymoma, choroid plexus carcinoma, and xanthogranuloma of the choroid plexus. Up to one fifth of papillomas seed the CSF, and this is more common with the malignant form of the disease.

The treatment of these tumors is an attempted gross surgical removal. Their intraventricular location and vascularity present a challenge to the neurosurgeon. With smaller tumors, en-bloc removal following isolation of the choroidal blood supply may be possible, but frequently the tumors are large, requiring piecemeal removal. The present operative mortality rates range between 10% and 24%, and between 27% and 72% of patients require a shunt postoperatively despite tumor removal.[23,82,101,184,230] Subdural fluid collections may develop because of a persisting ventriculosubdural fistula after a transcortical procedure, requiring further treatment.[23] For treating lesions subtotally resected, the issue regarding the necessity of radiation therapy remains unresolved. McGirr and colleagues[146] reported the long-term follow-up review of 10 patients with tumors that were subtotally resected, of whom 8 received postoperative radiation therapy. Half of those patients had died of recurrent disease at follow-up 6 to 40 months later, whereas 2 of 10 patients treated without radiation therapy were alive at 6 and 8 years postsurgery.

Those patients with malignant choroid plexus papillomas have a poor prognosis. Dohrmann and Collias,[56] in a review of 22 cases, reported mean survivals of 9 months for 16 children and 3.5 years in six adults. All patients with malignant tumors should undergo staging of the craniospinal axis to rule out leptomeningeal disease. It is our practice to treat malignant forms with low-dose CSI and a focal boost to the tumor, in combination with nitrosourea-based chemotherapy.

MEDULLOBLASTOMAS

Medulloblastomas account for approximately 4% of tumors in all ages and between 14% to 23% of all brain tumors in children.[39,90,131,171] The majority of these tumors (70% to 80%) occur in patients of less than 16 years of age, with a peak incidence in children between 5 and 6 years; they rarely are found in patients aged less than 1 year and older than 40.[39] In most series, male patients outnumber female patients from 1.3 : 1 to 2 : 1. These tumors have been classified as undifferentiated primitive neuroectodermal tumors; two histologic types, classical and desmoplastic variants, are described.[15,30] In children the most common location for the tumor is in the cerebellar vermis (65%), followed by lateral cerebellar hemispheric (19.6%) and paramedian locations (13.6%).[90] Less than 1% of tumors in adults are medulloblastomas, and in adults these tumors are equally distributed between vermian and hemispheric locations.[97]

Children with medulloblastoma present with a short clinical history, usually less than 3 months, and more than 80% have the symptom complex of headaches, nausea and vomiting, papilledema, and gait disturbance.[39] There may be associated hydrocephalus. At the time of diagnosis, between 16% and 46% of patients have evidence of CSF metastases.[39,49] These patients with CSF spread are more likely to develop systemic metastases, the most common sites being bone, lymph nodes, lung, and liver.[97] CT scans reveal a round, well-circumscribed lesion that is usually isodense or slightly hyperdense on noncontrast studies, with relatively homogeneous enhancement after the administration of contrast agents. On T_1-weighted MRI, these tumors are of low signal intensity and of increased signal intensity on T_2 studies. Gadolinium-enhanced T_1-weighted images are superior to CT scans for evaluating these posterior fossa tumors. Studies in the sagittal and axial planes reveal invasion of the floor of the fourth ventricle, which occurs in 33% of patients.[39]

The mortality associated with the operative removal of medulloblastomas has declined over the years and is close to zero in the experienced surgeon's hands.[90,171] Associated hydrocephalus is managed with ventriculostomy at the time of posterior fossa craniotomy, with ventriculoperitoneal shunting reserved for those patients who have persisting hydrocephalus following surgical resection. Choux and associates[39] in their extensive review observed that gross total resection gives the best short-term and long-term survival. The extent of surgical resection is one of the criteria defining good-risk and poor-risk patients.[36,39,99,171] Good-risk patients are those with greater than 75% removal, no evidence of leptomeningeal or systemic metastases at diagnoses, and age greater than 2 years.[131] Staging of the craniospinal axis is done approximately 2 weeks after surgery with radiologic imaging and analysis of CSF cytology. In our early experience with MRI of the spine, we observed one patient in whom subdural blood mimicked leptomeningeal tumor on an early postoperative enhanced scan.

Radiation therapy is the most effective treatment for this disease, but the long-term physical, intellectual, and endocrine sequelae are now well known. Growth hormone disturbance occurs in 60% to 70% and intellectual deficits in 33% of patients after CSI.[39] Although local tumor control is best achieved with a dose greater than 50 Gy to the posterior fossa, it is now becoming evident that lower doses to the craniospinal axis can be used without an increased risk of recurrence outside of the primary site.[24,99,131,229] Levin and associates[131] treated 47 patients with preirradiation procarbazine followed by craniospinal radiation in combination with hydroxyurea, with a dose of 55 Gy to the posterior fossa, 25 Gy to 35 Gy to the whole brain, and 25 Gy to the spinal cord. The overall 5-year survival rate was 66%, and only one patient had an isolated spinal recurrence. The authors concluded that for good-risk patients, reduced doses to the spinal axis and whole brain did not increase the risk of recurrence in these sites.

The addition of chemotherapy to radiation therapy appears to benefit some poor-risk patients.[4,135,173,177] Two large prospective studies comparing radiation therapy alone with radiation plus adjuvant chemotherapy suggested an increased survival rate in the group treated with chemotherapy, although this difference was not statistically significant.[4] Packer and co-workers[173] reported on the preliminary results of postoperative chemotherapy in 26 poor-risk patients who received vincristine, cisplatin, and CCNU. The 2-year survival rate for those receiving chemotherapy was 96% as compared with 59% for a similar control group treated with radiation therapy alone. Chemotherapy at recurrence may result in objective responses, and Pendergrass and colleagues[177] have documented a combined complete-partial response rate of 50% with the "8 in 1" protocol.

All patients with a medulloblastoma are treated with dexamethasone preoperatively, and obstructive hydrocephalus is managed with either preoperative or intraoperative ventriculostomy. Assessment of the need for a shunt is carried out after surgery. Current microsurgical instrumentation, namely ultrasonic aspirators and the carbon dioxide laser, have helped to reduce the morbidity and mortality of attempts at gross total resection. Within 3 to 7 days following surgery, depending on the patient's condition, a repeat CT/MR image of the posterior fossa is obtained to assess residual disease. Two weeks after surgery, staging of the craniospinal axis is undertaken, with imaging of the entire neural axis as well as assessment of CSF cytology. A gadolinium-enhanced MR image of the entire spine is done, and if this is negative, along with negative cytology findings, no myelogram is performed. If there are any questionable areas, most commonly seen posteriorly in the thoracic region, a myelogram is performed. Good-risk patients (age greater than 2 years, gross total resection of tumor, negative craniospinal axis staging) are treated in the manner previously reported by Levin and associates.[131] The dose to the posterior fossa is 55 Gy, and the dose to the craniospinal axis is 25 Gy. Poor-risk patients are treated with an experimental protocol combining neoadjuvant nitrosourea-based chemotherapy, craniospinal axis radiation, posterior fossa boost, and postradiation chemotherapy.

PRIMARY LYMPHOMA OF THE CENTRAL NERVOUS SYSTEM

In the past, primary CNS lymphoma was a rarely diagnosed tumor, but its incidence has risen with the increase of acquired immunotherapy deficiency syndrome (AIDS) and with medically induced compromise of the immune system for organ transplantation and the treatment of autoimmune diseases.[86,192] In the population that is not immunocomprised, however, the incidence has tripled in the past 10 years.[86,122,180,192] At present, primary CNS lymphoma accounts for 0.5% to 3% of all brain tumors and approximately 1.7% of all malignant lymphomas. Hochberg and Miller[86] have written an excellent review on the topic.

Primary CNS lymphoma is most common between the ages of 40 and 60 in the nonimmunocompromised state. The most common symptoms at presentation are personality change, focal weakness, and headache. Thirty percent of patients may present with an atypical syndrome mimicking dementia, encephalitis, or demyelinating disease.[21]

The disease may involve multiple brain sites in 30% to 50%, CSF in 10% to 25%, and the vitreous in 10% to 20%. Lymphoma occurs most commonly in the basal ganglia, thalamus, corpus callosum, and frontal and parietal lobe periventricular white matter.[86] Approximately 15% occur in the posterior fossa.

The neurosurgical management of CNS lymphoma relies primarily on establishing the diagnosis by stereotaxic or ultrasound-directed biopsy. On nonenhanced CT scans the tumor may be hyperdense, although hemorrhage is unusual. With contrast enhancement, lesions within the white matter are either solid and homogeneously enhancing, diffuse and periventricular in location, or diffuse and nonenhancing.[21] Such tumors were previously described by a number of different terms, but it is now clear that the majority of them are of a monoclonal B cell origin. The patient's survival has been related to the histopathologic cell subtype. The median survival for the small-cell cleaved variety is 36.5 months, and it is 11.2 months for the large-cell immunoblastic types.[86] These cells may gain access to the CNS from the subarachnoid space or choroid plexus through Virchow-Robin spaces.[218] Although 10% of patients have systemic spread following failure of treatment for their CNS lesions, it is very unusual for patients who present with intra-axial versus leptomeningeal lymphoma to have synchronous systemic disease. We agree with Hochberg and Miller[86] that extensive systemic workups are not warranted, but all patients with CNS lymphoma should have a detailed ophthalmologic examination and analysis of CSF cytology.

Primary CNS lymphoma, like systemic lymphoma, may respond dramatically to oral steroid medications and radiation therapy. However, median survivals are still on the order of 13 months to 15 months.[86,122,180] Recent reports have noted the efficacy of single and multiple drug combinations as effective primary therapy for CNS lymphoma, reserving radiation therapy for therapeutic failures.[70,147,180] Intensive systemic chemotherapy is contraindicated in patients with AIDS or immunocompromised patients because of the high risk of overwhelming infection.

UPDATE ON THERAPY

Radiosurgery

Radiosurgery is a technique by which a large radiation dose is delivered to a tumor in a single fraction using small and well-collimated beams. Leksell[127] has had the greatest experience with this technique using the gamma knife, a 179 cobalt 60 (^{60}Co) source machine, for treating arteriovenous malformations and acoustic neuromas. Recently, Lunsford and associates[138] have described the operating system and early clinical experience with a 201 ^{60}Co gamma knife at the University of Pittsburgh. Their series of 52 patients included 4 with intra-axial malignant neoplasms up to 18 mm in diameter, with treatment times on the order of 10 to 12 minutes and procedural times of 3 to 5 hours. With the linear accelerator, single-plane, multiple noncoplanar converging arcs or dynamic rotation have been developed for radiosurgery performed with the patient in a stereotaxic head frame.[179,222,248] Using this technique, single doses of 20 to 30 Gy can be used to treat lesions 1 to 3.5 cm in diameter within a short time.

Patients suitable for radiosurgery include those with small (1- to 2.5-cm) tumors in surgically inaccessible areas, those with conditions that preclude anesthesia and a conventional surgical approach, and those patients refusing open operation. Volumes larger than 3.5 cm have less favorable isodose curves and are therefore not as well suited to this technique. Cerebral metastases, with their well-defined borders, are ideal targets. The total treatment time is approximately 1 hour, and procedural time is 3 to 4 hours. Further recommendations await the results of clinical trials.

Surgical Therapies

Laser Surgery

Lasers, neurosurgical instrumentation since the 1970s, have three functions: photocoagulation, photovaporization of tissue, and photoactivation of sensitizing agents such as hematoporphyrin derivatives (HpD).[59] They are not, however, a panacea for brain tumors. They are useful for those tumors located centrally with only a narrow corridor of approach available and for tough, fibrotic recurrent tumors.

The currently available systems include the carbon dioxide laser, the neodymium-YAG (NG-YAG) laser, and argon lasers. The carbon dioxide and ND-YAG lasers have received widest neurosurgical application.[59,227] The carbon dioxide laser is safer, based on its maximal absorption of light and minimal dispersion of energy into the surrounding tissues. With a focused beam it can be used as a cutting instrument. Salcman,[202] in evaluating a series of patients operated on with or without a laser, found that blood loss, length of hospital stay, and morbidity and mortality rates were the same for both groups; the only significant difference was the length of operation, which was 299 minutes with a laser and 237 minutes without one. The ND-YAG laser is used primarily as a coagulating tool because its long wavelength and diffuse scatter within tissues produce heating and coagulation.

The selective uptake of HpD by tumors and its activation by the argon laser makes photoradiation therapy theoretically attractive. The mediators of cell destruction include singlet oxygen, hydrogen peroxide, and hydroxyl radicals generated by the action of laser light on HpD.[104] The initial results with this technique were disappointing. Limitations related to the photosensitizing agent and the depth of tumor illumination have been reviewed by Kaye and associates.[104] Muller and Wilson[157] have recently reported experience in 40 patients with malignant gliomas who received either HpD or dihematoporphyrin ether preoperatively; intraoperative activation was obtained by illumination from the argon dye pump laser. The median survival in this group of patients was 259 days, with a 1-year and 2-year survival rate of 30% and 13%, respectively. The efficacy of this technique awaits further testing with newer radiation sensitizers and light delivery systems.

Computer-Assisted Removal

Computer-assisted stereotaxic removal of intra-axial neoplasms is a complicated technique requiring integration of data from three different imaging modalities, a three-dimensional coordinate system for localizing the tumor in the operating room, and special microsurgical instruments and operating equipment. The group at the Mayo Clinic[105-107] has published the results of computer-assisted stereotaxic removal by using this technique for a variety of lesions, and at present it is their preferred method for any intra-axial lesion not located in frontal, temporal, occipital poles, or superficially in the posterior fossa.

Since 1980 this system has been used for 267 computer-assisted craniotomies on 258 patients, with morbidity and mortality rates of 10.4% and 1.1%, respectively.[105] Most of these tumors were considered unresectable by conventional techniques. There were 141 patients with gliomas, of which 62 were malignant. In the group of malignant tumors with gross total resection, using this technique, the median survival was 42 weeks, which is comparable to results with conventional techniques for tumors in accessible locations. Those patients with histologically well-circumscribed and noninfiltrating, deep-seated or centrally located tumors, such as juvenile pilocytic astrocytomas, are said to derive the most benefit from this procedure.[106] The authors pointed out that the system has been many years in development and requires expensive equipment and specially trained support staff. The operating surgeon also needs special training to understand the system and to work effectively and safely with the necessary special instruments. Until information is available that clearly demonstrates superior results with this system as compared with conventional treatment for gliomas (and considering that the system is costly), it is unlikely that stereotactic resection will become widely used.

Biologic Response Modifiers

Biologic response modifiers are agents that act on either the host or the tumor, with a demonstrated antitumor effect. This group includes a number of drugs, the interferons, monoclonal antibodies, lymphokines, and lymphokine-activated killer (LAK) cells. Examples of the clinical results with some of these agents are presented below.

Polyamine Inhibitors

Polyamines are ubiquitous intracellular compounds essential for cell growth and proliferation. The drugs α-difluoromethylornithine (DFMO), an inhibitor of ornithine decarboxylase, and mitoguazone (MGBG), an inhibitor of S-adenosylmethionine, inhibit cell growth in culture. These drugs have demonstrated clinical activity in the treatment of recurrent anaplastic astrocytomas. Levin and associates[128] evaluated 33 patients with recurrent tumors, of whom 19 had anaplastic astrocytoma. In this group of patients 21% had a clear response, 53% had disease stabilization, and 26% showed tumor progression after one cycle of treatment. There was no significant activity against glioblastomas. A subsequent study by Prados and colleagues[182] combining BCNU and DFMO demonstrated a 57% response rate in recurrent anaplastic astrocytomas, with a median survival of 56 weeks and little response in glioblastoma multiforme. A phase II randomized trial comparing DFMO alone to DFMO-MGBG for the treatment of recurrent malignant gliomas is underway.[181]

Monoclonal Antibodies

Hybridoma technology has allowed the development of monoclonal antibodies (MABs) against a variety of lymphoid differentiation and neuroectodermal tumor-associated antigens. A variety of MABs have been developed for immunohistochemistry in neuropathology; more recently, in defining the proliferative potential of tumors with Ki-67, they have been directed against nuclear antigens expressed by proliferating cells in all phases of the cell cycle.[26,167,259] For clinical practice the hope is that an antibody with affinity for glioma-associated antigens will permit the delivery of drugs and radionuclides selectively directed against the tumor mass. Researchers have been hampered by problems of cross-reactivity, the blood-brain-barrier, the host immune response to the antibody itself, and tumor antigen heterogeneity. Although tumor antigen heterogeneity is an inherent characteristic of malignant gliomas, a degree of specificity to glioma-associated antigens has been demonstrated in both subcutaneous and intracranial xenograft models.[123,124] Lee and associates[123] demonstrated in nude mice harboring an intracranial glioma xenograft that treatment with the ^{131}I-labeled MAB 81C6 resulted in a significant prolongation of survival in the treated group as compared with controls.

Experimentally, the intracarotid administration of MABs increases delivery to the tumor by 20%. An even larger dose can be delivered if intracarotid administration is preceded by an even greater opening of the blood-brain-barrier.[27] Reducing the size of MABs by cleaving the Fc portion may assist in the penetration and clearance of Fab fragments while maintaining binding affinity.[43] The problems of nonspecific binding in other tissues and host immune reactions may as well be reduced by cleaving the Fc portion.

Clinical work with MABs for imaging and treatment has already begun. Preliminary results in patients with leptomeningeal metastases indicate activity using MABs after other forms of treatment have failed.[118] Further work with these agents may improve our ability to control, and possibly eliminate, malignant intra-axial tumors.

Interferons

The interferons (IFNs) are cytokines that have an antiproliferative effect on tumor cells and an immunomodulatory effect on normal host tissues. Three different types have been identified. Interferons alfa and beta are made by virtually all cells, and gamma are made by T lymphocytes and large granular lymphocytes. All prolong the cell cycle and may activate or enhance cell-mediated immunity.[183] Alfa and beta interferon have shown the most activity against glioma cell lines in vitro, and all three have

been used in the treatment of recurrent malignant gliomas (Table 16–5).[52,139,141,257]

Preliminary results of a multicenter phase I-II nonrandomized trial of beta IFN for recurrent malignant gliomas indicate that, of 65 evaluable patients, the combined response stabilization rate was approximately 50%. The MTTP for both anaplastic astrocytomas and glioblastoma multiforme was 11 weeks.[181] The major toxicity in this and other series relates to the systemic side effects of fever and chills, as well as a reversible dementia. Further work with these agents will involve combinations of IFNs with radiation and other chemotherapeutic agents.

Adoptive Immunotherapy

Adoptive immunotherapy refers to the passive transfer to the host of immune cells with antitumor activity. Previous reports[189] demonstrated the potential effectiveness of this treatment in patients with metastatic cancer using LAK cells and interleukin-2 (IL-2). LAK cells, produced by incubating peripheral blood lymphocytes (PBL) with IL-2, lyse allogenic and autogenic tumor cells but not normal cells. Although patients with malignant gliomas have impaired cell-mediated immunity and reduced levels of circulating PBLs, when stimulated with IL-2 their PBLs demonstrate the same cytotoxicity against glioma cells as do those from healthy volunteers.[22]

The finding that long-term survival was associated with heavy lymphocytic infiltration in malignant gliomas gave support to the notion that cell-mediated immunity was active in patients with malignant gliomas.[53,176] Although in one study only 11.5% of tumors showed definite lymphocytic infiltration, experimental work has since revealed that the majority of these

TABLE 16–5. RESULTS OF RECENT SERIES USING INTERFERONS FOR THE TREATMENT OF RECURRENT MALIGNANT GLIOMAS

Series	n	Interferon	Response	Median Survival (d)
Mahaley, et al[141]	17	alfa	7/17	511
Duff, et al[57a]	12	beta	1/12	165
Mahaley, et al[139]	14	gamma	1/14	168

TABLE 16-6. **RESULTS OF TRIALS USING ADOPTIVE IMMUNOTHERAPY FOR RECURRENT MALIGNANT GLIOMAS**

Series	n	Treatment	Response (%)	CNS Toxicity	Median Survival (wk)
Young, et al[256]	17	Single intratumoral (IT) injection of PBLs*	47	Occasional ICP (10 mL injected)	22.5
Merchant, et al	13	9-IT LAK†+IL-2; then IL-2 alone via Ommaya 4-IT LAK + IL-2 × 2	38	100%‡	23
Merchant, et al	20§	IT LAK + IL-2; then IL-2 alone via Ommaya	40	100%¶	21.5
Yoshida, et al[254]	23	IT LAK + IL-2 via Ommaya	26	none	NA**
Barba, et al[13]	9	IT LAK + IL-2 via Ommaya	11	100%	18

* Peripheral blood lymphocytes.
†Lymphokine activated killer cells.
§Five patients no prior treatment.
¶ICP; aseptic meningitis.
**Not stated.

cells as T lymphocytes. Young and associates[256] assessed the feasibility of harvesting and transferring PBLs and injecting them into the tumor cavity of patients with recurrent gliomas as a form of treatment. The combination of LAK and IL-2 injected directly into the tumor cavity has since been tried in several phase I studies of patients with recurrent gliomas (Table 16-6).[13,100,149,150,254] In most studies, there has been significant toxicity related to an increase in cerebral edema and an increase in ICP. It is likely that the increase in cerebral edema is related to IL-2 and may be a mechanism similar to the capillary leak syndrome seen with high-dose systemic IL-2. In none of these early studies has adoptive immunotherapy had a significant impact on survival.

Recently, interest has shifted to tumor-infiltrating (TIL cells) as an effector of tumor cell kill. Rosenberg and colleagues[190] have reported that TIL cells are 50 to 100 times more effective in their potency against murine sarcoma and adenocarcinoma cell lines. TIL cells may be harvested from gliomas.[116,151,152,198,206] There is hope that clonal expansion of these cells may provide a population of cells with more effective

glioma cell killing, such that the amount of IL-2 necessary to sustain an antitumor effect may be reduced, thereby avoiding the side effect of cerebral edema. To this point, TIL cells have not been cultured for longer than 6-to-8-week intervals, nor have enough cells been generated to produce the numbers required for therapy.[151,207]

FUTURE PROSPECTS

Further gains in the treatment of malignant neuroepithelial tumors will likely come through a well-coordinated multimodality approach. Surgery of these intra-axial neoplasms will improve with the increased availability and use of some of the techniques discussed in this chapter. The results of current trials using different modes of administration of radiation will be forthcoming in the next few years. The possibilities for the in vitro assessment of sensitivity of individual tumors to various chemotherapeutic agents should increase their effectiveness.[110,210] The most exciting areas for further research — immunobiology and molecular genetics — should provide the pathway to a better understanding of these tumors and the potential for curative interventions.

REFERENCES

1. Abernathey, CD, Camacho, A, and Kelly, PJ: Stereotaxic suboccipital transcerebellar biopsy of pontine mass lesions. J Neurosurg 70:195–200, 1989.
2. Albright, AL, Guthkelch, AN, Packer, RJ, Price, RA, and Rourke, LB: Prognostic factors in pediatric brain stem gliomas. J Neurosurg 65:751–755, 1986.
3. Albright, AL, Price, RA, and Guthkelch, AN: Brain stem gliomas of children: A clinicopathological study. Cancer 52:2313–2319, 1983.
4. Allen, JC, Bloom, J, Ertel, I, Hammond, D, Jones, H, Levin, V, Jenkin, D, Sposto, R, and Wara, W: Brain tumors in children: Current cooperative and institutional chemotherapy trials in newly diagnosed and recurrent disease. Semin Oncol 13:110–122, 1986.
5. Ammirati, M, Galicich, JH, Arbit, E, and Liao, Y: Reoperation in the treatment of recurrent intracranial malignant gliomas. Neurosurgery 21:607–614, 1987.
6. Ammirati, M, Vick, N, Liao, Y, Ciric, I, and Mikhael, M: Effect of the extent of surgical resection on survival and quality of life in patients with supratentorial glioblastomas and anaplastic astrocytomas. Neurosurgery 21: 201–206, 1987.
7. Annual Cancer Statistics Review (1987). NIH Publ No 882789. National Cancer Institute, Bethesda, MD, 1988, p 20.
8. Apuzzo, ML: Surgery of intracranial tumors: Aspects of operating room design with integration and use of technical adjuvants. Clin Neurosurg 35:185–214, 1987.
9. Apuzzo, MLJ, Chandrasoma, PT, Cohen, D, Zee, CS, and Zelman, V: Computed imaging stereotaxy: Experience and perspective related to 500 procedures applied to brain masses. Neurosurgery 20:930–937, 1987.
10. Artigas, J, Ferszt, R, Brock, M, Kazner, E, and Cervos-Navarro, J: The relevance of pathological diagnosis for therapy and outcome of brain stem gliomas. Acta Neurochir Suppl (Wien) 42:166–169, 1988.
11. Bailey, P and Cushing, H: A Classification of Tumors of the Glioma Group. JB Lippincott Philadelphia, 1926.
12. Baram, TZ, Van Eys, J, Dowell, RE, Cangir, A, Pack, B, and Bruner, JM: Survival and neurologic outcome of infants with medulloblastoma treated with surgery and MOPP chemotherapy. Cancer 60:173–177, 1987.
13. Barba, D, Saris, SC, Holder, C, Rosenberg, SA, and Oldfield, EH: Intratumoral LAK cell and interleukin-2 therapy of human gliomas. J Neurosurg 70:175–182, 1989.
14. Bashir, R, Hochberg, FH, Linggold, RM, and Hott-

leman, K: Preirradiation internal carotid artery BCNU in treatment of glioblastoma multiforme. J Neurosurg 68:917–919, 1988.
15. Becker, LE and Hinton, D: Primitive neuroectodermal tumors of the central nervous system. Hum Pathol 14:538–550, 1983.
16. Berger, MS, Ojemann, GA, and Lettich, E: Intraoperative brain mapping techniques to maximize tumor resection: Experience with 96 adult and pediatric cases. Presented at the Annual Meeting of the American Association of Neurological Surgeons, Washington, 1989.
17. Bernstein, M and Gutin, PH: Interstitial irradiation of brain tumors: A review. Neurosurgery 9:741–750, 1981.
18. Bigner, DD and Pegram, CN: Virus induced experimental brain tumors and putative associations of viruses with human brain tumors: A review. Adv Neurol 15:57–83, 1976.
19. Bishop, JM: The molecular genetics of cancer. Science 235:305–311, 1987.
20. Black, PM and Ronner, SF: Cortical mapping for defining the limits of tumor resection. Neurosurgery 20:914–919, 1987.
21. Bogdahn, U, Bogdahn S, Mertens, HG, Dommasch, D, Wodarz, R, Wunsch, PH, Kuhl, P, and Richter, E: Primary non-Hodgkin's lymphomas of the CNS. Acta Neurol Scand 73:602–614, 1986.
22. Bosnes, V and Hirschberg, H: Comparison of in vitro glioma cell cytotoxicity of LAK cells from glioma patients and healthy subjects. J Neurosurg 69:234–238, 1988.
23. Boyd, MC and Steinbok, P: Choroid plexus tumors: Problems in diagnosis and management. J Neurosurg 66:800–805, 1987.
24. Brand, WN, Schneider, PA, and Tokars, RP: Long term results of a pilot study of low dose cranial-spinal irradiation for cerebellar medulloblastoma. Int J Radiat Oncol Biol Phys 13:1641–1645, 1987.
25. Bullard, DE: Role of stereotaxic biopsy in the management of patients with intracranial lesions. Neurol Clin 3:817–830, 1985.
26. Bullard, DE and Bigner, DD: Applications of monoclonal antibodies in the diagnosis and treatment of primary brain tumors. Review article. J Neurosurg 63:2–16, 1985.
27. Bullard, DE, Bourdon, M, and Bigner, DD: Comparison of various methods for delivering radiolabeled monoclonal antibody to normal rat brain. J Neurosurg 61:901–911, 1984.
28. Bullard, DE, Rawlings, CE, Phillips, D, Cox, EB, Schold, SC, Burger, P, and Halperin, EC: Oligodendroglioma: An analysis of the value of radiation therapy. Cancer 60:2179–2188, 1987.
29. Burger, PC: Pathologic anatomy and CT correlations in the glioblastoma multiforme. Appl Neurophysiol 46:180–187, 1983.
30. Burger, PC and Vogel, FS: Surgical Pathology of the Brain and its Coverings. John Wiley & Sons, New York, 1982.
31. Burger, PC, Vogel, FS, Green, SB, and Strike, TA:

Glioblastoma multiforme and anaplastic astrocytoma: Pathologic criteria and prognostic implications. Cancer 56:1106–1111, 1985.

32. Butler, AB, Brooks, WH, and Netsky, MG: Classification and biology of brain tumors. In Youmans, JR (ed): Neurological Surgery, ed 2, Vol 5. WB Saunders, Philadelphia, 1982, p 2659.

33. Cairncross, JG and MacDonald, DR: Successful chemotherapy for recurrent malignant oligodendroglioma. Ann Neurol 23:360–364, 1988.

34. Chandler, WF and Knake, JE: Intra-operative use of ultrasound in neurosurgery. Clin Neurosurg 31:550–563, 1984.

35. Chang, CH, Horton, J, Schoenfeld, D, Salazer, O, Perez-Tamayo, R, Kramer, S, Weinstein, A, Nelson, JS, and Tsukada, Y: Comparison of postoperative radiotherapy and combined postoperative radiotherapy and chemotherapy in the multidisciplinary management of malignant gliomas. Cancer 52:997–1007, 1983.

36. Chang, CH, Housepian, EM, and Herbert, C: An operative staging system and a megavoltage radiotherapeutic technic for cerebellar medulloblastoma. Radiology 93:1351–1359, 1969.

37. Chin, HW, Hazel, JJ, Kim, TH, and Webster, JH: Oligodendrogliomas. I. A clinical study of cerebral oligodendrogliomas. Cancer 45:1458–1466, 1980.

38. Cho, KG, Nagashima, T, Barnwell, S, and Hoshino, T: Flow cytometric determination of modal DNA population in relation to proliferative potential of human intracranial neoplasms. J Neurosurg 69:588–592, 1988.

39. Choux, M, Lena, G, and Hassoun, J: Prognosis and long-term follow-up in patients with medulloblastoma. Clin Neurosurg 30:246–277, 1983.

40. Ciric, I, Ammirati, M, Vick, N, and Mikhael, M: Supratentorial gliomas: Surgical considerations and immediate postoperative results. Neurosurgery 21:21–27, 1987.

41. Coffey, RJ and Lunsford, LD: Stereotactic surgery for mass lesions of the midbrain and pons. Neurosurgery 17:12–18, 1985.

42. Coffey, RJ, Lunsford, LD, and Taylor, FH: Survival after stereotactic biopsy of malignant gliomas. Neurosurgery 22:465–473, 1988.

43. Colapinto, EV, Humphrey, PA, Zalutsky, MR, Groothuis, DR, Friedman, HS, De Tribolet, N, Carrel, S, and Bigner, D: Comparative localization of murine monoclonal antibody Me1-14 F(ab')$_2$ fragment and whole IgG2a in human glioma xenografts. Cancer Res 48:5701–5707, 1988.

44. Colombo, F, Casentini, L, Zanusso, M, Danieli, D, and Benedetti, A: Validity of stereotactic biopsy as a diagnostic tool. Acta Neurochir 42:152–156, 1988.

45. Copeland, DD and Bigner, DD: Glial mesenchymal tropism of in vivo avian sarcoma virus

neuro-oncogenesis in rats. Acta Neuropathol 41:23–25, 1978.

46. Daumas-Duport, C, Scheithauer, B, O'Fallon, J, and Kelly, P: Grading of astrocytomas. A simple and reproducible method. Cancer 62:2152–2165, 1988.

47. Davis, LW: Presidential address: Malignant glioma—a nemesis which requires clinical and basic investigation in radiation oncology. Int J Radiat Oncol Biol Phys 16:1355–1365, 1989.

48. Davis, RL: Personal communication, June 1989.

49. Deutsch, M: Medulloblastoma: Staging and treatment outcome. Int J Radiat Oncol Biol Phys 14:1103–1107, 1988.

50. Deutsch, M, Green, SB, Strike, TA, Burger, PC, Robertson, JT, Selker, RG, Shapiro, WR, Mealey, J, Ransohoff, J, Paoletti, P, Smith, KR, Odom, GL, Hunt, WE, Young, B, Alexander, E, Walker, MD, and Pistenmaa, DA: Results of a randomized trial comparing BCNU plus radiotherapy, streptozocin plus radiotherapy, BCNU plus hyperfractionated radiotherapy, and BCNU following misonidazole plus radiotherapy in the postoperative treatment of malignant glioma. Int J Radiat Oncol Biol Phys 16:1389–1396, 1989.

51. Di Chiro, G, Oldfield, E, Wright, DC, De Michele, D, Katz, DA, Patronas, NJ, Doppman, JL, Larson, SM, Ito, M, and Kufta, CV: Cerebral necrosis after radiotherapy and/or intraarterial chemotherapy for brain tumors: PET and neuropathologic studies. AJR 150:189–197, 1988.

52. Dick, RS and Hubbell, HR: Sensitivities of human glioma cell lines to interferons and double-stranded RNAs individually and in synergistic combinations. J Neurooncol 5:331–338, 1987.

53. Di Lorenzo, N, Palma, L, and Nicole, S: Lymphocytic infiltration in long-survival glioblastomas: Possible host's resistance. Acta Neurochir (Wien) 39:27–33, 1977.

54. Di Marco, A, Campostrini, F, Pradella, R, Reggio, M, Palazzi, M, Grandinetti, A, and Garusi, GF: Postoperative irradiation of brain ependymomas: Analysis of 33 cases. Acta Oncol 27:261–267, 1988.

55. Dohrmann, GJ: Ependymomas. In Wilkins, RH and Rengachary, SS (eds): Neurosurgery, Vol 1. McGraw-Hill, New York, 1985, p 767.

56. Dohrmann, GJ and Collias, JC: Choroid plexus carcinoma: Case report. J Neurosurg 43:225–232, 1975.

57. Dohrmann, GJ, Farwell, JR, and Flannery, JT: Astrocytomas in childhood: A population based study. Surg Neurol 23:64–68, 1985.

57a. Duff, TA, Borden, E, Bay, J, Piepmeier, J, and Sielaff, K: Phase II trial of interferon-B for treatment of recurrent glioblastoma multiforme: J Neurosurg 64:408–413, 1986.

58. Earnest, F, Kernohan, JW, and Craig, WM: Oligodendrogliomas: A review of two hundred cases. Arch Neurol 63:964–976, 1950.

59. Edwards, MS, Boggan, JE, and Fuller, TA: The laser

in neurological surgery: Review article. J Neurosurg 59:555–566, 1983.

60. Edwards, MS, Levin, VA, and Wilson, CB: Brain tumor chemotherapy: An evaluation of agents in current use for phase II and phase III trials. Cancer Treat Rep 64:1179–1205, 1980.

61. Edwards, MS and Prados, M: Current management of brain stem gliomas. Pediatr Neurosci 13:309–315, 1987.

62. Edwards, MS, Wara, WM, Urtasun, RC, Prados, M, Levin, VA, Fulton, D, Wilson, CB, Hannigan, J, and Silver, P: Hyperfractionated radiation therapy for brain-stem glioma: A Phase I-II trial. J Neurosurg 70:691–700, 1989.

63. Epstein, F and McCleary, EL: Intrinsic brain-stem tumors of childhood: Surgical indications. J Neurosurg 64:11–15, 1986.

64. Epstein, F and Wisoff, J: Intra-axial tumors of the cervicomedullary junction. J Neurosurg 67:483–487, 1987.

65. Fazekas, JT: Treatment of grades I and II brain astrocytomas: The role of radiotherapy. Int J Radiat Oncol Biol Phys 2:661–666, 1977.

66. Francavilla, TL, Miletich, RS, Di Chiro, G, Patronas, NJ, Rizzoli, H, and Wright, DC: Positron emission tomography in the detection of malignant degeneration of low-grade gliomas. Neurosurgery 24:1–5, 1989.

67. Frank F, Fabrizi, AP, Frank-Ricci, R, Gaist, G, Sedan, R, and Peragut, JC: Stereotactic biopsy and treatment of brain stem lesions: Combined study of 33 cases (Bologna-Marseille). Acta Neurochir Suppl (Wien) 42:177–181, 1988.

68. Franzini, A, Allegranza, A, Melcarne, A, Giorgi, C, Ferraresi, S, and Broggi, G: Serial stereotactic biopsy of brain stem expanding lesions: Considerations on 45 consecutive cases. Acta Neurochir Suppl (Wien) 42:170–176, 1988.

69. Freeman, CR, Krischer, J, Sanford, RA, Burger, PC, Cohen, M, and Norris, D: Hyperfractionated radiotherapy in brain stem tumors: Results of a pediatric oncology group study. Int J Radiat Oncol Biol Phys 15:311–318, 1988.

70. Gabbal, AA, Hochberg, FH, Linggood, RM, Bashir, R, and Hotleman, K: High-dose methotrexate for non-AIDS primary central nervous system lymphoma: Report of 13 cases. J Neurosurg 70:190–194, 1989.

71. Garrett, PG and Simpson, WJK: Ependymomas: Results of radiation treatment. Int J Radiat Oncol Biol Phys 9:1121–1124, 1983.

72. Giunta, F, Marini, G, Grasso, G, and Zorzi, F: Brain stem expansive lesions: Stereotactic biopsy for a better therapeutic approach. Acta Neurochir Suppl (Wien) 42:182–186, 1988.

73. Gol, A: The relatively benign astrocytomas of the cerebrum. J Neurosurg 18:501–506, 1961.

74. Gordon, H: Oncogenes. Mayo Clin Proc 60:697–713, 1985.

75. Greenberg, HS, Chandler, WF, Diaz, RF, Ensminger, WD, Junck, L, Page, MA, Gebarski, SS, McKeever, P, Hood, TW, Stetson, PL, Litchter, AS, and Tankanow, R: Intra-arterial bromodeoxyuridine radiosensitization and radiation treatment of malignant astrocytomas. J Neurosurg 69:500–505, 1988.

76. Greenberg, HS, Ensminger, WD, Chandler, WF, Layton, PB, Junck, L, Knake, J, and Vine, AK: Intra-arterial BCNU chemotherapy for treatment of malignant gliomas of the central nervous system. J Neurosurg 61:423–429, 1984.

77. Guthrie, BL, Steinberg, GK, and Adler, JR: Posterior fossa stereotaxic biopsy using the Brown-Robert-Wells stereotaxic system: Technical note. J Neurosurg 70:649–652, 1989.

78. Gutin, PH, Leibel, SA, Wara, WM, Larson, D, Phillips, T, and Silver, P: Survival and quality of life following interstitial implantation of removable high activity iodine-125 sources for recurrent malignant gliomas (abstr). J Clin Oncol 8:84, 1989.

79. Gutin, PH, Phillips, TL, Wara, WM, Leibel, SA, Hosobuchi, Y, Levin, VA, Weaver, KA, and Lamb, S: Brachytherapy of recurrent malignant brain tumors with removable high-activity iodine-125 sources. J Neurosurg 60:61–68, 1984.

80. Harsh, GR, Levin, VA, Gutin, PH, Seager, M, Silver, P, and Wilson, CB: Reoperation for recurrent glioblastoma and anaplastic astrocytoma. Neurosurgery 21:615–621, 1987.

81. Harsh, GR and Wilson, CB: Neuroepithelial tumors of the adult brain. In Youmans, JR (ed): Neurological Surgery, ed 3, Vol 5. WB Saunders, Philadelphia, 1990, pp 3040–3136.

82. Hawkins, JC: Treatment of choroid plexus papillomas in children: A brief analysis of twenty years experience. Neurosurgery 6:380–384, 1980.

83. Healy, ME, Hesselink, JR, Press, GA, and Middleton, MS: Increased detection of intracranial metastases with intravenous Gd–DTPA. Radiology 165:619–624, 1987.

84. Hirakawa, K, Naruse, S, Higuchi, T, Horikawa, Y, Tanaka, C, and Ebisu, T: The investigation of experimental brain tumors using ^{31}P-MRS and ^{1}H-MRI. Acta Neurochir Suppl (Wien) 43:140–144, 1988.

85. Hirsch, JR, Rose, CS, Pierre-Kahn, A, Pfister, A, and Hoppe-Hirsch, E: Benign astrocytic and oligodendrocytic tumors of the cerebral hemispheres in children. J Neurosurg 70:568–572, 1989.

86. Hochberg, FH and Miller, DC: Primary central nervous system lymphoma: Review article. J Neurosurg 68:835–853, 1988.

87. Hochberg, FH and Pruitt, A: Assumptions in the radiotherapy of glioblastoma. Neurology 30:907–911, 1980.

88. Hochberg, FH, Pruitt, AA, Beck, DO, DeBrun, G, and Davis, K: The rationale and methodology for intra-arterial chemotherapy with BCNU as treatment for glioblastoma. J Neurosurg 63:876–880, 1985.

89. Hoffman, HJ, Becker, L, and Craven, MA: A clinically and pathologically distinct group of benign brain stem gliomas. Neurosurgery 7: 243–248, 1980.
90. Hoffman, HJ, Hendrick, EB, and Humphreys, RP: Management of medulloblastoma in childhood. Clin Neurosurg 30:226–245, 1983.
91. Hood, TW, Gebarski, SS, McKeever, PE, and Venes, JL: Stereotaxic biopsy of intrinsic lesions of the brain stem. J Neurosurg 65:172–176, 1986.
92. Horm, JW, Asire, AJ, Young, JL, and Pollak, ES (eds): SEER Program: Cancer Incidence and Mortality in the United States 1973–1981. National Cancer Institute, Bethesda, MD, 1984, p 53.
93. Hoshino, T: A commentary on the biology and growth kinetics of low-grade and high-grade gliomas. J Neurosurg 61:895–900, 1984.
94. Hoshino, T, Barker, M, Wilson, CB, Boldrey, EB, and Fewer, D: Cell kinetics of human gliomas. J Neurosurg 37:15–26, 1972.
95. Hoshino T, Rodriguez, LA, Cho, KG, Lee, KS, Wilson, CB, Edwards, MSB, Levin, VA, and Davis, RL: Prognostic implications of the proliferative potential of low-grade astrocytomas. J Neurosurg 69:839–842, 1988.
96. Hoshino, T and Wilson, CB: Cell kinetic analysis of human malignant brain tumors (gliomas). Cancer 44:956–962, 1979.
97. Hubbard, JL, Scheithauer, BW, Kispert, DB, Carpenter, SM, Wick, MR, and Laws, ER: Adult cerebellar medulloblastomas: The pathological, radiographic, and clinical disease spectrum. J Neurosurg 70:536–544, 1989.
98. Hubesch, B, Sappey-Marinier, DS, Roth, K, Meyerhoff, DJ, Matson, GB, and Weiner, MW: ^{31}P NMR spectroscopy of normal human brain and brain tumors. Radiology 174(2):401–409, 1990.
99. Hughes, EN, Shillito, J, Sallan, SE, Loeffler, JS, Cassady, JR, and Tarbell, N: Medulloblastoma at the Joint Center for Radiation Therapy between 1968 and 1984. Cancer 61:1992–1998, 1988.
100. Jacobs, SK, Wilson, DJ, Kornblith, PL, and Grimm, EA: Interleukin-2 autologous lymphokine-activated killer cell treatment of malignant glioma: Phase 1 trial. Cancer Res 46:2101–2104, 1986.
101. James, H: Choroid plexus papillomas. In Wilkins, JH and Rengachary, SS (eds): Neurosurgery, Vol 1. McGraw-Hill, New York, 1985, p 783.
102. Jenkin, RDT, Boesel, C, Ertel, I, Evans, A, Hittle, R, Ortega, J, Sposto, R, Wara, WM, Wilson, CW, Anderson, J, Leikin, S, and Hammond, D: Brain tumors in childhood: A prospective randomized trial of irradiation with and without adjuvant CCNU, VCR, and prednisone. A report of the Childrens Cancer Study Group. J Neurosurg 66:227–233, 1987.
103. Johnson, DW, Parkinson, D, Wolpert, SM, Kasdon, DL, Kwan, ES, Laucella, M, and Anderson, ML: Intracarotid chemotherapy with 1,3-bis-(2-chloroethyl)-1-nitrosourea (BCNU) in 5% dextrose in water in the treatment of malignant glioma. Neurosurgery 20:577–583, 1987.
104. Kaye, AH, Morstyn, G, and Apuzzo, MLJ: Photoradiation therapy and its potential in the management of neurological tumors: Review article. J Neurosurg 69:1–14, 1988.
105. Kelly, P: Stereotactic technology in tumor surgery. Clin Neurosurg 35:215–253, 1987.
106. Kelly, P: Volumetric stereotactic surgical resection of intra-axial brain mass lesions. Mayo Clin Proc 63:1186–1198, 1988.
107. Kelly, PJ and Alker, GJ: A stereotactic approach to deep-seated central nervous system neoplasms using the carbon dioxide laser. Surg Neurol 15:331–334, 1981.
108. Kelly, PJ, Daumas-Duport, C, Scheithauer, BW, Kall, BA, and Kispert, DB: Stereotactic correlations of computed tomography– and magnetic resonance imaging–defined abnormalities in patients with glial neoplasms. Mayo Clin Proc 62:450–459, 1987.
109. Kernohan, JW, Mabon, RF, Svien, HJ, and Adson, AW: A simplified classification of gliomas. Mayo Clin Proc 24:71–75, 1949.
110. Kimmel, DW, Shapiro, JR, and Shapiro, WR: In-vitro drug sensitivity testing in human glioma: Review article. J Neurosurg 66:161–171, 1987.
111. Kinzler, KW, Bigner, SH, Bigner, DD, Trent, JM, Law, ML, O'Brien, SJ, Wong, AJ, and Vogelstein, B: Identification of an amplified, highly expressed gene in a human glioma. Science 236:70–73, 1987.
112. Knake, JE, Chandler, WF, Gabrielsen, TO, Latack, JT, and Gebarski, SS: Intraoperative sonographic delineation of low-grade neoplasms defined poorly by computed tomography. Radiology 151:735–739, 1984.
113. Kornblith, PL and Walker, M: Chemotherapy for malignant gliomas: Review article. J Neurosurg 68:1–17, 1988.
114. Kucharczyk, W, Brant-Zawadzki, M, Sobel, D, Edwards, MB, Kelly, WM, Norman, D, and Newton, TH: Central nervous system tumors in children: Detection by magnetic resonance imaging. Radiology 155:131–136, 1985.
115. Kum, LE, Kovnar, EH, and Sanford, RA: Ependymomas in children. Pediatr Neurosci 14:57–63, 1988.
116. Kuppner, MC, Hamou, MF, and De Tribolet, N: Immunohistological and functional analyses of lymphoid infiltrates in human glioblastomas. Cancer Res 48:6926–6932, 1988.
117. Kurland, LT, Schoenberg, BS, and Anneger, JF: The incidence of primary intracranial neoplasms in Rochester, Minnesota. Ann NY Acad Sci 381:6–16, 1982.
118. Lashford, LS, Davies, G, Richardson, RB, Bourne, SP, Bullimore, JA, Eckert, H, Kemshead, JT, and Coakham, HB: A pilot study of I-131 monoclonal antibodies in the therapy of leptomeningeal tumors. Cancer 61:857–868, 1988.
119. Launay, M, Fredy, D, Merland, JJ, and Bories, J: Narrowing and occlusion of arteries by intra-

cranial tumors. Neuroradiology 14:117–126, 1977.

120. Laws, ER, Taylor, WF, Bergstralh, EJ, Okazaki, H, and Clifton, MB: The neurosurgical management of low-grade astrocytomas. Clin Neurosurg 33:575–588, 1985.

121. Laws, ER, Taylor, WF, Clifton, MB, and Okazaki, H: Neurosurgical management of low-grade astrocytoma of the cerebral hemispheres. J Neurosurg 61:665–673, 1984.

122. Leavens, ME, Manning, JT, Wallace, S, Maor, MH, and Velasquez, WS: Primary lymphoma of the central nervous system. In Wilkins, RH and Rengachary, SS (eds): Neurosurgery, Vol 1. McGraw-Hill, New York, 1985, p 1022.

123. Lee, Y, Bullard, DE, Humphrey, PA, Colapinto, EV, Friedman, HS, Zalutsky, MR, Coleman, RE, and Bigner, DD: Treatment of intracranial human glioma xenografts with ^{131}I-labeled anti-tenascin monoclonal antibody 81C6. Cancer Res 48:2904–2910, 1988.

124. Lee, Y, Bullard, DE, Zalutsky, MR, Coleman, RE, Wikstrand, CJ, Friedman, HS, Colapinto, EV, and Bigner, DD: Therapeutic efficacy of antiglioma mesenchymal extracellular matrix ^{131}I-radiolabeled murine monoclonal antibody in human glioma xenograft model. Cancer Res 48:559–566, 1988.

125. Leibel, SA and Sheline, GE: Radiation therapy for neoplasms of the brain: Review article. J Neurosurg 66:1–22, 1987.

126. Leibel, SA, Sheline, GE, Wara, WM, Boldrey, EB, and Nielsen, SL: The role of radiation therapy in the treatment of astrocytomas. Cancer 35:1551–1557, 1975.

127. Leksell, L: Stereotactic radiosurgery. J Neurol Neurosurg Psychiatry 46:797–803, 1983.

128. Levin, VA, Chamberlain, MC, Prados, MD, Choucair, AK, Berger, MS, Silver, P, Seager, M, Gutin, PH, Davis, RL, and Wilson, CB: Phase I–II study of eflornithine and mitoguazone combined in the treatment of recurrent primary brain tumors. Cancer Treat Rep 71:459–464, 1987.

129. Levin, VA, Edwards, MS, Wara, WM, Allen, J, Ortega, J, and Vestnys, P: 5-Fluorouracil and 1 - (2 - chloroethyl) - 3 - cyclohexyl - 1 - nitrosourea (CCNU) followed by hydroxyurea, misonidazole, and irradiation for brain stem gliomas: A pilot study of the Brain Tumor Research Center and the Childrens Cancer Group. Neurosurgery 14:679–681, 1984.

130. Levin, VA, Kabra, PM, and Freeman-Dove, MA: Pharmacokinetics of intracarotid artery ^{14}C-BCNU in the squirrel monkey. J Neurosurg 48:587–593, 1978.

131. Levin, VA, Rodriguez, LA, Edwards, MSB, Wara, WM, Liu, HC, Fulton, D, Davis RL, Wilson, CB, and Silver, P: Treatment of medulloblastoma with procarbazine, hydroxyurea, and reduced radiation doses to whole brain and spine. J Neurosurg 68:383–387, 1988.

132. Levin, VA, Wilson, CB, Davis, R, Wara, WM, Pischer, TL, and Irwin, L: A phase III comparison of BCNU, hydroxyurea, and radiation therapy to BCNU and radiation therapy for the treatment of primary malignant gliomas. J Neurosurg 51:526–532, 1979.

133. Lindegaard, KF, Mork, SJ, Eide, G, Halvorsen, TB, Hatlevoli, R, Solgaard, T, Dahl, O, and Ganz, J: Statistical analysis of clinicopathologic features, radiotherapy, and survival in 170 cases of oligodendroglioma. J Neurosurg 67:224–230, 1987.

134. Liu, HC, Davis, RL, Vestnys, P, Resser, KJ, and Levin, VA: Correlation of survival and diagnosis in supra-tentorial malignant gliomas (abstr). J Neurooncol 2:268, 1984.

135. Loeffler, JS, Kretschmar, CS, Sallan, SE, LaVally, BL, Winston, KR, Fischer, EG, and Tarbell, NJ: Pre-radiation chemotherapy for infants and poor prognosis children with medulloblastoma. Int J Radiat Oncol Biol Phys 15:177–181, 1988.

136. Loew, F and Papavero, L: The intraarterial route of drug delivery in the chemotherapy of malignant brain tumors. Adv Tech Stand Neurosurg 16:53–79, 1988.

137. Ludgate, CM, Douglas, BG, Dixon, PF, Steinbok, P, Jackson, SM, and Goodman, GB: Superfractionated radiotherapy in grade III, IV intracranial gliomas. Int J Radiat Oncol Biol Phys 15:1091–1095, 1988.

138. Lunsford, LD, Flickinger, J, Linder, G, and Maitz, A: Stereotactic radiosurgery of the brain using the first United States 201 cobalt-60 source gamma knife. Neurosurgery 24:151–159, 1989.

139. Mahaley, MS, Bertsch, L, Cush, S, and Gillespie, GY: Systemic gamma-interferon therapy for recurrent gliomas. J Neurosurg 69:826–829, 1988.

140. Mahaley, MS, Hipp, SW, Dropcho, EJ, Bertsch, L, Cush, S, Tirey, T, and Gillespie, GY: Intracarotid cisplatin chemotherapy for recurrent gliomas. J Neurosurg 70:371–378, 1989.

141. Mahaley, MS, Urso, M, Whaley, RA, Blue, M, Williams, TE, Guaspari, A, and Selker, RG: Immunobiology of primary intracranial tumors. Part 10: Therapeutic efficacy of interferon in the treatment of recurrent gliomas. J Neurosurg 63:719–725, 1985.

142. Mallya, KB, Galicich, JH, Arbit, E, and Krol, G: The role of CT-documented gross total resection in the combined modality treatment of malignant gliomas (abstr). Can J Neurol Sci 16:237, 1989.

143. Margetts, JC and Kalyan-Raman, UP: Giant-celled glioblastoma of the brain: A clinico-pathological and radiological study of ten cases (including immunohistochemistry and ultrastructure). Cancer 63:524–531, 1989.

144. McDonald, JD and Dohrmann, GJ: Molecular biology of brain tumors. Neurosurgery 23:537–544, 1988.

145. McGahan, JP, Ellis, WG, Budenz, RW, Walter, JP, and Boggan, J: Brain gliomas: Sonographic

characterization. Radiology 159:485–492, 1986.

146. McGirr, SJ, Ebersold, MJ, Scheithauer, BW, Quast, LM, and Shaw, EG: Choroid plexus papilloma: Long-term follow-up results in a surgically treated series. J Neurosurg 69:843–849, 1988.

147. McLaughlin, P, Velasquez, WS, Redman, JR, Yung, WKA, Hagemeister, FB, Rodriguez, MA, and Cabanillas, F: Chemotherapy with dexamethasone, high-dose cytarabine, and cisplatin for parenchymal brain lymphoma. J Natl Cancer Inst 80:1408–1412, 1988.

148. Medberry, CA, Straus, KL, Steinberg, SM, Cotelingam, JD, and Fisher, WS: Low-grade astrocytomas: Treatment results and prognostic variables. Int J Radiat Oncol Biol Phys 15:837–841, 1988.

149. Merchant, RE, Grant, AJ, Merchant, LH, and Young, HF: Adoptive immunotherapy for recurrent glioblastoma multiforme using lymphokine activated killer cells and recombinant interleukin-2. Cancer 62:665–671, 1988.

150. Merchant, RE, Merchant, LH, Cook, SHS, McVicar, DW, and Young, HF: Intralesional infusion of lymphokine-activated killer (LAK) cells and recombinant interleukin-2 (rIL-2) for the treatment of patients with malignant brain tumor. Neurosurgery 23:725–732, 1988.

151. Miescher, S, Whiteside, TL, De Tribolet, N, and Von Fliedner, V: In situ characterization, clonogenic potential, and antitumor cytolytic activity of T lymphocytes infiltrating human brain cancers. J Neurosurg 68:438–448, 1988.

152. Miyatake, SI, Kikuchi, H, Iwasaki, K, Yamashita, J, Li, Y, Namba, Y, and Hawaoka, M: Specific cytotoxic activity of T lymphocyte clones derived from a patient with gliosarcoma. J Neurosurg 69:751–759, 1988.

153. Morantz, RA: Radiation therapy in the treatment of cerebral astrocytoma. Neurosurgery 20:975–982, 1987.

154. Mork, SJ, Lindegaard, KF, Halvorsen, TB, Lehmann, EH, Solgaard, T, Hatlevoll, R, Harvel, S, and Ganz, J: Oligodendroglioma: Incidence and biological behavior in a defined population. J Neurosurg 63:881–889, 1985.

155. Mork, SJ and Loken, AC: Ependymoma: A follow-up study of 101 cases. Cancer 40:907–915, 1977.

156. Mukai, N and Kobayashi, S: Human adenovirus–induced medulloepitheliomatous neoplasms in Sprague-Dawley rats. Am J Pathol 73:671–690, 1973.

157. Muller, PJ and Wilson, BC: Photodynamic therapy of malignant brain tumors (abstr). Can J Neurol Sci 16:260, 1989.

158. Muller, W, Afra, D, and Schroder, R: Supratentorial recurrences of gliomas: Morphological studies in relation to time intervals with as-trocytoma. Acta Neurochir (Wien) 37:75–91, 1977.

159. Nagashima, T, Hoshino, T, Cho, KG, Edwards, MSB, Hudgins, RJ, and Davis, RL: The proliferative potential of human ependymomas measured by in situ bromodeoxyuridine labeling. Cancer 61:2433–2438, 1988.

160. Nelson, DF, Diener-West, M, Weinstein, AS, Schoenfeld, D, Nelson, JS, Sause, WT, Chang, CH, Goodman, R, and Carabell, S: A randomized comparison of misonidazole sensitized radiotherapy plus BCNU and radiotherapy plus BCNU for the treatment of malignant glioma after surgery: Final report of an RTOG study. Int J Radiat Oncol Biol Phys 12:1793–1800, 1986.

161. Nelson, DF, Urtasun, RC, Saunders, WM, Gutin, PH, and Sheline, GE: Recent and current investigations of radiation therapy of malignant gliomas. Semin Oncol 13:46–55, 1986.

162. Nelson, JS, Tsukada, Y, Schoenfield, D, Fulling, K, Lamarche, J, and Peress, N: Necrosis as a prognostic criterion in malignant supratentorial, astrocytic gliomas. Cancer 52:550–554, 1983.

163. Neuwelt, EA: Therapeutic potential for blood-brain barrier modification in malignant brain tumor. Prog Exp Tumor Res 28:51–60, 1984.

164. Newman, HFV, Bleehen, NM, Ward, R, and Workman, P: Hypoxic cell radiosensitizers in the treatment of high grade gliomas: A new direction using combined RO 03-8799 (pimonidazole) and SR 2508 (etanidazole). Int J Radiol Oncol Biol Phys 15:677–684, 1988.

165. Niizuma, H, Otsuki, T, Yonemitsu, T, Kitahara, M, Katakura, R, and Suzuki, J: Experience with CT-guided stereotaxic biopsies in 121 cases. Acta Neurochir (Wien) 42:157–160, 1988.

166. Nishio, S, Tashima, T, Takeshima, I, and Fukui, M: Intraventricular neurocytoma: Clinicopathological features of six cases. J Neurosurg 68:665–670, 1988.

167. Nishizaki, T, Orita, T, Furutani, Y, Ikeyama, Y, Aoki, H, and Sasaki, K: Flow-cytometric DNA analysis and immunohistochemical measurement of Ki-67 and BUDR labeling indices in human brain tumors. J Neurosurg 70:379–384, 1989.

168. Nister, M, Heldin, CH, Wasteson, A, and Westermark, B: A glioma derived analogue to platelet derived growth factor: Demonstration of receptor competing activity and immunological cross reactivity. Proc Natl Acad Sci U S A 81:926–930, 1984.

169. O'Brien, MS and Johnson, MM: Brain stem gliomas. In Wilkins, RH and Rengachary, SS (eds): Neurosurgery, Vol 1. McGraw-Hill, New York, 1985, p 762.

170. Oldfield, EH, Clark, WC, Dedrick, RL, Egorin, MJ, Austin, HA, DeVroom, HD, Joyce, KM, and Doppman, JL: Reduced systemic drug expo-

sure by combining intraarterial cis-diamine-dichloroplatinum (II) with hemodialysis of regional venous drainage. Cancer Res 47: 1962–1967, 1987.

171. Packer, RJ and Finlay, JL: Medulloblastoma: Presentation, diagnosis and management. Oncology 2:35–49, 1988.

172. Packer, RJ, Littman, PA, Sposto, RM, D'Angio, G, Priest, JR, Heideman, RL, Bruce, DA, and Nelson, DF: Results of a pilot study of hyperfractionated radiation therapy for children with brain stem gliomas. Int J Radiat Oncol Biol Phys 13:1647–1651, 1987.

173. Packer, RJ, Siegel, KR, Sutton, LN, Evans, AE, D'Angio, G, Rorke, LB, Bunin, GR, and Schut, L: Efficacy of adjuvant chemotherapy for patients with poor risk medulloblastoma: A preliminary report. Ann Neurol 24:503–508, 1988.

174. Packer, RJ, Zimmerman, RA, Luerssen, TG, Sutton, LN, Bilaniuk, LT, Bruce, DA, and Schut, L: Brain stem gliomas of childhood: Magnetic resonance imaging. Neurology 35:397–401, 1985.

175. Palma, L, Celli, P, Maleci, A, Di Lorenzo, N, and Cantore, G: Malignant monstrocellular brain tumors: A study of 42 surgically treated cases. Acta Neurochir (Wien) 97:17–25, 1989.

176. Palma, L, Di Lorenzo, N, and Guidetti, B: Lymphocytic infiltrates in primary glioblastomas and recidivous gliomas. J Neurosurg 49: 854–861, 1978.

177. Pendergrass, TW, Milstein, JM, Geyer, JR, Mulne, AF, Kosnik, EJ, Morris, JD, Heideman, RL, Ruymann, FB, Stuntz, JT, and Bleyer, WA: Eight drugs in one day chemotherapy for brain tumors: Experience in 107 children and rationale for preradiation chemotherapy. J Clin Oncol 5:1221–1231, 1987.

178. Piepmeier, JM: Observations on the current treatment of low-grade astrocytic tumors of the cerebral hemispheres. J Neurosurg 67:177–181, 1987.

179. Podgorsak, EB, Pike, GB, Olivier, A, Pla, M, and Souhami, L: Radiosurgery with high energy photons beams: A comparison among techniques. Int J Radiat Oncol Biol Phys 16:857–865, 1989.

180. Pollack, IF, Lunsford, LD, Flickinger, JC, and Dameshek, HL: Prognostic factors in the diagnosis and treatment of primary central nervous system lymphoma. Cancer 63:939–947, 1989.

181. Prados, M: Personal communication, June 1989.

182. Prados, M, Rodriguez, L, Chamberlain, M, Silver, P, and Levin, VA: Treatment of recurrent gliomas with 1,3-bis(2-chloroethyl)-1-nitrosourea and alpha-difluoromethylornithine. Neurosurgery 24:806–809, 1989.

183. Prados, MD, Levin, VA, Hoshino, T, and Wilson, CB: Chemotherapy of brain tumors. In Youmans, JR (ed): Neurological Surgery, ed 3, Vol 5. WB Saunders, Philadelphia 1990, pp 3412–3425.

184. Raimondi, AJ and Gutierrez, FA: Diagnosis and surgical treatment of choroid plexus papillomas. Child's Nerv Syst 1:81–115, 1975.

185. Rawlings, CE, Giangaspero, F, Burger, PC, and Bullard, DE: Ependymomas: A clinicopathologic study. Surg Neurol 29:271–281, 1988.

186. Ringertz, N: Grading of gliomas. Acta Pathol Microbiol Scand 27:51–64, 1950.

187. Rorke, LB: Relationship of morphology of ependymoma in children to prognosis. Prog Exp Tumor Res 30:170–174, 1987.

188. Rosen, N, Reynolds, CP, Thiele, CJ, Biedler, JL, and Israel, MA: Increased n-myc expression following progressive growth of human neuroblastoma. Cancer Res 46:4139–4142, 1986.

189. Rosenberg, SA, Lotze, MT, Muul, LM, Chang, AE, Avis, FP, Leitman, S, Linehan, M, Robertson, CN, Lee, RE, Rubin, JT, Seipp, CA, Simpson, CG, and White, DE: A progress report on the treatment of 157 patients with advanced cancer using lymphokine-activated killer cells and interleukin-2 or high dose interleukin-2 alone. N Engl J Med 316:889–897, 1987.

190. Rosenberg, SA, Spiess, P, and Lafreniere, R: A new approach to the adoptive immunotherapy of cancer with tumor infiltrating lymphocytes. Science 233:1318–1321, 1986.

191. Rosenblum, ML, Berens, ME, and Rutka, JT: Recent perspectives in brain tumor biology and treatment. Clin Neurosurg 35:314–335, 1987.

192. Rosenblum, ML, Levy, RM, and Bredesen, DE: Overview of AIDS and the nervous system. In Rosenblum, ML, Levy, RM, and Bredesen, DE (eds): AIDS and the Nervous System. Raven Press, New York, 1988, p 1.

193. Ross, GW and Rubinstein, LJ: Lack of histopathological correlation of malignant ependymomas with postoperative survival. J Neurosurg 70:31–36, 1989.

194. Russell, DS and Rubinstein, LJ: Pathology of Tumors of the Nervous System, ed 5. Williams & Wilkins, Baltimore, 1989.

195. Rutka, JT, Apodaca, G, Stern, R, and Rosenblum, M: The extracellular matrix of the central and peripheral nervous systems: Structure and function. Review article. J Neurosurg 69:155–170, 1988.

196. Rutka, JT, Giblin, JR, Apodaca, G, De Armond, ST, Stern, R, and Rosenblum, ML: Inhibition of growth and induction of differentiation in a malignant human glioma cell line by normal leptomeningeal extracellular matrix proteins. Cancer Res 47:3515–3522, 1987.

197. Rutten, EHJM, Kazem, I, Slooff, JL, and Walder, AHD: Post operative radiation therapy in the management of brain astrocytomata: Retrospective study of 142 patients. Int J Radiat Oncol Biol Phys 7:191–195, 1981.

198. Saito, T, Tanaka, R, Yoshida, S, Washiyama, K, and Kumanishi, T: Immunohistochemical analysis of tumor-infiltrating lymphocytes and

major histocompatibility antigens in human gliomas and metastatic brain tumors. Surg Neurol 29:435–442, 1988.

199. Salazar, OM, Castro-Vita, H, VanHoutte, P, Rubin, P, and Aygun, C: Improved survival in cases of intracranial ependymoma after radiation therapy. J Neurosurg 59:652–659, 1983.

200. Salcman, M: Resection and reoperation in neuro-oncology: Rationale and approach. Neurol Clin 3:831–842, 1985.

201. Salcman, M: Supratentorial gliomas: Clinical features and surgical therapy. In Wilkins, RH and Rengachary, SS (eds): Neurosurgery, Vol 1. McGraw-Hill, New York, 1985, p 579.

202. Salcman, M: Surgical decision making for malignant brain tumors. Clin Neurosurg 35:285–313, 1987.

203. Salcman, M, Kaplan, RS, Ducker, TB, Abdo, H, and Montgomery, E: Effect of age and reoperation on survival in the combined modality treatment of malignant astrocytoma. Neurosurgery 10:454–463, 1982.

204. Sanford, RA, Freeman, CR, Burger, P, and Cohen, ME: Prognostic criteria for experimental protocols in pediatric brainstem gliomas. Surg Neurol 30:276–280, 1988.

205. Sano, K: Integrative treatment of gliomas. Clin Neurosurg 30:93–124, 1983.

206. Sawamura, Y, Abe, H, Aida, T, Hosokawa, M, and Kobayashi, H: Isolation and in vitro growth of glioma-infiltrating lymphocytes and an analysis of their surface phenotypes. J Neurosurg 69:745–750, 1988.

207. Scanlon, PW and Taylor, WF: Radiotherapy of intracranial astrocytomas: Analysis of 417 cases treated from 1960 through 1969. Neurosurgery 5:301–308, 1979.

208. Schmidek, HH: The molecular genetics of nervous system tumors: Review article. J Neurosurg 67:1–16, 1987.

209. Schold, SC, Brent, TP, Von Hofe, E, Friedman, HS, Mitra, S, Bigner, DD, Swenberg, JA, and Kleihues, P: O⁶-alkylguanine-DNA alkyltransferase and sensitivity to procarbazine in human brain tumor xenografts. J Neurosurg 70:573–577, 1989.

210. Seeger, RC, Brodeur, GM, Sather, H, Dalton, A, Siegel, SSE, Wong, KY, and Hammond, D: Association of multiple copies of the n-myc oncogene with rapid progression of neuroblastoma. N Engl J Med 313:1111–1116, 1985.

211. Segebarth, CM, Baleriaux, DF, Arnold, DL, Luyten, PR, and Hollander, JA: MR image-guided P-31 MR spectroscopy in the evaluation of brain tumor treatment. Radiology 165:215–219, 1987.

212. Shapiro, WR and Green, SB: Letter to the Editor. J Neurosurg 66:313–315, 1987.

213. Shapiro, WR, Green, SB, Burger, PC, Mahaley, MS, Selker, RG, Van Gilder, JC, Robertson, JT, Ransohoff, J, Mealey, J, Strike, TA, and Pistenmaa, DA: Randomized trial of 3 chemotherapy regimens and 2 radiotherapy regimens in postoperative treatment of

malignant glioma. Brain Tumor Cooperative Trial 8001. J Neurosurg 71:1–9, 1989.

214. Shaw, EG, Daumas-Duport, C, Schithauer, BW, Gilbertson, DT, O'Fallon, JR, Earle, JD, Laws, ER, and Okazaki, H: Radiation therapy in the management of low-grade supratentorial astrocytomas. J Neurosurg 70:853–861, 1989.

215. Shaw, EG, Evans, RG, Scheithauer, BW, Ilstrup, DM, and Earle, JD: Postoperative radiotherapy of intracranial ependymoma in pediatric and adult patients. Int J Radiat Oncol Biol Phys 13:1457–1462, 1987.

216. Shaw, EG, Scheithauer, BW, Gilbertson, DT, Nichols, DA, Laws, ER, Earle, JD, Daumas-Duport, C, O'Fallon, J, and Dinapoli, RP: Postoperative radiotherapy of supratentorial low-grade gliomas. Int J Radiat Oncol Biol Phys 16:663–668, 1988.

217. Sheline, GE and Wara, WM: Radiation therapy of brain tumors. In Youmans, JR (ed): Neurological Surgery, Vol 5. WB Saunders, Philadelphia, 1982, p 3096.

218. Shibata, S: Sites of origin of primary intracerebral malignant lymphoma. Neurosurgery 25:14–19, 1989.

219. Silverman, C and Marks, JE: Prognostic significance of contrast enhancement in low-grade astrocytomas of the adult cerebrum. Radiology 139:211–213, 1981.

220. Soffietti, R, Chio, A, Giordana, MT, Vasario, E, and Schiffer, D: Prognostic factors in well-differentiated cerebral astrocytomas in the adult. Neurosurgery 24:686–692, 1989.

221. Stroink, AR, Hoffman, HJ, Hendrick, EB, Humphreys, RP, and Davidson, G: Transependymal benign dorsally exophytic brain stem gliomas in childhood: Diagnosis and treatment recommendations. Neurosurgery 20:439–444, 1987.

222. Sturm, V, Kober, B, Hover, KH, Schlegel, W, Boesecke, R, Pastyr, O, Hartmann, GH, Schabbert, S, Winkel, KZ, Kunze, S, and Lorenz, W: Stereotactic percutaneous single dose irradiation of brain metastases with a linear accelerator. Int J Radiat Oncol Biol Phys 13:279–282, 1987.

223. Sun, ZM, Genka, S, Shitara, N, Akanuma, A, and Takakura, K: Factors possibly influencing the prognosis of oligodendroglioma. Neurosurgery 22:886–891, 1988.

224. Sutherland, GR, Florell, R, Louw, D, Choi, NW, and Sima, AAF: Epidemiology of primary intracranial neoplasms in Manitoba, Canada. Can J Neurol Sci 14:586–592, 1987.

225. Swenberg, JA: Chemical induction of brain tumors. Adv Neurol 15:85–99, 1976.

226. Sze, G, Shin, J, Krol, G, Johnson, C, Liu, D, and Deck, MDF: Intraparenchymal brain metastases: MR imaging versus contrast-enhanced CT. Radiology 168:187–194, 1988.

227. Tew, JM and Tobler, WD: The laser: History, biophysics and neurosurgical applications. Clin Neurosurg 31:506–549, 1984.

228. Thomsen, C, Jensen, KE, Achten, E, and Henrik-

sen, O: In vivo magnetic resonance imaging and ^{31}P spectroscopy of large human brain tumors at 1.5 Tesla. Acta Radiol 29:77–82, 1988.

229. Tomita, T and McLone, DG: Medulloblastoma in childhood: Results of radical resection and low-dose neuraxis radiation therapy. J Neurosurg 64:238–242, 1986.

230. Tomita, T, McLone, DG, and Flannery, AM: Choroid plexus papillomas of neonates, infants and children. Pediatr Neurosci 14:23–30, 1988.

231. Tsuda, T, Obara, M, Hirano, H, Gotoh, S, Kubomura, S, Higashi, K, Kuroiwa, A, Nakagawara, A, Nagahara, N, and Shimizu, K: Analysis of n-myc amplification in relation to disease stage and histologic types in human neuroblastoma. Cancer 60:820–826, 1987.

232. University of California, San Francisco, Cancer Program Annual Report, 1988.

233. Urtasun, RC, Fulton, D, Huyser-Wierenga, D, Scott-Brown, I, Shin, K, Geggie, P, and Hanson, J: Dose intensity in radiotherapy: "Is more better" for patients with malignant gliomas (abstr). J Clin Oncol 8:84, 1989.

234. Valk, PE, Budinger, TF, Levin, VA, Silver, P, Gutin, PH, and Doyle, WK: PET of malignant cerebral tumors after interstitial brachytherapy: Demonstration of metabolic activity and correlation with clinical outcome. J Neurosurg 69:830–838, 1988.

235. Velema, JP and Percy, CL: Age curves of central nervous system tumor incidence in adults: Variation of shape by histologic type. J Natl Cancer Inst 79:623–629, 1987.

236. Walker, AE, Robins, M, and Weinfeld, FD: Epidemiology of brain tumors: The national survey of intracranial neoplasms. Neurology 35:219–226, 1985.

237. Walker, MD, Alexander, E, Hunt, WE, MacCarty, CS, Mahaley, MS, Mealey, J, Norrell, HA, Owens, G, Ransohoff, J, Wilson, CB, Gehan, EA, and Strike, TA: Evaluation of BCNU and/or radiotherapy in the treatment of anaplastic gliomas. J Neurosurg 49:333–343, 1978.

238. Walker, MD, Green, SB, Byar, DP, Alexander, E, Batzdorf, U, Brooks, WH, Hunt, WE, MacCarty, CS, Mahaley, MS, Mealey, J, Owens, G, Ransohoff, J, Robertson, JT, Shapiro, WR, Smith, KR, Wilson, CB, and Strike, TA: Randomized comparisons of radiotherapy and nitrosoureas for the treatment of malignant glioma after surgery. N Engl J Med 303: 1323–1329, 1980.

239. Walker, MD, Strike, TA, and Sheline, GE: An analysis of dose-effect relationship in the radiotherapy of malignant gliomas. Int J Radiat Oncol Biol Phys 5:1725–1731, 1979.

240. Wallner, KE, Galicich, JH, Kroll, G, Arbit, E, and Malkin, MG: Patterns of failure following treatment for glioblastoma multiforme and anaplastic astrocytoma. Int J Radiat Biol Phys 16:1405–1409, 1989.

241. Wallner, KE, Gonzales, M, and Sheline, G: Treatment of oligodendrogliomas with or without postoperative irradiation. J Neurosurg 68: 684–688, 1988.

242. Wallner, KE, Gonzales, MF, Edwards, MSB, Wara, WM, and Sheline, GE: Treatment results of juvenile pilocytic astrocytoma. J Neurosurg 69:171–176, 1988.

243. Wara, WM: Radiation therapy for brain tumors. Cancer 55:2291–2295, 1985.

244. Weir, B: The relative significance of factors affecting postoperative survival in astrocytomas, grades 3 and 4. J Neurosurg 38:448–452, 1978.

245. Weir, B and Elvidge, AR: Oligodendrogliomas: An analysis of 63 cases. J Neurosurg 29:500–505, 1968.

246. Weir, B and Grace, M: The relative significance of factors affecting postoperative survival in astrocytomas, grades one and two. Can J Neurol Sci 3:47–50, 1976.

247. Wilson, CB, Boldrey, EB, and Enot, KJ: 1,3-bis(2-chloroethyl)-1-nitrosourea (NSC-409962) in the treatment of brain tumors. Cancer Treat Re 54:273–281, 1970.

248. Winston, KR and Lutz, W: Linear accelerator as a neurosurgical tool for stereotactic radiosurgery. Neurosurgery 22:454–464, 1988.

249. Wise, RJS, Thomas, DGT, Lammertsua, AA, and Rhodes, CG: PET scanning of human brain tumors. Prog Exp Tumor Res 27:154–169, 1984.

250. Wolff, SN, Phillips, GL, and Herzig, GP: High-dose carmustine with autologous bone marrow transplantation for the adjuvant treatment of high-grade gliomas of the central nervous system. Cancer Treat Rep 71:183–185, 1987.

251. Woo, SY, Donaldson, SS, and Cox, RS: Astrocytomas in children: 14 years' experience at Stanford University Medical Center. J Clin Oncol 6:1001–1007, 1988.

252. Wood, CC, Spencer, DD, Allison, T, McCarthy, G, Williamson, PD, and Goff, WR: Localization of human sensorimotor cortex during surgery by cortical surface recording of somatosensory evoked potentials. J Neurosurg 68:99–111, 1988.

253. Yasargil, MG: Surgical approaches to inaccessible tumors. Clin Neurosurg 34:42–110, 1986.

254. Yoshida, S, Tanaka, R, Takai, N, and Ono, K: Local administration of autologous lymphokine-activated killer cells and recombinant interleukin-2 to patients with malignant brain tumors. Cancer Res 48:5011–5016, 1988.

255. Young, B, Oldfield, EH, Markesbery, WR, Haack, D, Tibbs, PA, McCombs, P, Chin, HW, Maruyama, Y, and Meacham, WF: Reoperation for glioblastoma. J Neurosurg 55:917–921, 1981.

256. Young, H, Kaplan, A, and Regelson, W: Immunotherapy with autologous white cell infusions ("lymphocytes") in the treatment of recurrent glioblastoma multiforme: A preliminary report. Cancer 40:1037–1044, 1977.

257. Yung, WKA, Steck, PA, Kelleher, PJ, Moser, RP, and Rosenblum, MG: Growth inhibitory effect of recombinant alpha and beta interferon on human glioma cells. J Neurooncol 5:323–330, 1987.

258. Zaprianov, Z and Christov, K: Histologic grading, DNA content, cell proliferation and survival of patients with astroglial tumors. Cytometry 9:380–386, 1988.

259. Zuber, P, Hamou, MF, and De Tribolet, N: Identification of proliferating cells in human gliomas using the monoclonal antibody Ki-67. Neurosurgery 22:364–368, 1988.

260. Zuccarello, M, Sawaya, R, and deCourten-Myers, G: Glioblastoma occurring after radiation therapy for meningioma: Case report and review of literature. Neurosurgery 19:114–119, 1986.

261. Zulch, KJ: Histologic typing of tumors of the central nervous system. International Histological Classification of Tumors, No 21. WHO, Geneva, 1979, p 15.

CHAPTER 17

• •

THE MANAGEMENT OF A SINGLE CNS METASTASIS

Lisa M. DeAngelis, M.D.

A quarter of patients with systemic malignancies will have brain metastases, and half of these will be single. Thus, managing a patient with a single brain metastasis is a common problem.

DeAngelis advocates what could be considered an aggressive approach: all patients with single metastases should be considered for surgery at the time of diagnosis, even those with disseminated systemic disease. Moreover, all patients, regardless of whether suitable for surgery or not, should receive radiotherapy.

The author makes a persuasive case that this approach improves the quality of life for the majority of patients. The dilemma arises if the metastases recur. DeAngelis advocates "further surgery, whole brain radiotherapy or possibly chemotherapy. . . ." I am not so sure.

VCH

Brain metastases are one of the most frequent and ominous neurologic complications of systemic cancer. The majority of patients who develop brain metastases have a relatively short survival, despite the fact that initial treatment is often effective. The short survival is usually a result of the patient's advanced systemic cancer, and consequently, brain metastases are often approached with therapeutic nihilism by the physician. Although for some patients effective palliation is transient or not possible, other patients with metastatic brain disease do well for prolonged periods with a vigorous therapeutic approach. For the most part, these are patients with a single cerebral metastasis, and it is important to identify these patients at diagnosis because they demand such a different therapeutic approach.

EPIDEMIOLOGY

Intracerebral metastases are common, found in 24% of autopsied patients at Memorial Sloan-Kettering Cancer Center.[34] Sixty-three percent of these patients had brain metastases, accounting for 15% of all patients with systemic cancer who die here. The vast majority of these patients were symptomatic from their neurologic disease, although there are patients who have brain metastases discovered at autopsy that were not suspected in life. Lung cancer is the most common cause of brain metastases, although the exact percentage varies greatly among the different sources (Table 17–1). This high incidence is a direct reflection of both the frequency of lung cancer in the population and the fact that tumor in the

TABLE 17–1. **PRIMARY TUMOR IN PATIENTS WITH BRAIN METASTASES**

Primary Tumor	Posner and Chernick[34] (N = 168)	Zimm, et al.[48] (N = 191)	Delattre, et al.[12] (N = 288)
Lung	61 (36%)	122 (64%)	144 (50%)
Breast	33 (20%)	26 (14%)	43 (15%)
Melanoma	50 (30%)	8 (4%)	30 (10%)
Unknown	—	16 (8%)	32 (11%)
Colon	6 (4%)	6 (3%)	—
Renal	11 (7%)	4 (2%)	—
Other	7 (4%)	9 (5%)	39 (14%)

lung provides a direct route to the brain via hematogenous dissemination. Other tumors, particularly melanoma, have a greater propensity to produce intracerebral metastases, and brain metastases are found with a greater frequency in patients harboring these primary neoplasms (Table 17–2).

About half of all brain metastases are single; both autopsy and computed tomography–(CT) based studies confirm that 47% to 51% of parenchymal brain metastases are single.[7,12,34] Zimm and associates[48] reported a marked difference in the incidence of single metastasis diagnosed premortem compared with autopsy findings; however, the use of high-resolution CT and MRI (magnetic resonance imaging) has reduced this discrepancy. Single metastases are more common with certain tumor types than others (Table 17–3). Renal and pelvic-abdominal tumors produce single brain metastasis with greater frequency than lung or melanoma primaries, but even melanoma leads to single lesions in one third of patients.

Occasionally, neurologic symptoms are the patient's first indication of an underlying malignancy. In patients who present with brain metastases, about half have their primary tumor identified, usually by history/physical examination and chest x-ray.[25,43] In the remaining patients, the primary neoplasm is rarely found, even at autopsy. Lung cancer is the most frequent primary identified, but any primary can present as a brain metastasis.

PATHOPHYSIOLOGY

Most brain metastases are believed to arise by hematogenous dissemination of tumor from the primary neoplasm.[11] Patients with lung cancer have a high incidence of brain metastases, and patients with other primaries have a 70% incidence of lung metas-

TABLE 17–2. **INCIDENCE OF BRAIN METASTASES IN AUTOPSIED PATIENTS ACCORDING TO PRIMARY TUMOR***

Primary Tumor	Incidence (%)
Lung	21
Breast	10
Melanoma	40
Renal	21
Testis	46
Colon	5
Ovary	5

*Source: Modified from Posner and Chernik.[34]

TABLE 17–3. **PROPORTION OF SINGLE METASTASIS BY PRIMARY TUMOR TYPE**

Primary Tumor	%	Reference
Lung	41–48	7,12,34
Melanoma	25–41	7,12,34,48
Breast	56–59	7,12,34
Renal*	50–91	7,34,48
Colon	33–36	7,34
Ovarian	100	34
Testis	82	7

* 69%, all pelvic and abdominal primaries; Delattre, et al.[12]

tases when secondary brain tumors are identified.[12] Tumor cells are thought to embolize to the nervous system, and therefore should form brain metastases in regions of the brain proportional to its blood supply. In general this is true, but recent work shows the watershed regions of brain to be overrepresented in their share of cerebral metastases.[12] This supports the tumor embolization theory, with cells lodging in vessels of smallest caliber. There are rare circumstances when a tumor embolus is of sufficient size to cause a strokelike episode by occluding an artery.[30]

There are a few circumstances in which nonspecific hematogenous spread does not explain the observed distribution of brain metastases. Pelvic and abdominal tumors have a predilection to form posterior fossa metastases far in excess of what the proportion of blood supply to this region would predict.[11] Dissemination by way of Batson's plexus has long been invoked to explain this phenomenon; however, not all pelvic tumors — for example, renal cancer — form a disproportionate number of posterior fossa metastases. In addition, the expected increase in spinal and skull metastases in patients bearing posterior fossa metastases has not been observed, although these structures are also drained by Batson's plexus. Therefore, preferential access to the posterior fossa is not an adequate explanation of the observed discrepancy.

It has long been known that circulating tumor cells may travel throughout the body, but metastases tend to form in particular organs.[15] The "soil and seed" hypothesis of metastasis formation is supported by a growing body of evidence that demonstrates that the organ microenvironment (the "soil"), and the adhesive and invasive capabilities of the metastasizing tumor cell (the "seed") must be matched for a metastasis to develop. This is true for the brain as well. Experimentally it has been shown that subgroups of melanoma can preferentially metastasize to the brain, and indeed to specific regions of the brain.[4] The microenvironment of areas of the brain that permit metastases to develop is poorly understood but is likely an important factor for the localization of metastatic disease to specific areas.

DIAGNOSIS

The clinical presentation of a cerebral metastasis is similar to the presentation of any intracranial mass lesion. Headaches and focal motor and sensory signs are frequent.[33,48] Seizures occur in about 15% to 20% of patients. Occasionally, a patient may develop acute neurologic symptoms suggestive of a stroke, and this may be due to hemorrhage into a preexisting metastasis. Encephalopathy in the absence of significant focal signs may be a presentation of multiple metastases but is rarely the sole clinical finding with single brain metastasis. The diagnosis of brain metastasis has been dramatically simplified with CT scanning. Currently, a cranial MRI scan with gadolinium contrast enhancement is the best screening test for patients who develop cerebral symptoms and, if available, should be the diagnostic test of choice. There are no pathognomonic radiographic features that distinguish a brain metastasis on CT or MRI without reference to the clinical context; however, a peripheral location, ring enhancement with prominent peritumoral edema, and multiple lesions all suggest metastatic disease. These characteristics are helpful but not diagnostic; if the primary tumor is unknown, tissue should be obtained to confirm the diagnosis.

If a CT scan is performed and a single lesion identified, MRI with gadolinium contrast enhancement is essential to confirm that no additional lesions are evident before deciding on a surgical approach to treatment.[42] Although additional lesions are detected in the minority of patients, their presence can alter the therapeutic plan, and preoperative MRI is the most important test prior to sending a patient for craniotomy. If MRI is unavailable, a double-dose delayed contrast CT scan can identify lesions not seen on the usual CT study; however, there are examples of cases with negative double-dose CT studies, but positive MRI scans (Fig. 17–1).

TREATMENT

Treatment of patients with brain metastases can be divided into two areas: sympto-

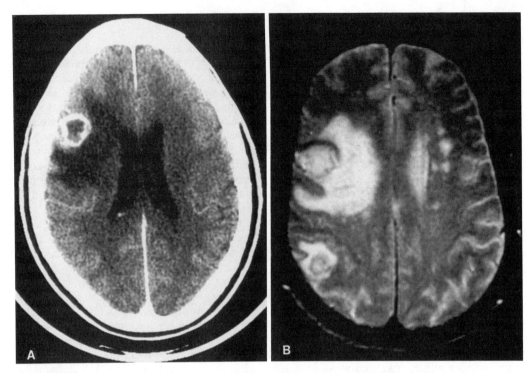

FIGURE 17-1. *A*, Contrast-enhanced CT scan demonstrating a single metastasis from renal carcinoma. *B*, T_2-weighted MRI scan on the same patient performed at the same time revealing two separate lesions. Small foci of hyperintensity in the white matter of the left hemisphere are thought to represent ischemic changes.

matic therapy and definitive therapy. Symptomatic measures are usually instituted immediately and are the same for patients with single or multiple metastases; they include corticosteroids for control of cerebral edema and anticonvulsants for seizure control. Definitive therapy is directed against the tumor itself and is designed to eradicate or at least diminish the malignancy; radiotherapy and surgical extirpation are the most commonly used treatments for this purpose. We will discuss each separately.

Corticosteroids

Corticosteroids are an invaluable tool for the management of the associated edema that surrounds most metastatic brain tumors. Reduction of edema and the consequent reduction of the total mass effect caused by edema plus tumor can produce prompt and dramatic clinical improvement,

usually within hours.[44] Steroids usually improve the patient's level of alertness and reduce or eliminate focal deficits, and they can be life-saving in situations where the brain is herniating from a large combined mass effect. Without definitive therapy, however, the benefit of corticosteroids is temporary. Improvement may last for weeks or even a few months, but eventually, edema or tumor growth will necessitate increasing doses of corticosteroid to maintain the patient's functional status.

The mechanisms of brain tumor–induced cerebral edema are multifactorial and have been an area of active research. Blood vessels within tumor do not have a blood-brain barrier (BBB) and are inherently more permeable than normal cerebral vessels. Hence, tumor vessels will permit normally restricted materials and fluid to enter the cerebral interstitial space. In addition, it is postulated that tumors can secrete vasoactive substances that alter capillary permeability, allowing fluid to leak out of the vasculature and into the surrounding tissue.[3] The production of vasoactive substances may explain why some tumors have a great deal of associated edema and others much less, depending on their ability to synthesize and secrete these factors. The mechanism of corticosteroid effect in cerebral edema remains unclear, although it is thought to restore this disrupted capillary integrity. Despite the efficacy of corticosteroids, control of cerebral edema can be difficult and can cause the patient's demise even in the absence of obvious tumor growth.

Most neurologists use dexamethasone as the corticosteroid of choice, largely because of its minimal mineralocorticoid effect. The usual starting dose is 16 mg/d of dexamethasone, but any corticosteroid is effective if given in equipotent doses. If this dose is inadequate, increasing the dexamethasone is often effective, and doses as high as 100 mg/d have been used, although this is rarely necessary. Side effects from corticosteroids are frequent and can contribute to disability. Acutely, patients may experience personality changes, particularly hypomania and, less commonly, depression. Steroid myopathy, hyperglycemia, hypertension, weight gain with cushingoid features, and reduced mineralization of bone are common when the drug is given chronically, particularly in high doses. Once cerebral edema is under control and definitive therapy completed, every effort should be made to gradually reduce the dose of corticosteroid to the minimum requirement, which for the majority of patients means that they can come off the drug completely. Unfortunately, this is often overlooked, and frequently patients remain on stable and disabling doses of corticosteroids long after they are necessary.

Anticonvulsants

Anticonvulsants are used as a matter of course for patients who have had a seizure. The role of prophylactic anticonvulsants remains controversial, because no prospective study has been performed. However, retrospective data are accumulating which suggest that prophylactic anticonvulsants

are not effective in preventing seizures, particularly because the dosages are not maintained within the therapeutic range.[20,40] Although 25% of patients with brain metastases have or develop seizures during their illness, the vast majority of these occur at the time of diagnosis. Few late seizures develop in these patients unless they experience a recurrence of tumor in the nervous system. In addition, side effects from anticonvulsants are common and can be potentially life-threatening in this population.[13] Consequently, we do not recommend prophylactic anticonvulsants for patients with brain metastases. Patients with cerebral metastases from melanoma may be unique because they have an unusually high incidence of seizures (50%);[5] however, even in these patients, the role of prophylactic medication has not been defined.[20] If prophylactic anticonvulsants are used, careful attention to blood levels is necessary because patient compliance may be poor when the drug is used for preventive purposes.

Cranial Radiotherapy

Whole brain radiotherapy (WBRT) is the major treatment for cerebral metastases. Radiotherapy is delivered to the whole brain in all patients. Those with multiple metastases require WBRT, but even patients with single brain metastases receive WBRT because of the concern that microscopic metastases exist below the resolution of CT or MRI. In addition, if a focal port of RT is used to treat a single lesion, it becomes technically difficult to treat recurrent disease that falls outside the original focal field.

For all patients with brain metastases, median survival is 3 to 6 months with the use of cranial irradiation.[2,5,7,17,24,29,33,38,48] The majority of patients with brain metastases are effectively palliated with WBRT, with substantial reduction in neurologic signs and symptoms, but few are cured.[6] The short survival reflects the high percentage of patients who have disseminated systemic disease, and many die of progressive systemic tumor despite adequately controlled neurologic disease.

Regardless of the primary tumor type, WBRT is usually delivered in a standard schedule designed to achieve rapid and effective palliation. A series of studies performed by the Radiation Therapy Oncology Group (RTOG) demonstrated that a variety of fractionation schedules, ranging from 1000 cGy in one dose to 4000 cGy delivered in 20 fractions, produced comparable improvement in neurologic function and survival.[2,17] However, very high daily fractions, such as 1000 cGy/d, can produce severe neurologic side effects during treatment, and early recurrence.[21,47] Neurologic deterioration during RT leading to cerebral herniation has been seen, particularly in patients with substantial mass effect from their metastasis. Because a variety of RT schedules appear to be equally efficacious and patients with brain metastases generally have a short survival, WBRT should be delivered quickly but safely to permit a rapid return home. For these reasons, a common schedule is 300 cGy/d for 10 days to a total dose of 3000 cGy WBRT. Unfortunately, radiosensitizers have not improved the response rate or survival over WBRT alone.[1]

Patients with radiosensitive malignancies, such as breast cancer, usually fare better than those with relatively radioresistant primaries, such as the colon or melanoma; patients with renal carcinoma, which is highly radioresistant even to total doses of RT in excess of 4000 cGy, have a poor response rate to WBRT.[29] Accordingly, median survival time varies depending on tumor type, for patients treated with similar WBRT regimens, but differences in survival are also a reflection of the availability of effective systemic therapy for the underlying primary tumor.

Acute toxicities of WBRT when administered in a standard regimen are few, and the treatment is well tolerated. Cranial irradiation causes alopecia in all patients, although hair does grow back several months after treatment is completed. Fatigue is a common side effect of cranial RT; most patients experience it to some degree, and occasionally it can be debilitating. Reassurance that it will resolve after completion of WBRT is usually all that is necessary. Headaches, nausea, and vomiting may be seen during the course of WBRT, and they tend to occur in patients with raised intracranial pressure and significant mass effect from the metas-

tasis. Corticosteroids often prevent or ameliorate these symptoms, although this benefit was not observed in the RTOG studies. We always maintain patients on a minimum of 6 mg/d dexamethasone during WBRT.

Early delayed reactions from cranial irradiation occur a few weeks to months after completion of radiotherapy; the most common cerebral early delayed reaction is the somnolence syndrome seen in children receiving prophylactic cranial irradiation for acute lymphoblastic leukemia, but it can occur in any patient undergoing WBRT.[26] Clinically, it can mimic tumor progression, and patients usually experience a reappearance or exacerbation of their focal neurologic deficits, often accompanied by nausea, vomiting, and lethargy. CT or MRI scan may demonstrate increased enhancement and edema, but both the clinical and radiologic features of early delayed reactions are temporary, and patients usually recover fully within a few weeks. Corticosteroids can be useful to reduce symptoms. The early delayed reaction is thought to be a demyelinating process, and recovery is attributed to remyelination. Early delayed toxicity is rare after cranial radiotherapy and does not predict which patients will develop the late delayed complications of radiotherapy.

Delayed neurologic toxicity is seen in only a small minority of patients treated with WBRT alone, because most patients do not survive long enough to be at risk for the permanent sequelae of cranial irradiation. However, it has been observed in some patients successfully treated with standard WBRT regimens who become long-term survivors.[9] Most patients develop symptoms about 1 year after WBRT, but a latency of 5 to 36 months has been reported. Clinically, late toxicity can appear as radionecrosis, which can act as a mass lesion and have the identical CT/MRI appearance of tumor recurrence, or as radiation-induced dementia, which is associated with ataxia and urinary incontinence.[9,41] Any patient who develops focal neurologic signs and a contrast-enhancing lesion on CT/MRI 1 to 2 years after successful treatment of a metastatic brain tumor with WBRT should be considered for a biopsy to establish a diagnosis of recurrent tumor or radionecrosis. The progressive dementia can respond to ventriculoperitoneal shunting in some patients, although its benefit may be temporary and incomplete.

Patients who have a good response to WBRT may respond well to a second course of cranial irradiation if they develop recurrent metastatic disease.[23] Although the potential for delayed radiation toxicity is often raised as an argument against re-irradiating patients who have received 3000 to 4000 cGy of WBRT, the issue is of little importance because most patients are unlikely to survive long enough to develop neurotoxicity. However, they may achieve further neurologic palliation for a short time.

Surgery

Surgery has been used in the treatment of metastatic brain tumors for decades, but its role remains controversial. Many older surgical series, prior to the availability of CT or even nuclear brain scan, report a significant percentage of patients who survive 1 year or longer after surgical resection (Table 17–4). These figures are comparable and often better than the 1-year survival figures after WBRT alone. However, it is often difficult to compare surgical and nonsurgical series because patients selected to undergo craniotomy are usually in good condition and are the same patients likely to do well with nonsurgical therapy. This remains a problem even with more recent literature, and the issue of patient selection has remained the single most important obstacle to an objective interpretation of the surgical data. However, a recent case-controlled retrospective comparison of complete resection of a single brain metastasis from non–small-cell lung cancer followed by WBRT versus WBRT alone has shown convincing data to support surgical extirpation in selected patients; Those treated with surgery plus WBRT had a median survival of 19 months compared with 9.0 months with WBRT alone.[31] Furthermore, all patients appeared to benefit from surgery, even those with disseminated systemic disease at the time of craniotomy.

These highly suggestive data are now being confirmed with randomized prospective studies that are ongoing in several institutions. Preliminary data show that patients who have a complete resection followed by WBRT live longer and in better neurologic condition than identical patients who receive WBRT alone.[32] Accordingly, surgery should be considered in every patient with a single brain metastasis at diagnosis. Surgery is often reserved for patients with limited or no systemic disease at the time of brain metastasis, and these patients do fare best with vigorous treatment; however, even patients with disseminated systemic disease may be candidates for extirpation if their disease is controllable (e.g., bone metastases from breast cancer) or if their primary neoplasm is radioresistant and unlikely to respond to WBRT alone (e.g., renal cancer). In these situations, patients can obtain significant functional improvement and have an improved quality of life even if their life is not prolonged by surgery.

This approach can be justified when experienced neurosurgeons are available to perform the craniotomy. In our institution patients are hospitalized for only 7 to 10 days for resection, and in the prospective study mentioned above, 30-day mortality was identical for operated and unoperated patients who received WBRT alone.[32]

TABLE 17–4. **SURGICAL TREATMENT OF BRAIN METASTASIS**

Author	No. of Patients	Median	1-Yr Survival
Lang and Slater[24]	284	4.2 mo	22%
Haar and Patterson[19]	167	6 mo	22%
Winston, et al[46]	79	5 mo	22%
Magilligan, et al[28]	22	14 mo (mean)	45%
Ransohoff[36]	100	—	38%
Galicich, et al[16]	78	6 mo	29%
White, et al[45]	122	7 mo	35%

Complete excision of a metastasis is the goal of surgery. However, occasionally a subtotal resection is performed or only one of several metastases is removed because it is immediately life-threatening; in these circumstances postoperative radiotherapy is necessary to treat the remaining disease. Most patients who undergo a complete excision of a single brain metastasis also receive postoperative WBRT, although its value has not been established. Postoperative WBRT is administered to treat any residual disease left by the surgeon or microscopic disease that may reside elsewhere in the brain undetected by preoperative CT or MRI scans. This is a logical approach, but its contribution to survival or control of neurologic disease has not been determined with certainty. Three retrospective studies have examined this issue, all with different conclusions. Dosoretz and colleagues[14] found that postoperative WBRT did not improve survival or reduce neurologic recurrence, whereas data summarizing the Mayo Clinic experience showed that WBRT reduced subsequent relapse in the nervous system and improved survival.[39] A recent review of our experience at Memorial Sloan-Kettering Cancer Center demonstrated that postoperative WBRT prolonged the interval to neurologic relapse but had no impact on survival because patients continued to die of their systemic disease.[10] Furthermore, long-term survivors who were irradiated had a significant incidence (11%) of radiation-induced dementia. This was associated with RT schedules adopted from the standard treatment of patients with brain metastases who receive WBRT alone using high daily fractions for rapid palliation; however, patients selected for resection have a high likelihood of long-term survival, with almost 50% living 1 year or longer. These patients are vulnerable to the late toxicities of cranial irradiation. Until a randomized prospective study is completed that clarifies the role and dose of postoperative WBRT, we recommend that postoperative RT be administered in daily fractions not to exceed 200 cGy and that the total dose should be tumoricidal, 4000 to 5000 cGy, that is, that the patients be treated with curative intent.

Brachytherapy

Radioactive seed implantation, or brachytherapy, delivers high doses of focal radiation to a tumor by implanting radioactive seeds directly into the tumor bed. Because high doses of radiation are delivered to the tumor bed alone, the surrounding brain is spared the consequences of WBRT. Thus brachytherapy can be used not only as first treatment but also when metastatic disease recurs after WBRT. In the nervous system, brachytherapy has been used primarily in the treatment of malignant gliomas, where it doubles the median survival from 36 to 74 weeks for patients with recurrent tumor.[18] Currently, its role in the initial treatment of primary brain tumors is being studied in several ongoing cooperative protocols. The isotope used for all these studies is iodine 125 because of its high energy and rapid fall-off of activity.

Experience with brachytherapy for metastatic brain disease is limited, but preliminary work suggests it can be useful in selected patients. Most patients who have received radioactive implants have had single brain metastases with limited or no active systemic tumor. Implantation at the time of recurrence, usually after failure of WBRT, has achieved prolonged survival with a median of 80 weeks for 14 patients treated in this fashion.[35] This is far superior to repeated courses of WBRT. Furthermore, the effectiveness of brachytherapy has not been limited to patients harboring radiosensitive tumors, but has also proved useful in the treatment of metastases from relatively radioresistant primary neoplasms, such as melanoma, because of the high local doses achieved.

Radionecrosis can form at the tumor site months after implantation. In 50% of patients with primary brain tumors, it becomes symptomatic and can mimic tumor recurrence clinically and radiographically. When this occurs, surgical resection is usually necessary for both diagnosis and treatment. In the majority of patients the resected material is a combination of radionecrosis and recurrent tumor, but removal of this tissue improves the patient's clinical condition. The possibility of late radionecrosis is one of the potentially limiting factors in patient selection for brachytherapy, because the metastasis must be in a surgically accessible location. Therefore, patients who are likely to be good candidates for brachytherapy are the same patients who are good candidates for surgical resection. No comparative data exist on which to base a specific recommendation; further experience is necessary to define the role of brachytherapy in patients with metastatic brain disease. Brachytherapy may include the implantation of more than one lesion; implanting lesions that cannot be resected, such as deep tumors; or the use of permanent low-activity seeds.

Chemotherapy

The use of chemotherapy for the treatment of brain metastases has been disappointing. Most systemically administered agents do not penetrate the BBB adequately enough to be effective even though the BBB is not normal in the region of the tumor. Furthermore, very small metastases probably have a normal BBB, and brain tumors may develop while patients are taking a chemotherapeutic regimen that is effective against their systemic disease.[27] Only those agents or regimens likely to be efficacious in the periphery have a chance of being effective in the nervous system, and any chemotherapeutic drug that is known to be inactive against the systemic neoplasm is likely to be ineffective against its cerebral metastases. Therefore, brain metastases that originate from primary neoplasms that are chemosensitive, such as breast and testicular cancers, respond best to systemic therapy.[22,27,37] When WBRT and surgery have failed, and a patient has a chemoresponsive primary

MANAGEMENT OF BRAIN METASTASES

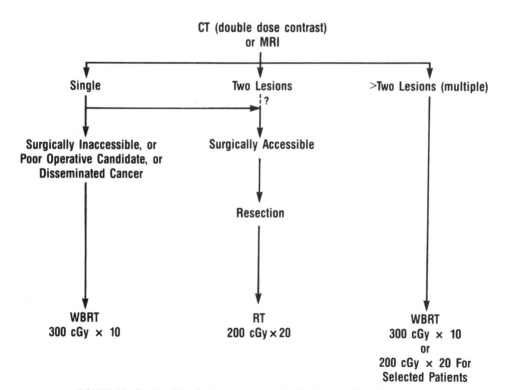

FIGURE 17–2. Algorithm for the management of patients with brain metastases.

tumor, it is reasonable to try systemic chemotherapy for treatment of brain metastases. There is no role for adjuvant chemotherapy after WBRT and/or surgical resection to prevent or delay neurologic recurrence of disease.

There is no distinction in the use of chemotherapy for the treatment of single or multiple brain metastases, and there is no difference in response rate. In an effort to circumvent the BBB, intra-arterial carmustine (BCNU) was tried for the treatment of brain metastases with limited success; however, there were a few patients who had regression of tumor in the distribution of the perfused artery, whereas lesions elsewhere in the brain progressed, suggesting this approach has merit in some patients.[8] Theoretically, patients with single brain metastases would be the best candidates for regional chemotherapy if the appropriate agent were chosen.

SUMMARY

A significant proportion of patients with malignancy develop brain metastases, and half of the metastases are single. All patients with single metastases should be considered for surgical resection at the time of diagnosis, even those with disseminated systemic disease (Fig. 17 – 2). A vigorous therapeutic approach with extirpation followed by tumoricidal doses (4000 to 5000 cGy) of postoperative WBRT in low daily fractions (<200 cGy/d) will prolong life and improve the quality of life for the majority of patients. Furthermore, the patient's risk of delayed neurologic toxicity from WBRT will be minimized without compromising the efficacy of the treatment. Those patients who are not surgical candidates should receive WBRT in a regimen designed for safe and rapid palliation of neurologic symptoms (e.g., 300 cGy/d × 10). Recurrence of cerebral metastases may be treated with further surgery, WBRT, or possibly chemotherapy, if appropriate to the underlying neoplasm. Brachytherapy may be useful in selected patients, but additional clinical research is necessary to define its role in the treatment of metastatic brain disease.

REFERENCES

1. Aiken, R, Leavengood, JM, Kim, J-H, Deck, MDK, Thaler, HT, and Posner, JB: Metronidazole in the treatment of metastatic brain tumors. J Neurooncol 2:105–111,1984.
2. Borgelt, B, Gelber, R, Kramer, S, Brady, LW, Chang, CH, Davis, LW, Perez, CA, and Hendrickson, FR: The palliation of brain metastases: Final results of the first two studies by the radiation therapy oncology group. Int J Radiat Oncol Biol Phys 6:9, 1980.
3. Bruce, JN, Criscuolo, GR, Merrill, MJ, Moquin, RR, Blacklock, JB, and Oldfield, EH: Vascular permeability induced by protein product of malignant brain tumors. Inhibition of dexamethasone. J Neurosurg 67:880–884, 1987.
4. Brunson, KW, Beattie, G, and Nicolson, GL: Selections and altered properties of brain colonizing metastatic melanoma. Nature 272:543–544, 1978.
5. Byrne, TN, Cascino, TL, Posner, JB: Brain metastasis from melanoma. J Neurooncol 1:313–317, 1983.
6. Cairncross, JG, Chernik, NL, Kim, J-H, and Posner, JB: Sterilization of cerebral metastases by radiation therapy. Neurology 29:1195–1202, 1979.
7. Cairncross, JG, Kim, J-H, and Posner, JB: Radiation therapy for brain metastases. Ann Neurol 7:529–541, 1980.
8. Cascino, TL, Byrne, TN, Deck, MDF, and Posner, JB: Intra-arterial BCNU in the treatment of metastatic brain tumors. J Neurooncol 1:211–218, 1983.
9. DeAngelis, LM, Delattre, J-Y, Posner, JB: Radiation-induced dementia in patients cured of brain metastases. Neurology 39:789–796, 1989.
10. DeAngelis, LM, Mandell, LR, Thaler, HT, Kimmel, DW, Galichich, JH, Fuks, Z, and Posner, JB: The role of postoperative radiotherapy after resection of single brain metastases. Neurosurgery 24:798–805, 1989.
11. Del Regato, JA: Pathways of metastatic spread of malignant tumors. Seminars in Oncology 4:33–38, 1977.
12. Delattre, JY, Krol, G, Thaler, HT, Posner, JB: Distribution of brain metastases. Arch Neurol 45:741–744, 1988.
13. Delattre, Y-V, Safai, B, Posner, JB: Erythema multiforme and Stevens-Johnson syndrome in patients receiving cranial irradiation and phenytoin. Neurology 38:194–198, 1988.
14. Dosoretz, DE, Blitzer, PH, Russell, AH, and Wang, CC: Management of solitary metastasis to the brain: The role of elective brain irradiation following complete surgical resection. Int J Rad Oncol Biol Phys 6:1727–1730, 1980.
15. Fidler, IJ: Origin of cancer metastases and its implications for therapy. Isr J Med Sci 24:456–463, 1988.
16. Galicich, JH, Sundaresan, N, Arbit, E, and Passe S: Surgical treatment of single brain metastasis: Factors associated with survival. Cancer 45:381–386, 1980.

17. Gelber, RD, Larson, M, Borgelt, BB, and Kramer, S: Equivalence of radiation schedules for the palliative treatment of brain metastases in patients with favorable prognosis. Cancer 48:1749–1753, 1981.
18. Gutin, PH, Leibel, SA, Wara, WM, Choucair, A, Levin, VA, Philips, TL, Silver, P, DaSilva, V, Edwards, MSB, Davis, RL, Weaver, KA, and Lamb, S: Recurrent malignant gliomas: Survival following interstitial brachytherapy with high-activity iodine-125 sources. J Neurosurg 67:864–873, 1987.
19. Haar, F and Patterson, RH: Surgery for metastatic intracranial neoplasm. Cancer 30:1241–1245, 1972.
20. Hagen, NA, Cirrincione, C, Thaler, HT, and DeAngelis, LM: The role of whole brain radiotherapy following resection of cerebral metastasis from melanoma. Neurology 40:158–160, 1990.
21. Hindo, WA, DeTrana, FA, Lee, M-S, and Hendrickson, FR: Large dose increment irradiation in treatment of cerebral metastases. Cancer 26:138–141, 1970.
22. Kolaric, K, Roth, A, Jelicic, I, and Matkovic, A: Phase II clinical trial of cis-dichlorodiammine platinum (Cis DDP) in metastatic brain tumors. J Cancer Res Clin Oncol 104:287–293, 1982.
23. Kurup, P, Reddy, S, and Hendrickson, FR: Results of re-irradiation for cerebral metastases. Cancer 46:2587–2589, 1980.
24. Lang, EF and Slater, J: Metastatic brain tumors. Results of surgical and nonsurgical treatment. Surg Clin North Am 44:865–872, 1964.
25. Le Chevalier, T, Smith, FP, Caille, P, Constans, JP, and Rouesse, JG: Sites of primary malignancies in patients presenting with cerebral metastases. Cancer 56:880–882, 1985.
26. Leibel, SA and Sheline, GE: Tolerance of the central and peripheral nervous system to therapeutic irradiation. In Lett, JT and Altman, KI (eds): Advances in Radiation Biology. Academic Press, New York, 1987, pp 257–288.
27. Lester, SF, Morphis II, JG, Hornback, NB, Williams, SD, and Einhorn, LH: Brain metastases and testicular tumors: Need for aggressive therapy. J Neurooncol 2:1397–1403, 1984.
28. Magillian, DJ, Rogers, JS, Knighton, RS, and Davila, JC: Pulmonary neoplasm with solitary cerebral metastasis. J Thorac Cardiovasc Surg 72:690–696, 1976.
29. Maor, MH, Frias, AE, and Oswald, MJ: Palliative radiotherapy for brain metastases in renal carcinoma. Cancer 62:1912–1917, 1988.
30. O'Neill, BP, Dinapoli, RP, and Okazaki H: Cerebral infarction as a result of tumor emboli. Cancer 60:90–95, 1987.
31. Patchell, RA, Cirrincione, C, Thaler, HT, Galicich, JH, Kim, J-H, and Posner, JB: Single brain metastases: Surgery plus radiation or radiation alone. Neurology 34:447–453, 1986.
32. Patchell, RA, Tibbs, PA, Walsh, JW, Dempsey, RJ,

Maruyama, Y, Kryscio, RJ, McDonald, JS, and Young, AB: Surgical treatment of single brain metastases: A prospective randomized trial. Proc Am Soc Clin Oncol 3:85, 1989.
33. Posner, JB: Management of central nervous system metastases. Semin Oncol 4:81–91, 1977.
34. Posner, JB and Chernick, NL: Intracranial metastases from systemic cancer. Adv Neurol 19:579–592, 1978.
35. Prados, M, Leibel, S, Barnett, CM, and Gutin, P: Interstitial brachytherapy for metastatic brain tumors. Cancer 63:657–660, 1989.
36. Ransohoff, J: Surgical management of metastatic tumors. Semin Oncol 2:21–27, 1975.
37. Rosner, D, Nemoto, T, Pickren, J, and Lane, W: Management of brain metastases from breast cancer by combination chemotherapy. J Neurooncol 1:131–137, 1983.
38. Sheline, GE and Brady, LW: Radiation therapy for brain metastases. J Neurooncol 4:219–225, 1987.
39. Smalley, SR, Schray, MF, Laws, ER Jr, O'Fallon, JR: Adjuvant radiation therapy after surgical resection of solitary brain metastasis: Association with pattern of failure and survival. Int J Radiat Oncol Biol Phys 13:1611–1616, 1987.
40. Strauss, CG, Silver, LD, and Recht, L: Should prophylactic anticonvulsants be administered to patients with newly-diagnosed cerebral metastases? A retrospective analysis. J Clin Oncol 6:1621–1624, 1988.
41. Sundaresan, N, Galicich, JH, Deck, MDF, and Tomita, T: Radiation necrosis after treatment of solitary intracranial metastases. Neurosurgery 8:329–333, 1981.
42. Sze, G, Shin, J, Krol, G, Johnson, C, Liu, D, and Deck, MDF: Intraparenchymal brain metastatses: MR imaging versus contrast-enhanced CT. Radiology 168:187–194, 1988.
43. Voorhies, RM, Sundaresan, N, and Thaler, HT: The single supratentorial lesion: An evaluation of preoperative diagnostic tests. J Neurosurg 53:364–368, 1980.
44. Weinstein, JD, Toy, FJ, Jaffe, ME, and Goldberg, HI: The effect of dexamethasone on brain edema in patients with metastatic brain tumors. Neurology 23:121–129, 1972.
45. White, KT, Fleming, TR, and Laws, ER: Single metastasis to the brain: Surgical treatment in 122 consecutive patients. Mayo Clin Proc 56:424–428, 1981.
46. Winston, KR, Walsh, JW, and Fischer, EG: Results of operative treatment of intracranial metastatic tumors. Cancer 45:2639–2645, 1980.
47. Young, DF, Posner, JB, Chu, F, and Nisce, L: Rapid-course radiation therapy of cerebral metastases: Results and complications. Cancer 34:1069–1076, 1974.
48. Zimm, S, Wampler, GL, Stablein, D, Hazra, T, and Young, HF: Intracerebral metastases in solid-tumor patients: Natural history and results of treatment. Cancer 48:384–394, 1981.

CHAPTER 18

• •

MANAGEMENT OF MULTIPLE BRAIN METASTASES

Edward J. Dropcho, M.D.

It is a tribute to the progress in neurooncology that a credible chapter can be written on the active management of patients with multiple brain metastases.

Dropcho thinks that with the exception of patients with widespread systemic cancer whose predicted survival is extremely short, radiotherapy and/or chemotherapy should be offered to all patients with brain metastasis, including those with "radioresistant" tumors.

While aggressive treatment may prolong the life of those who need to settle their affairs or finish something precious, like Ulysses S. Grant completing his memoirs while dying of throat cancer, all patients eventually reach the point where survival may prove more grievous than death.

VCH

SIGNIFICANCE

Brain metastases are the most common of brain tumors in adults and are also the most common "direct effect" of systemic cancer on the nervous system. Parenchymal brain metastases are present in 10% to 20% of cancer patients at autopsy,[56,72,73] and it has been estimated that the metastases in 60% to 75% of these patients are symptomatic during life.[12] In the United States the incidence of clinically evident brain metastases is at least 20,000 and perhaps as high as 100,000 cases annually, a figure that far exceeds the incidence of primary brain tumors such as meningiomas or glioblastoma multiforme.[91,93] The incidence of symptomatic brain metastases seems to be increasing for a variety of tumors, including sarcomas[59] and carcinomas of the breast,[70] ovary,[23,87] and testis.[82] For at least some of these patients the central nervous system (CNS) is be-

lieved to be a "sanctuary" from chemotherapy, so that brain metastases appear as patients survive for longer periods following improved control of the systemic tumor.

Brain metastases derive their clinical importance not only from their frequency but also from their terrible impact on patients' quality of life and, in some cases, on the length of survival. The occurrence of brain metastases usually represents another debilitating blow to patients who already have progressive, widespread disease, but in a significant number of patients (most commonly with lung cancer) the brain lesions occur as the solitary site of metastases when the primary tumor is under control. As will be discussed, most patients with brain metastases die of their systemic cancers, but patients whose brain lesions do not respond to therapy often die of uncontrolled intracranial hypertension or of the medical complications of severe neurologic disability.

269

TABLE 18–1. ORIGIN OF BRAIN
METASTASES BY PRIMARY
TUMOR TYPE

Primary Tumor	Reported Incidence
Bronchogenic carcinoma	23–64%
Breast carcinoma	10–24%
Malignant melanoma	5–17%
Colorectal carcinoma	3–11%
Renal carcinoma	2–8%
Unknown primary site	4–20%

PATHOPHYSIOLOGY

Any malignant neoplasm is capable of metastasizing to the brain, but only a handful of tumor types account for the great majority of patients with brain metastases. Bronchogenic carcinoma, breast carcinoma, and malignant melanoma (in that order) are the most common sources of parenchymal brain metastases in modern series (Table 18–1) and together account for approximately 75% of affected patients.[11,26,69,94] In a significant percentage of patients the brain metastases arise from an undetected primary source; bronchogenic carcinoma is subsequently found in many of these patients, but in 50% or more the primary tumor is never discovered during life.[31] Radiographically evident multiple metastases are present in 50% to 70% of patients, whereas the incidence of multiple metastases approaches 70% to 80% in autopsy studies; in melanoma patients this figure is even higher.[11,18,56,69,94] Solitary metastases are relatively more common with cancers of the lung, gastrointestinal tract, and genitourinary system than with other primary tumors.[26,94]

The overwhelming majority of parenchymal brain metastases arise from embolization of tumor cells through the arterial circulation. The occurrence of metastases in different locations of the brain is roughly proportional to their relative mass (and blood flow); for example, 10% to 15% of metastases (in most but not all series) occur in the cerebellum or brainstem, as would be predicted from their relative mass.[18,26,72,90] Brain metastases most often appear to originate at the junction of the hemispheric gray and white matter[56,79] and are overrepresented in "watershed" areas of the brain,[26] consistent with the origin of metastases from tumor cell emboli carried to terminal arterioles.

The "cascade" theory of cancer metastasis postulates that most tumors follow a predictable stepwise pattern of metastasizing to various organs and that brain metastases arise not from the primary tumor itself but from other metastases in "key generalizing sites"; for the great majority of solid tumors this site is the lung.[7,18] The cascade theory is supported by the fact that brain metastases tend to arise relatively early in the course of lung cancer, and are often the sole site of metastasis, whereas patients with other solid tumors generally develop brain metastases later in the course and in the setting of disseminated disease.[26,94] For example, up to 85% of patients with brain metastases from colorectal carcinoma also have grossly evident lung metastases.[15] Although a significant minority of patients with brain metastases do not have radiographically detectable lung lesions, a practical corollary of the cascade theory is that efforts at finding the primary tumor in patients with brain metastases "of unknown origin" should concentrate on the lungs.[31,94]

The concept of a cascade process in the origin of brain metastases is useful but does not explain the remarkable differences in the propensity of primary tumors to spread to the brain parenchyma (Table 18–2). Melanoma, choriocarcinoma, and other germ cell tumors carry the highest incidence of brain metastases.[48,72,82] Symptomatic brain metastases occur in 20% to 45% of melanoma patients,[1,47] and 70% to 90% of melanoma patients harbor brain metastases at autopsy.[1,18,24] Melanoma is also unusual in its predilection to metastasize to the cerebral cortex and basal ganglia rather than to the gray-white matter junction.[9,24] There is evidence that specific interactions between melanoma cells and the brain microenvironment enable the tumor cells to form symptomatic metastases in the brain without having to pass through intermediate metastatic sites such as the liver or lungs.[24,72] Among primary lung cancers, small-cell carcinomas are the most likely, squamous cell tumors

TABLE 18-2. RELATIVE PROPENSITY OF PRIMARY TUMORS TO METASTASIZE TO THE BRAIN

High	Intermediate	Low
Melanoma	Breast carcinoma	Colorectal carcinoma
Choriocarcinoma	Non-small-cell lung carcinomas	Prostatic carcinoma
Small-cell lung carcinoma	Renal carcinoma	Sarcomas
Germ cell tumors		Lymphomas
		Ovarian tumors

the least likely, and adenocarcinomas or large-cell tumors intermediate in their likelihood to metastasize to the brain.[33,44,86] Burkitt's lymphoma and lymphoblastic lymphomas are much more likely to spread to the brain than are other non-Hodgkin's or Hodgkin's lymphomas.[58,60] Brain metastases arising from cancers of the prostate and the gastrointestinal tract are distinctly uncommon despite the high prevalence of these tumors. Interestingly, thyroid cancers and sarcomas frequently spread to the lungs but only rarely metastasize to the brain, lending further support to the notion of differential "neurotropism."[69]

Several series have indicated that primary tumors arising in the abdomen or pelvis give rise to a disproportionately high number of metastases in the brainstem and cerebellum.[12,15,26,72] The conventional explanation for this observation is that tumor cells enter Batson's vertebral venous plexus and gain access to the posterior fossa without having to enter the arterial circulation. If, however, Batson's plexus were a common route for tumor spread, it would be predicted that patients with brain metastases from colorectal or genitourinary tumors would also have a high incidence of epidural metastases in the spine and cranium. With the exception of prostate tumors this is apparently not the case.[26]

CLINICAL FEATURES

The signs and symptoms of brain metastases derive mainly from their specific location and do not differ greatly from those of other expanding intracranial lesions, although several clinical features deserve mention. Headache is a presenting symptom of brain metastases in 40% to 50% of patients, but only a minority of these patients have the "classic" headache associated with intracranial hypertension.[69,74,94] Papilledema is present in only 15% to 25% of patients.[12] Fifteen percent to 20% of patients present with focal or generalized seizures. Another 5% to 10% of patients have an acute "strokelike" onset of symptoms, including patients with acute intratumoral hemorrhage (especially from melanoma or choriocarcinoma).[9,48,62] At initial diagnosis 50% to 75% of patients have altered mental status or impaired cognition, particularly those patients with multiple small metastases and/or increased intracranial pressure.[74] These patients may or may not have accompanying focal symptoms and often resemble "metabolic encephalopathy."

DIAGNOSIS

Magnetic resonance imaging (MRI) is generally believed to be more sensitive than computed tomography (CT) in detecting intraparenchymal metastases, particularly in demonstrating posterior fossa lesions or multiple punctate metastases. Contrast-enhanced CT may occasionally detect lesions not clearly visualized by unenhanced MRI; small metastases may be masked in unenhanced MR images by high signal from the edema surrounding a larger, nearby metastasis. These small lesions are more easily visualized with gadolinium-enhanced MRI.[43,79,88] Another potential difficulty with MRI is that in elderly patients, punctate lesions restricted to the white matter may represent small vessel ischemic disease rather than metastases. At this time, gadolinium-enhanced imaging is recommended for all patients who are candidates for surgical resection of an apparently single metastasis as seen on CT or unenhanced MR images. Where MRI is not available, the use of double-dose contrast material and delayed scanning improves the sensitivity of CT.

A histologic confirmation of brain metastases is seldom necessary for patients with a proven diagnosis of systemic cancer, especially those with progressive disease, and with "typical" abnormalities on CT or MR scans. It should be emphasized, however, that CT or MRI cannot absolutely differentiate brain metastases from primary brain tumors or nonneoplastic conditions. Serious consideration should be given to biopsying cerebral lesions that have an atypical radiographic appearance or lesions that arise in patients with well-controlled systemic cancer, particularly if a long interval has elapsed since the initial cancer diagnosis. In the age of stereotaxic brain biopsy, there is never a justification for irradiating presumed brain metastases without a histologic diagnosis of cancer.

TREATMENT

General Considerations

Before discussing specific treatment modalities for brain metastases, it is useful to review the criteria by which treatment results are evaluated. This is important not only for practical patient management but also for designing and interpreting clinical therapy trials. Improvement in neurologic function is obviously a prime goal of treatment, but patients' neurologic status can be affected by corticosteroid dose and concurrent medical problems, and its evaluation is subject to bias on the part of physician and patient. More objective ways of evaluating treatment include performing serial imaging studies (CT or MRI) and documenting decreases in corticosteroid requirements. Surprisingly, there are very few reports in the literature that use improvement on imaging studies as a criterion of response to radiation therapy or other treatments.[11,12] The duration of survival after diagnosis of brain metastases is an objective and easily determined way of evaluating treatment re-

sponse, but the usefulness of survival time as a treatment endpoint is complicated by the fact that most patients with brain metastases die from effects of their systemic cancer burden and not from their neurologic disease (see p. 274). Survival is clearly prolonged in some patients (particularly those with relatively little tumor burden outside the nervous system) by successful treatment of brain metastases, but if the length of survival is used as a measure of treatment efficacy, the cause of death of patients ("neurologic" or "nonneurologic") should also be specified.

Corticosteroids

The use of dexamethasone to control cerebral edema has improved, even if only temporarily, the quality of life of countless patients with brain metastases. Up to 75% of patients with brain metastases show marked clinical improvement within 24 to 72 hours after beginning dexamethasone;[12,73] "generalized" symptoms such as headache and altered mental status tend to improve more dramatically than focal symptoms. When used as the sole form of treatment, dexamethasone produces about a 1-month "remission" of symptoms and slightly increases the 4- to 6-week median survival of patients who receive no treatment at all.[11,64]

The use of corticosteroids must be individualized for each patient, but several general guidelines apply. Dexamethasone is usually begun at a (somewhat arbitrary) dose of 16 mg/d in divided doses and should be started prior to beginning radiation therapy (RT). The dose should be increased if a satisfactory response is not seen within 48 hours. Patients who are obtunded or have severe intracranial hypertension should receive high-dose dexamethasone (24 to 100 mg/d) for 48 to 72 hours before beginning RT. It is advisable to continually attempt to reduce the dose once definitive treatment is underway and patients have stabilized; patients who respond well can often be completely weaned off steroids within several weeks, whereas approximately 25% of patients require long-term dexamethasone to maintain neurologic function.[12] A prolonged requirement for corticosteroids is an objective indicator of poor response to anti-tumor therapy. Steadily escalating doses of dexamethasone may be given as a final effort to preserve quality of life for as long as possible in patients whose brain metastases recur or fail to respond to other treatments.

Anticonvulsants

As mentioned earlier, seizures are a presenting symptom of brain metastases in 15% to 20% of patients and occur in a total of 28% to 40% of patients during the course of their illness.[12,20,69] Retrospective reviews have not shown prophylactic anticonvulsants to be effective in preventing late seizures,[20] but unfortunately a prospective randomized study of prophylactic anticonvulsants (with diligent monitoring of blood levels) has never been done. One significant problem associated with anticonvulsant therapy in these patients is that there are mutual interactions between the metabolism of dexamethasone and phenytoin (or most other anticonvulsants). This often results in difficulties in maintaining therapeutic blood levels on conventional doses of anticonvulsants. In addition, patients on anticonvulsants may require unexpectedly high doses of corticosteroids to control cerebral edema.[12,17] Erythema multiforme and Stevens-Johnson syndrome have recently been reported as apparently rare but life-threatening complications in patients taking phenytoin and tapering doses of dexamethasone during or shortly after receiving cranial RT.[27] Unless solid evidence to the contrary becomes available, the consensus is that anticonvulsants should be withheld in patients with brain metastases until a seizure occurs. Patients with metastatic melanoma are an exception to this approach; the high incidence of seizures in these patients (up to 50%) justifies prophylactic anticonvulsants.[9,12,27]

Radiation Therapy

Whole brain radiation therapy (WBRT) remains the mainstay of treatment for brain metastases. The most frequently used WBRT regimen delivers a total dose of 3000 cGy in 10 to 15 daily fractions. The whole brain is irradiated even in patients with seemingly localized lesions, because CT and MRI probably fail to detect a significant number of small metastases, and it is difficult to give a second course of treatment following focal RT. WBRT is sometimes supplemented by a "coned-down" focal dose of RT to the area of a single or prominent metastasis, but this has not been shown to yield better results than conventional WBRT alone. Several large studies, including those sponsored by the Radiation Therapy Oncology Group (RTOG), have shown that a number of WBRT regimens using different fraction sizes and total doses (2000 to 5000 cGy) produced equivalent response rates and duration of improvement, although patients appeared to respond more quickly when the RT was delivered over a 2-week period, compared with longer regimens.[6,84] Doses exceeding 3000 cGy have not yielded better response rates or duration of improvement, even in patients who are believed to have a relatively favorable prognosis for survival.[37,51] Recent evidence regarding neurotoxicity of RT suggests that the daily dose fractionation of WBRT should be modified according to individual patients' survival prognosis (see below).

The results of RT vary significantly among various primary tumor types (Table 18–3) and also vary, somewhat unpredictably, between individuals with similar tumors. Overall, from 30% to 80% of all patients with brain metastases respond to WBRT by clinical and/or CNS imaging criteria.[11,12,84] Lymphomas are generally quite radiosensitive, as are germ cell tumors,[57,82] breast cancer,[11] and small-cell lung carcinoma.[4,39]

TABLE 18–3. **RELATIVE RESPONSIVENESS OF BRAIN METASTASES TO CRANIAL IRRADIATION**

More Responsive	*Less Responsive*
Lymphomas	Melanoma
Small-cell lung carcinoma	Non–small-cell
Breast carcinoma	lung carcinomas
Germ cell tumors	Colorectal carcinoma
	Renal carcinoma

The response rates of brain metastases from non–small-cell lung cancers and other solid tumors are lower,[11,76] but some patients with radioresistant tumors such as colorectal and renal carcinomas show significant objective responses to RT.[11,15,36,63]

The responsiveness of melanoma to RT is somewhat controversial. WBRT produced "symptomatic improvement" in 76% of metastatic melanoma patients in RTOG studies,[13] but the results of other published series are much less favorable.[1,47,94] In one series only 13% of patients showed objective improvement on follow-up CT scans, and 84% of patients remained dependent on corticosteroids until death.[9] Various reports have suggested that brain metastases from melanoma respond better to total WBRT doses exceeding 300 cGy,[50] to daily dose fractions greater than 400 cGy,[47] or to hyperfractionated (twice daily) WBRT,[19] but definitive prospective comparisons have not been done.

Two thirds of patients irradiated for brain metastases maintain an improved level of neurologic function until death is caused by systemic disease; these patients represent clinical neurologic "cures."[11,12] Autopsy-proved cases of total eradication of brain metastases by RT have been reported, but most patients whose metastases disappear on imaging studies are found to have residual microscopic tumor deposits at autopsy.[10,11] Approximately one third of patients who initially respond to RT suffer a "CNS relapse," whether progression of preexisting lesions or the appearance of new metastatic foci; most relapses occur within 6 months of RT.[6,11]

The median survival of patients following WBRT is 3 to 6 months, with only 10% to 20% of patients surviving 1 year.[11,84,94] Among patients with solid tumors, breast cancer tends to carry the best 1-year survival outlook, whereas melanoma patients have a particularly poor prognosis.[11,28] As discussed, these statistics may be misleading because the main determinant of survival is patients' systemic cancer and not the brain lesions. Only in metastatic melanoma do a majority of patients die neurologic deaths,[9,11,84] although progressive neurologic disability in nonresponders with any primary tumor may contribute to early mortality.

WBRT is widely considered a "one-time" therapy, but a second course of WBRT has been reported to benefit 30% to 75% of patients with recurrent brain metastases.[42,52,94] Retreatment with RT should be reserved for patients who clearly (objectively) responded to the initial course of irradiation. Patients who survive longer than several months after re-irradiation are probably at significant risk for developing diffuse cerebral damage (see below), but when other treatment options are severely limited this risk may not be an overriding consideration.

The neurotoxicity of cranial RT is traditionally classified according to its time of onset into acute, early delayed, and late forms.[55,85] Acute effects are the most common and usually consist of headache, nausea, somnolence, and worsening of preexisting focal symptoms early in the course of RT.[11] The symptoms tend to occur more frequently and to be more severe in patients with many metastases or increased intracranial pressure and in patients who receive large (greater than 3000 cGy) daily WBRT fractions.[85] Acute toxicity generally responds well to increased doses of dexamethasone.[12] Early delayed toxicity appears 1 to 4 months after the completion of WBRT and usually consists of transient somnolence and deterioration in preexisting deficits.[73] The sparse pathologic studies of this entity have implicated myelin as the primary site of damage.[85] This demyelination is apparently reversible, in that patients improve with or without corticosteroids.

The most disturbing form of RT-associated neurotoxicity occurs several months to years after WBRT and can take the form of either focal necrosis or diffuse cerebral atrophy. The risk of developing focal brain necrosis has been estimated at less than 5% following 5000 to 6000 cGy given in conventional fractionation;[55] this is a rare occurrence after RT for brain metastases, because patients generally receive lower doses and few patients survive long enough to be at risk. On the other hand, as many as 50% of patients who survive more than 1 year after WBRT for metastases develop diffuse cerebral atrophy, ventricular enlargement, and hypodensity of the periventricular white matter on serial CT scans.[3,11] The white matter abnormalities are detected with increased sensitivity by MRI and appear as increased periventricular signal intensity on T_2-weighted images.[35]

These characteristic changes on CNS imaging studies appear to be asymptomatic in the majority of patients, although there are few published studies of careful neurologic and neuropsychologic examinations. A minority of patients develop a fairly characteristic picture of dementia, psychomotor retardation, and gait disturbance, with an insidious onset approximately 6 to 18 months after WBRT and progression to severe disability.[3,25,35] The few autopsies reported on these patients have found diffuse injury to myelin sheaths with relative preservation of axons and blood vessels.[3,25] Ventriculoperitoneal shunting has been reported to produce an incomplete and temporary improvement in some patients, but there is apparently no clear way to predict which patients may benefit from a shunt.[3,25]

The incidence of RT-induced dementia has been estimated at 2% to 5% of all brain metastasis patients and as high as 19% of patients who survive 1 year or more after WBRT.[25] Closer analysis reveals that nearly all reported patients with clinically evident RT dementia received high daily dose fractions (more than 300 cGy).[25,35] This has led to the recommendation that patients who are anticipated to have a long survival should receive 4000 to 4500 cGy in daily dose fractions of 180 to 200 cGy, rather than the conventional short-duration WBRT of 3000 cGy given in ten 300 cGy fractions. Even this fractionation scheme, however, does not guarantee against the occurrence of diffuse cerebral injury.[3]

Chemotherapy

Chemotherapy has so far played a very minor role in the treatment of brain metastases. The most important limiting factor for chemotherapy is probably the inherent resistance of many of the primary tumors to currently available agents. Among the solid tumors that commonly metastasize to the brain, only breast cancer and small-cell lung cancer respond well to chemotherapy, while the limited responsiveness of melanoma, colon cancer, and non–small-cell lung cancer to chemotherapy also applies to brain metastases from these tumors. In addition, the tendency for brain metastases to occur late in the course of the disease often means that patients have already failed chemotherapy and are less able to tolerate intensive treatment. Finally, the entry of drugs into the brain is limited by local blood flow and by the integrity of the blood-brain (blood-tumor) barrier. The ability to achieve cytotoxic drug concentrations probably varies among primary tumor types, among individual patients, and even among different regions within a single metastasis. There are well-documented cases of brain metastases failing to respond to, or arising in the setting of, chemotherapy that produces a good response outside the CNS. It is difficult to know in individual patients whether the brain is a sanctuary protecting the metastases from chemotherapy or whether there are differences in chemosensitivity between the primary tumor and subpopulations of metastatic tumor cells.

Despite the theoretical and practical problems in chemotherapy for brain metastases, recent reports have indicated its usefulness in a number of settings. The best results have been reported for brain metastases from germ cell tumors: combinations of vincristine, bleomycin, methotrexate, and cisplatin have produced durable responses in metastatic nonseminomatous tumors. Several of these patients have had long-lasting, complete radiographic disappearance of their cerebral lesions without ever having received WBRT.[81] Given the high level of chemosensitivity of these tumors and the anticipated long duration of survival, a case can be made for using chemotherapy as the front line treatment for brain metastases and reserving WBRT for chemotherapy failures. A similar approach has been advocated for gestational trophoblastic tumors.[67]

In one study,[78] combination chemotherapy including cyclophosphamide and 5-fluorouracil produced objective improvement on serial CT scans in 50% of patients with brain metastases from breast cancer. The median duration of remission in the responders was 7 months, and 37% of initial responders benefited from "second-line" chemotherapy after relapse of the brain metastases. These results are somewhat difficult to reconcile with the fact that brain metastases from breast cancer often arise while patients are actively receiving systemic chemotherapy.[28] The relative benefits and toxicities of WBRT versus chemotherapy for brain metastases from breast cancer have not been explored in any direct comparison studies.

Several reports indicate the effectiveness (temporarily) of etoposide (VP-16) or teniposide (VM-26) in some patients with small-cell lung carcinoma whose brain metastases recurred after WBRT.[38,41] A small proportion of patients with metastatic melanoma respond temporarily to cisplatin or to a nitrosourea.[75]

Intra-arterial (IA) chemotherapy has received considerable attention for primary brain tumors, because it is theoretically capable of producing high concentrations of cytotoxic drugs in a local area without increasing systemic toxicity. There are only a few small published studies of IA chemotherapy for brain metastases, and most patients were treated after failing RT, so that it is difficult to get an accurate idea of response rates. Fewer than one third of reported patients with non–small-cell lung cancer had an objective response to IA BCNU, and the response rate of metastatic melanoma is probably less than 10%.[14,61] There are anecdotal reports of responses to intracarotid cisplatin in metastatic melanoma, germ cell tumors, and small-cell lung cancer.[32] Despite the generally disappointing results of IA chemotherapy, in occasional patients with bilateral brain metastases the lesion(s) ipsilateral to the IA BCNU or cisplatin infusion responded, whereas lesions in the contralateral hemisphere showed progression despite being exposed to the drug via the systemic circulation.[14,32,92] Aside from the logistic problem of infusing several arteries in patients with multiple brain metastases, the toxicity of IA chemotherapy is considerable and may include local pain, vision loss, and stroke.[30]

Interest in IA BCNU has greatly faded following reports of severe and often fatal leukoencephalopathy occurring in the infused territory in patients with malignant gliomas. Intracarotid cisplatin has thus far not been associated with long-term neurologic toxicity but can cause hearing loss, seizures, or acute, occasionally life-threatening neurologic deterioration.[30] Until the efficacy and toxicity of IA chemotherapy are better clarified, this form of treatment should be restricted to the research setting.

The assumption that inadequate drug delivery across the blood-brain barrier (BBB) is a major determinant of clinical therapeutic resistance has led to studies of hyperosmotic BBB disruption prior to IA chemotherapy. BBB disruption followed by IA methotrexate (as well as systemic cyclophosphamide and procarbazine) produced occasional responses and relatively little acute toxicity in a pilot study of patients with multiple brain metastases,[65] but it is not at all clear whether the BBB disruption actually improved the effect that would be seen with IA chemotherapy alone. Serious objections to this type of treatment have been raised on the basis of several animal models demonstrating that the proportional increase in drug delivery to surrounding normal brain after BBB disruption is far greater than the increase in delivery to the tumor itself.[34] The unanswered question is whether the potentially severe neurotoxicity caused by BBB disruption and IA chemotherapy would outweigh any increment in antitumor activity.

Immunotherapy

Selective cytotoxicity for tumor cells but not for normal tissue is probably more critical for successful therapy of brain tumors than for any other neoplasms. Immunotherapy has therefore received special interest in neurooncology, because it holds the promise, at least theoretically, of acting on tumor cells while sparing the normal brain. Various forms of immunotherapy have been applied to primary brain tumors, but to date the only work on brain metastases has involved passive serotherapy with monoclonal antibodies (MABs), mostly with metastatic melanoma. The major obstacles blocking the practical use of MABs are (1) the paucity of highly specific antitumor MABs that do not react with normal brain antigens, (2) the heterogeneous expression of antigens between tumor cells and individual tumors, and (3) the problems associated with delivering macromolecules in effective concentrations into brain tumors. As to the problem of MAB delivery, hyperosmotic disruption of the BBB probably has more promise for MAB therapy than for chemotherapy, since there would be less concern over the effects of increased MAB delivery to the surrounding normal brain. Increased delivery of antimelanoma MABs into brain metastases following BBB disruption has been reported in a pilot study.[66]

PROPHYLACTIC THERAPY

The morbidity caused by brain metastases and the often disappointing results of their current treatment have understandably led to efforts at preventing their occurrence by prophylactic cranial irradiation (PCI). Most of the studies of PCI have concentrated on small-cell lung carcinoma (SCLC), owing to the high incidence of brain metastases in the face of improved systemic treatment: 25% to 45% of all patients develop symptomatic brain metastases, and the risk of brain metastases increases steadily with prolonged survival (up to 60% to 80% of 2-year survivors).[29,44,49,68,83] In some of these patients the brain metastases represent the sole apparent site of metastasis.[39,68,77]

Several studies have shown that PCI (2000 to 3000 cGy of WBRT) in SCLC patients significantly decreases the overall incidence of brain metastases (from an average of 25% to between 5% and 8%), delays the median time of appearance of brain metastases, and reduces the incidence of brain metastases as a solitary site of relapse.[2,8,49,71,83] The benefits of PCI are more evident for patients who achieve a complete response to systemic therapy than patients who are less than complete responders; it is likely that "reseeding" of the CNS occurs in the latter group.[2,77] None of the randomized studies of PCI has demonstrated a significant survival advantage for the irradiated group, as the length of survival was mainly deter-mined by systemic relapse; some studies have seen a trend toward increased survival for the subgroup of patients who received PCI after attaining a complete remission from systemic therapy.[77] Given the relatively high rate of responsiveness of brain metastases from SCLC to RT (50% to 80%),[4,39,68] the consensus approach is to reserve PCI for those patients who achieve a complete systemic response and to defer RT in incomplete responders until symptomatic brain metastases occur. The optimal dose, fractionation, and timing of PCI in relation to chemotherapy have not been established.

There is increasing evidence that PCI itself is not without risk. Mild-to-moderate diffuse cerebral atrophy and abnormal hemispheric white matter have been found on CT and MRI scans in a majority of SCLC patients who survive 1 year or more after PCI.[16,22,46,54] These abnormalities are detectable 6 to 18 months after PCI and frequently show progressive worsening on serial imaging studies. Most of these patients do not have gross neurologic deficits, but a majority of patients tested have impairment of memory and cognitive functions, and a few develop a progressive dementing illness indistinguishable from that which occurs following therapeutic WBRT.[16,22,35,46,53] There is some evidence that overt neurotoxicity is more likely to occur when patients receive high daily RT fractions and/or concomitant systemic chemotherapy during PCI.[5,35,46,54,71] As with the WBRT treatment of symptomatic brain metastases, these findings have initiated a trend toward giving lower daily RT doses.

PCI also appears to reduce but not eliminate the incidence of brain metastases from non–small-cell lung carcinomas (NSCLC), particularly from adenocarcinoma, and to reduce the occurrence of brain metastases as the first site of relapse, without affecting the duration of survival.[21,40,45,89] Irradiating all patients with NSCLC would probably provide a survival benefit for only a very small subset of patients; in a recent study only 4% of NSCLC patients died of solitary brain metastases.[33] The unresolved controversy revolves around whether sparing some NSCLC patients (probably less than 20%) the morbidity of brain metastases justifies the inconvenience and toxicity caused by giving PCI to all patients. For now the general belief is that until better systemic treatment for NSCLC is available, PCI should be considered only in patients with limited stage disease.

CONCLUSION

The pessimism that the diagnosis of brain metastases often engenders is largely due to the frequent occurrence of brain metastases in the setting of progressive systemic cancer and to the regrettably limited options for treating them. Although it is true that many patients fail to respond to treatment and that most patients die within a relatively short time even after "successful palliation" of brain metastases, physicians should not be led to a nihilistic attitude regarding treatment. Timely diagnosis and proper treatment result in a gratifying improvement in the neurologic condition and quality of life for most patients affected by brain metastases. In patients with an otherwise limited extent of metastatic disease, successful management of brain metastases also has a significant impact on the duration of survival. With the exception of patients with widespread systemic cancer whose predicted survival is extremely short, RT and/or chemotherapy should be offered to all patients with brain metastases, including those with "radioresistant" tumors.

REFERENCES

1. Amer, MH, Al-Sarraf, M, Baker, LH, and Vaitkevicius, VK: Malignant melanoma and central nervous system metastases: Incidence, diagnosis, treatment and survival. Cancer 42:660–668, 1978.
2. Aroney, RS, Aisner, J, Wesley, MN, Whitacre, MY, and Van Echo, DA: Value of prophylactic cranial irradiation given at complete remission in small cell lung carcinoma. Cancer Treat Rep 67:675–682, 1983.
3. Asai, A, Matsutani, M, Kohno, T, Nakamura, O, and Tanaka, H: Subacute brain atrophy after radiation therapy for malignant brain tumor. Cancer 63:1962–1974, 1989.
4. Baglan, RJ and Marks, JE: Comparison of symptomatic and prophylactic irradiation of brain metastases from oat cell carcinoma of the lung. Cancer 47:41–45, 1981.
5. Bleyer, WA: Hobson's choice in the CNS radioprophylaxis of small cell lung cancer. Int J Radiat Oncol Biol Phys 15:783–785, 1988.
6. Borgelt, B, Gelber, R, Kramer, S, Brady, LW, and Chang, CH: The palliation of brain metastases: Final results of the first two studies by the Radiation Therapy Oncology Group. Int J Radiat Oncol Biol Phys 6:1–9, 1980.
7. Bross, ID: The role of brain metastases in cascade processes. In Weiss, L, Gilbert, HA, and Posner, JB (eds): Brain Metastases. Martinus Nijhoff, Boston, 1980, pp 66–80.
8. Bunn, PA, Nugent, JL, and Matthews, MJ: Central nervous system metastases in small cell bronchogenic carcinoma. Semin Oncol 5(3):314–322, 1978.
9. Byrne, TN, Cascino, TL, and Posner, JB: Brain metastasis from melanoma. J Neurooncol 1:313–317, 1983.
10. Cairncross, JG, Chernik, NL, Kim, JH, and Posner, JB: Sterilization of cerebral metastases by radiation therapy. Neurology 29:1195–1202, 1979.
11. Cairncross, JG, Kim, JH, and Posner, JB: Radiation therapy for brain metastases. Ann Neurol 7:529–541, 1980.
12. Cairncross, JG and Posner, JB: The management of brain metastases. In Walker, MD (ed): Oncology of the Nervous System. Martinus Nijhoff, Boston, 1983, pp 342–377.
13. Carella, RJ, Gelber, R, Hendrickson, F, Berry, HC, and Cooper, JS: Value of radiation therapy in the management of patients with cerebral metastases from malignant melanoma. Cancer 45:679–683, 1980.
14. Cascino, TL, Byrne, TN, Deck, MD, and Posner, JB: Intra-arterial BCNU in the treatment of metastatic brain tumors. J Neurooncol 1:211–218, 1983.
15. Cascino, TL, Leavengood, JM, Kemeny, N, and Posner, JB: Brain metastases from colon cancer. J Neurooncol 1:203–209, 1983.
16. Catane, R, Schwade, JG, Yarr, I, Lichter, AS, and Tepper, JE: Follow-up neurological evaluation in patients with small cell lung carcinoma treated with prophylactic cranial irradiation and chemotherapy. Int J Radiat Oncol Biol Phys 7:105–109, 1981.
17. Chalk, JB, Ridgeway, K, Brophy, T, Yelland, J, and Eadie, MJ: Phenytoin impairs the bioavailability of dexamethasone in neurological and neurosurgical patients. J Neurol Neurosurg Psychiatry 47:1087–1090, 1984.
18. Chason, JL, Walker, FB, and Landers, JW: Metastatic carcinoma in the central nervous system and dorsal root ganglia: A prospective autopsy study. Cancer 16:781–787, 1963.
19. Choi, KN, Withers, HR, and Rotman, M: Metastatic melanoma in the brain: Rapid treatment or large dose fractions. Cancer 56:10–15, 1985.
20. Cohen, N, Strauss, G, Lew, R, Silver, D, and Recht, L: Should prophylactic anticonvulsants be administered to patients with newly diagnosed cerebral metastases? A retrospective analysis. J Clin Oncol 6:1621–1624, 1988.

21. Cox, JD, Stanley, K, Petrovich, Z, Paig, C, and Yesner, R: Cranial irradiation in cancer of the lung of all cell types. JAMA 245:469–472, 1981.

22. Craig, JB, Jackson, DV, Moody, D, Cruz, JM, and Pope, EK: Prospective evaluation of changes in computed cranial tomography in patients with small cell lung carcinoma treated with chemotherapy and prophylactic cranial irradiation. J Clin Oncol 2:1151–1156, 1984.

23. Dauplat, J, Nieberg, RK, and Hacker, NF: Central nervous system metastases in epithelial ovarian carcinoma. Cancer 60:2559–2562, 1987.

24. De la Monte, SM, Moore, GW, and Hutchins, GM: Patterned distribution of metastases from malignant melanoma in humans. Cancer Res 43:3427–3433, 1983.

25. DeAngelis, LM, Delattre, JY, and Posner, JB: Radiation-induced dementia in patients cured of brain metastases. Neurology 39:789–796, 1989.

26. Delattre, JY, Krol, G, Thaler, HT, and Posner, JB: Distribution of brain metastases. Arch Neurol 45:741–744, 1988.

27. Delattre, JY, Safai, B, and Posner, JB: Erythema multiforme and Stevens-Johnson syndrome in patients receiving cranial irradiation and phenytoin. Neurology 38:194–198, 1988.

28. DiStefano, A, Yap, HY, Hortobagyi, GN, and Blumenschein, GR: The natural history of breast cancer patients with brain metastases. Cancer 44:1913–1918, 1979.

29. Doyle, TJ: Brain metastases in the natural history of small cell lung cancer. Cancer 50:752–754, 1982.

30. Dropcho, EJ and Mahaley, MS: Chemotherapy for malignant gliomas in adults. In Thomas, DG (ed): Neuro-oncology: Primary malignant brain tumours. Edward Arnold, London, 1990, pp 222–241.

31. Eapen, L, Vachet, M, Catton, G, Danjoux, C, and McDermot, R: Brain metastases with an unknown primary: A clinical perspective. J Neurooncol 6:31–35, 1988.

32. Feun, LG, Wallace, S, Stewart, DJ, Chuang, VP, and Yung, WA: Intracarotid infusion of cisplatin in the treatment of recurrent malignant brain tumors. Cancer 54:794–799, 1984.

33. Figlin, RA, Piantadosi, S, and Feld, R: Intracranial recurrence of carcinoma after complete surgical resection of Stage I, II, and III non–small-cell lung cancer. N Engl J Med 318:1300–1305, 1988.

34. Fishman, RA: Is there a therapeutic role for osmotic breaching of the blood-brain barrier? Ann Neurol 22:298–299, 1987.

35. Frytak, S, Earnest, F, O'Neill, BP, Lee, RE, Creagan, ET, and Trautmann, JC: Magnetic resonance imaging for neurotoxicity in long-term survivors of carcinoma. Mayo Clin Proc 60:803–812, 1985.

36. Gay, PC, Litchy, WJ, and Cascino, TL: Brain metastases in hypernephroma. J Neurooncol 5:51–56, 1987.

37. Gelber, RD, Larson, M, Borgelt, BB, and Kramer, S:

38. Giaccone, G, Donadio, M, Bonardi, GM, Testore, F, and Calciati, A: Teniposide (VM-26): An effective treatment for brain metastases of small cell carcinoma of the lung. Eur J Cancer 24:629–631, 1988.

39. Giannone, L, Johnson, DH, Hande, KR, and Greco, FA: Favorable prognosis of brain metastases in small cell lung cancer. Ann Int Med 106:386–389, 1987.

40. Griffin, BR, Livingston, RB, Stewart, GR, Higano, C, and Russell, KJ: Prophylactic cranial irradiation for limited non–small cell lung cancer. Cancer 62:36–39, 1988.

41. Haaxma-Reiche, H, Berendsen, HH, and Postmus, PE: Podophyllotoxins for brain metastases of small cell lung cancer. J Neurooncol 6:231–232, 1988.

42. Hazuka, MB and Kinzie, JJ: Brain metastases: Results and effects of re-irradiation. Int J Rad Oncol Biol Phys 15:433–437, 1988.

43. Healy, ME, Hesselink, JR, Press, GA, and Middleton, MS: Increased detection of intracranial metastases with intravenous Gd-DTPA. Radiology 165:619–624, 1987.

44. Hirsch, FR, Paulson, OB, Hansen, HH, and Vraa-Jensen, J: Intracranial metastases in small cell carcinoma of the lung: Correlation of clinical and autopsy findings. Cancer 50:2433–2437, 1982.

45. Jacobs, RH, Awan, A, Bitran, JD, Hoffman, PC, and Little, AG: Prophylactic cranial irradiation in adenocarcinoma of the lung: A possible role. Cancer 59:2016–2019, 1987.

46. Johnson, BE, Becker, B, Goff, WB, and Petronas, N: Neurologic, neuropsychologic, and computed cranial tomography scan abnormalities in 2- to 10-year survivors of small cell lung cancer. J Clin Oncol 3:1659–1667, 1985.

47. Katz, HR: The relative effectiveness of radiation therapy, corticosteroids, and surgery in the management of melanoma metastatic to the central nervous system. Int J Radiat Oncol Biol Phys 7:897–906, 1981.

48. Kobayashi, T, Kida, Y, Yishida, J, Shibuya, N, and Kageyama, N: Brain metastases of choriocarcinoma. Surg Neurol 17:395–403, 1980.

49. Komaki, R, Cox, JD, and Whitson, W: Risk of brain metastases from small cell carcinoma of the lung related to the length of survival and prophylactic irradiation. Cancer Treat Rep 65:9–10, 1981.

50. Konefal, JB, Emami, B, and Pilepich, MV: Analysis of dose fractionation in the palliation of metastases from malignant melanoma. Cancer 61:243–246, 1988.

51. Kurtz, JM, Gelber, R, Brady, LW, Carella, RJ, and Cooper, JS: The palliation of brain metastases in a favorable patient population: A randomized clinical trial by the Radiation Therapy Oncology Group. Int J Radiat Oncol Biol Phys 7:891–895, 1981.

52. Kurup, P, Reddy, S, and Hendrickson, FR: Results

Equivalence of radiation schedules for the palliative treatment of brain metastases in patients with favorable prognosis. Cancer 45:1749–1753, 1981.

of re-irradiation for cerebral metastases. Cancer 46:2587–2589, 1980.

53. Laukkanen, E, Klonoff, H, Allan, B, Graeb, D, and Murray, N: The role of prophylactic brain irradiation in limited stage small cell lung cancer: Clinical, neuropsychologic, and CT sequelae. Int J Radiat Oncol Biol Phys 14:1109–1117, 1988.

54. Lee, JS, Umsawasdi, T, Lee, YY, Barkley, HT, and Murphy, WK: Neurotoxicity in long-term survivors of small cell lung cancer. Int J Radiat Oncol Biol Phys 12:313–321, 1986.

55. Leibel, SA and Sheline, GE: Radiation therapy for neoplasms of the brain. J Neurosurg 66:1–22, 1987.

56. Lesse, S and Netsky, MG: Metastasis of neoplasms to the central nervous system and meninges. Archives of Neurology and Psychiatry 72:133–153, 1954.

57. Lester, SG, Morphis, JG, Hornback, NB, Williams, SD, and Einhorn, LH: Brain metastases and testicular tumors: Need for aggressive therapy. J Clin Oncol 2:1397–1403, 1984.

58. Levitt, LJ, Dawson, DM, Rosenthal, DS, and Moloney, WC: CNS involvement in the non-Hodgkin's lymphomas. Cancer 45:545–552, 1980.

59. Lewis, AJ: Sarcoma metastatic to the brain. Cancer 61:593–601, 1988.

60. Mackintosh, FR, Colby, TV, Podolsky, WJ, Burke, JS, and Hoppe, RT: Central nervous system involvement in non-Hodgkin's lymphoma: An analysis of 105 cases. Cancer 49:586–595, 1982.

61. Madajewicz, S, West, CR, Park, HC, Ghoorah, J, and Avellanosa, AM: Phase II study of intra-arterial BCNU therapy for metastatic brain tumors. Cancer 47:653–657, 1981.

62. Mandybur, TI: Intracranial hemorrhage caused by metastatic tumors. Neurology 27:650–655, 1977.

63. Maor, MH, Frias, AE, and Oswald, MJ: Palliative radiotherapy for brain metastases in renal carcinoma. Cancer 62:1912–1917, 1988.

64. Markesbery, WR, Brooks, WH, Gupta, GD, and Young, AB: Treatment for patients with cerebral metastases. Arch Neurol 35:754–756, 1978.

65. Neuwelt, EA and Dahlborg, SA: Chemotherapy administered in conjunction with osmotic blood-brain barrier modification in patients with brain metastases. J Neurooncol 4:195–207, 1987.

66. Neuwelt, EA, Specht, HD, Barnett, PA, and Dahlborg, SA: Increased delivery of tumor-specific monoclonal antibodies to brain after osmotic blood-brain barrier modification in patients with melanoma metastatic to the central nervous system. Neurosurgery 20:885–895, 1987.

67. Newlands, ES: Chemotherapy for brain metastases. Prog Exp Tumor Res 29:167–176, 1985.

68. Nugent, JL, Bunn, PA, Matthews, MJ, Ihde, DC, and Cohen, MH: CNS metastases in small cell bronchogenic carcinoma: Increasing frequency and changing pattern with lengthening survival. Cancer 44:1885–1893, 1979.

69. Paillas, JE, and Pellet, W: Brain metastases. In Vinken, PJ and Bruyn, GW (eds): Handbook of Clinical Neurology, Vol 18. North-Holland, Amsterdam, 1975, pp 201–232.

70. Paterson, AH, Agarwal, M, Lees, A, Hanson, J, and Szafran, O: Brain metastases in breast cancer patients receiving adjuvant chemotherapy. Cancer 49:651–654, 1982.

71. Pedersen, AG, Kristjansen, PE, and Hansen, HH: Prophylactic cranial irradiation and small cell lung cancer. Cancer Treat Rev 15:85–103, 1988.

72. Pickren, JW, Lopez, G, Tsukada, Y, and Lane, WW: Brain metastases: An autopsy study. Cancer Treatment Symposia 2:295–313, 1983.

73. Posner, JB: Management of central nervous system metastases. Semin Oncol 4(1):81–91, 1977.

74. Posner, JB: Clinical manifestations of brain metastasis. In Weiss, L, Gilbert, H, and Posner, JB (eds): Brain Metastasis. Martinus Nijhoff, Boston, 1980, pp 189–207.

75. Retsas, S and Gershuny, AR: Central nervous system involvement in malignant melanoma. Cancer 61:1926–1934, 1988.

76. Robin, E, Bitran, JD, Golomb, HM, and Newman, S: Prognostic factors in patients with non-small cell bronchogenic carcinoma and brain metastases. Cancer 49:1916–1919, 1982.

77. Rosen, ST, Makuch, RW, Lichter, AS, Ihde, DC, and Matthews, MJ: Role of prophylactic cranial irradiation in prevention of central nervous system metastases in small cell lung cancer. Am J Med 74:615–624, 1983.

78. Rosner, D, Nemoto, T, and Lane, WW: Chemotherapy induces regression of brain metastases in breast carcinoma. Cancer 58:832–839, 1986.

79. Russell, DS, and Rubinstein, LJ: Pathology of Tumors of the Nervous System. Williams & Wilkins, Baltimore, 1972, pp 264–269.

80. Russell, EJ, Geremia, GK, Johnson, CE, and Huckman, MS: Multiple cerebral metastases: Detectability with Gd-DTPA–enhanced MR imaging. Radiology 165:609–617, 1987.

81. Rustin, GJ, Newlands, ES, Bagshawe, KD, Begent, RH, and Crawford, SM: Successful management of metastatic and primary germ cell tumors in the brain. Cancer 57:2108–2113, 1986.

82. Schold, SC, Vurgrin, D, Golbey, RB, and Posner, JB: Central nervous system metastases from germ cell carcinoma of testis. Semin Oncol 6(1):102–108, 1979.

83. Sculier, JP, Feld, R, Evans, WK, and DeBoer, G: Neurologic disorders in patients with small cell lung cancer. Cancer 60:2275–2283, 1987.

84. Sheline, GE and Brady, LW: Radiation therapy for brain metastases. J Neurooncol 4:219–225, 1987.

85. Sheline, GE, Wara, WM, and Smith, V: Therapeutic irradiation and brain injury. Int J Radiat Oncol Biol Phys 6:1215–1228, 1980.

86. Sorensen, JB, Hansen, HH, Hansen, M, and Dombernowsky, P: Brain metastases in adenocarcinoma of the lung: Frequency, risk groups, and prognosis. J Clin Oncol 6:1474–1480, 1988.

87. Stein, M, Steiner, M, Klein, B, and Beck, D: Involvement of the central nervous system by ovarian carcinoma. Cancer 58:2066–2069, 1986.

88. Sze, G, Shin, J, Krol, G, and Johnson, C: Intraparenchymal brain metastases: MR imaging versus contrast-enhanced CT. Radiology 168:187–194, 1988.

89. Umsawasdi, T, Valdivieso, M, Chen, TT, Barkley, HT, and Booser, DJ: Role of elective brain irradiation during combined chemoradiotherapy for limited disease non–small cell lung cancer. J Neurooncol 2:253–259, 1984.

90. Vieth, RG and Odom, GL: Intracranial metastases and their neurosurgical management. J Neurosurg 23:375–383, 1965.

91. Walker, AE, Robins, M, and Weinfeld, FD: Epidemiology of brain tumors: The national survey of intracranial neoplasms. Neurology 35:219–226, 1985.

92. Weiden, PL: Intracarotid cisplatin as therapy for melanoma metastatic to brain: Ipsilateral response and contralateral progression. Am J Med 85:439–440, 1988.

93. Wright, DC and Delaney, TF: Treatment of metastatic cancer to the brain. In DeVita, VT, Hellman, S, and Rosenberg, SA (eds): Cancer: Principles and Practice of Oncology, ed 3. JB Lippincott, Philadelphia, 1989, pp 2245–2261.

94. Zimm, S, Wampler, GL, Stablein, D, Hazra, T, and Young, HF: Intracerebral metastases in solid tumor patients: Natural history and results of treatment. Cancer 48:384–394, 1981.

INDEX

Note: Page numbers followed by "f" indicate figures; page numbers followed by "t" indicate tables.